D1525349

Advances in Veterinary Science
and Comparative Medicine

Volume 33

Vaccine Biotechnology

Advances in Veterinary Science and Comparative Medicine

Edited by

C. E. Cornelius
Department of Physiological Sciences
School of Veterinary Medicine
University of California
Davis, California

Michael Burridge
Department of Infectious Diseases
College of Veterinary Medicine
University of Florida
Gainesville, Florida

Advances in Veterinary Science
and Comparative Medicine

Volume 33

Vaccine Biotechnology

Edited by

James L. Bittle

Department of Molecular Biology
Scripps Clinic and Research Foundation
La Jolla, California

and

Frederick A. Murphy

Center for Infectious Diseases
Centers for Disease Control
Atlanta, Georgia

Academic Press, Inc.
Harcourt Brace Jovanovich, Publishers
San Diego   New York   Berkeley   Boston
London   Sydney   Tokyo   Toronto

ACADEMIC PRESS, INC.
San Diego, California 92101

United Kingdom Edition published by
ACADEMIC PRESS LIMITED
24-28 Oval Road, London NW1 7DX

LIBRARY OF CONGRESS CATALOG CARD NUMBER: 53-7098

ISBN 0-12-039233-X (alk. paper)

PRINTED IN THE UNITED STATES OF AMERICA
89 90 91 92   9 8 7 6 5 4 3 2 1

CONTENTS

Vaccines Produced by Conventional Means to Control Major Infectious Diseases of Man and Animals

JAMES L. BITTLE AND SUSIE MUIR

Poliovirus: Three-dimensional Structure of a Viral Antigen

JAMES M. HOGLE AND DAVID J. FILMAN

Immune Response to Vaccination

B. I. OSBURN AND J. L. STOTT

The Development of Biosynthetic Vaccines
Marc S. Collett

The Development of Chemically Synthesized Vaccines
F. Brown

Infectious Recombinant Vectored Virus Vaccines
Joseph J. Esposito and Frederick A. Murphy

Modern Approaches to Live Virus Vaccines
Erling Norrby

Live Bacterial Vaccines and Their Application as Carriers for Foreign Antigens

GORDON DOUGAN, LAURIE SMITH, AND FRED HEFFRON

Immunomodifiers in Vaccines

AMNON ALTMAN AND FRANK J. DIXON

Vaccines for Parasitic Infections

ANTHONY F. BARBET

Vaccines against Tumor Antigens

RALPH B. ARLINGHAUS

Human Immunodeficiency Virus: An Agent That Defies Vaccination

NEAL NATHANSON AND FRANCISCO GONZALEZ-SCARANO

Animal Virus Infections That Defy Vaccination: Equine Infectious Anemia, Caprine Arthritis-Encephalitis, Maedi-Visna, and Feline Infectious Peritonitis

NIELS C. PEDERSEN

PREFACE

The development of vaccines to prevent human and animal diseases is one of the great accomplishments of biomedical science. Although few diseases have been eliminated through the use of vaccines, there have been marked reductions in incidence, morbidity, and mortality. In fact, vaccines have been so successful in safeguarding humans from many of the great epidemic diseases that worldwide eradication, as in the case of smallpox, or regional elimination, as in the case of yellow fever and poliomyelitis, have become realities. Vaccines against the important diseases of livestock and poultry have also been used so successfully that they have allowed the development of the modern high-density husbandry systems now common to industrial agriculture. However, many infectious diseases of humans and animals still represent unresolved burdens to mankind; in each case, just as in the past, we continue to turn to vaccination for cost-effective, efficient approaches to disease control. For the foreseeable future, a solution lies in further development of the concept and practical application of vaccination.

This volume presents the most recent advances in the field of vaccinology and the most novel approaches in the development of vaccines. First is a review of the vaccines currently in use, followed by articles describing the many ways by which improvements are envisioned. As in most fields of endeavor, major developments follow certain basic advances in concept or technology. In vaccinology, today's application of recombinant-DNA technology represents such an advance. Improvements in safety, efficacy, stability, simplicity of production, and cost are forthcoming as more and more applications of recombinant-DNA technology unfold. This should mean wider availability and use of vaccines in the future. For example, the development of recombinant-DNA-derived hepatitis B vaccines may make it possible to control this disease in settings where the present plasma-derived vaccines are not being used. Similarly, foot-and-mouth disease vaccines developed either by peptide synthesis or by recombinant-DNA technology may, for the first time, eliminate this disease throughout Africa and South America.

The application of recombinant DNA technology to vaccine development is also advancing our understanding of the basic mechanisms of immunity: the nature of antigenic epitopes on infectious organisms, the presentation of such epitopes to the immune system, the complex set of effector responses involving the cellular and humoral arms of the immune system, and others.

Ultimately, understanding these mechanisms will further our overall comprehension of host–parasite interactions.

The thirteen chapters of this volume cover the diverse new technologies contributing to the improvement of vaccines. In this regard, the increasing role of structural analysis, molecular anatomy, in resolving the nature of antigenic epitopes and their presentation on the surfaces of infectious organisms is emphasized. Once identified, such epitopes may be reconstructed biosynthetically or chemically and then formulated into vaccines. Infectious viral or bacterial recombinant vectors are also being used to present antigenic epitopes in vaccines; this too is discussed.

In humans and in lower animals the most successful vaccines have been those containing attenuated living organisms. These include the human pediatric vaccines against measles, mumps, rubella, polio, and tuberculosis (BCG) and the animal vaccines against canine distemper, rinderpest, and Newcastle's disease. Yet all these vaccines produce some detrimental effects, usually caused by the growth and infectious processes of the inciting organism per se. New approaches reviewed in this volume, again dependent upon recombinant-DNA technology such as site-directed mutagenesis, promise to lead to safer vaccines made from living organisms.

Immunomodifiers will be important in improving the potency of new vaccines, as will improved adjuvants and delivery systems. Vaccines against parasitic infections and against tumors have proven particularly needful of such potentiation—subjects covered in this volume. Finally, it must be recognized that some classes of infectious diseases seem to defy our best efforts in vaccine development. Understanding these diseases, such as acquired immunodeficiency disease (AIDS) in humans, ungulate lentivirus infections, and feline infectious peritonitis, can also teach us much about the immune system and, perhaps, artificial stimulation of immune responsiveness when even natural means fail.

The purpose of this volume is to present developments in vaccinology in a comparative way, examining the lessons of human and veterinary medicine and sharing the successes and failures in each for the overall benefit of infectious disease control. We hope, therefore, that this volume will be of value to a broad cross section of medical, biomedical, and veterinary scientists.

JAMES L. BITTLE
FREDERICK A. MURPHY

Vaccines Produced by Conventional Means to Control Major Infectious Diseases of Man and Animals

JAMES L. BITTLE*[+] AND SUSIE MUIR[+]

*Johnson and Johnson Biotechnology Center, San Diego, California, and
[+]Department of Molecular Biology, Research Institute of Scripps Clinic, La Jolla, California

1

The publication by Jenner of "An Inquiry Into the Cause and Effects of Variolae Vaccinae" in 1798 is the first documented evidence for the use of vaccination. In the 190-year period since then, a number of vaccines have been developed to control the infectious diseases of man and animals. This chapter reviews the development of some of these vaccines and their use in controlling such major diseases as diphtheria, rinderpest, Newcastle disease, smallpox, pertussis, yellow fever, rabies, etc. Yet, infectious diseases are still a major problem in the world today, accounting for over 15 million human deaths annually in Africa, Asia, and South America alone (Warren, 1985) and untold numbers of animal deaths worldwide. Newer techniques will be needed to make vaccines safer and more effective and, most importantly, more available throughout the world. Other chapters in this book will describe these techniques, but for the present, it is the vaccines described in this chapter that are the key to disease control and prevention programs.

I. Vaccines for DNA Viruses

A. Parvoviridae

The most important animal parvoviruses are feline panleukopenia virus, mink enteritis virus, and canine parvovirus, all of which are serologically related, and the porcine parvovirus, which is serologically distinct. The parvovirus that infects mink, Aleutian disease virus, causes persistent infection leading to an unusual immune complex disease. Parvoviruses have been isolated from the feces, serum, and joints of man. The B-19 human parvovirus has been shown to cause Firth disease or erythema infectionsum, a rash on the limbs, with upper respiratory tract symptoms and arthralgia. Human parvoviruses have also been shown to be the principal cause of aplastic crisis in sickle cell anemia patients. Other members of the parvovirus genus that are less important are bovine parvovirus, avian parvovirus, goose parvovirus (which causes hepatitis), minute virus of mice, Kilham rat virus, and the adeno-associated viruses.

1. Feline Panleukopenia Virus

The first parvovirus shown to be a filterable agent was feline panleukopenia virus (Verge and Christoforoni, 1928), which was not characterized until much later (Johnson, 1967a,b; Johnson et al., 1967). The virus affects most members of the family Felidae, causing enteritis and bone marrow hypoplasia that results in severe leukopenia. The virus infects kittens in utero and postnatally causes cerebellar hypoplasia and ataxia (Kilham and Margolis, 1966).

Immunization. The first panleukopenia vaccines were produced by infecting susceptible cats and harvesting their tissues. Filtrates from these tissue suspensions were treated with chemical inactivants such as formalin. Two inoculations of this type of vaccine produced long-lasting protection (Leasure et al., 1934; Enders and Hammond, 1940). However, subsequent vaccines, produced in primary feline kidney cell culture and inactivated with formalin, proved safer and more effective (Bittle et al., 1970; Davis et al., 1970). An attenuated live-virus vaccine was also very effective in inducing immunity and protection (Slater and Kucera, 1966). Concern for the wide-scale use of an attenuated live-virus vaccine centers on the premise that shedding may spread the virus to other species, possibly allowing the emergence of pathogenic variants in these species. Attempts to immunize cats orally with attenuated live-virus vaccines have not been successful, but intranasal aerosol application has been effective (Scott and Glauberg, 1975; Schultz et al., 1973).

2. Canine Parvovirus

Three members of the parvovirus family are known to infect dogs: minute virus of canines, a defective canine adeno-associated virus, and the pathogenic canine parvovirus. Canine parvovirus is related to feline panleukopenia virus and may have originated from one of the mammalian parvoviruses. In young dogs, the virus causes leukopenia and severe intestinal disease with necrosis of crypt epithelium in the small intestine. Myocarditis occasionally develops, causing sudden heart failure in young dogs. In 1978 an epizootic of this disease occurred in the United States, causing high mortality (Eugester, 1978).

Immunization. Because of the close relationship between feline panleukopenia virus and canine parvovirus, inactivated feline panleukopenia vaccine initially was used to protect susceptible dog populations (Appel *et al.*, 1979a). Later, inactivated and attenuated vaccines produced with the canine virus proved to be much more effective (Pollack and Carmichael, 1983; Appel *et al.*, 1979b). These parvovirus vaccines have been formulated with other vaccines, including canine distemper and canine adenovirus vaccines, and are administered routinely to young dogs.

3. Porcine Parvovirus

Porcine parvovirus has a distant serologic relationship to other parvoviruses, but it causes disease only in swine. The virus, which is widespread, causes abortions, fetal death, and infertility in sows infected early in gestation. Immune sows reinfected during gestation give birth to normal piglets.

Immunization. Numerous reports have shown the effectiveness of inactivated porcine parvovirus vaccines in swine (Suzuki and Fujsaki, 1976; Mengeling *et al.*, 1979; Wratthal *et al.*, 1984; Fujisaki *et al.*, 1978; Joo and Johnson, 1977). For example, Mengeling *et al.* (1979) demonstrated the value of a vaccine in which the virus was inactivated with acetylethyleneimine.

An attenuated live-virus vaccine has been described (Paul and Mengeling, 1980) in which a porcine isolate was attenuated by 120–165 passages in a swine testicular cell line. This vaccine effectively induced antibodies and protected challenged animals. The vaccine virus did not cross the placenta; however, it did kill fetuses when inoculated *in utero*. The virus was shed in feces, and so could be transmitted to unvaccinated animals.

The inactivated vaccines now used in United States have been effective in controlling porcine parvovirus infection. Vaccination is recommended for gilts and sows before breeding.

B. ADENOVIRIDAE

Adenoviruses cause significant disease in dogs, foxes, and man, but have also been isolated from cattle, swine, goats, sheep, horses, turkeys, and chickens, where they produce mild infections, mainly associated with the respiratory and intestinal tracts.

There are at least 80 different adenoviruses, 43 of which occur in man. Each adenovirus has a narrow host range.

1. Canine Adenovirus

There are two canine adenoviruses. Canine adenoviruses 1 (CAV-1) causes infectious canine hepatitis, which at one time was widespread, but now has been controlled by vaccination. Infected dogs also develop corneal opacities following this infection, as a result of the formation of immune complexes and uveitis within the anterior chamber of the eye (Carmichael et al., 1975). In foxes, CAV-1 produces a rapidly fatal encephalitis.

Canine adenovirus 2 (CAV-2) causes respiratory disease in dogs, but neither hepatitis nor encephalitis in dogs or foxes. The respiratory disease varies depending on the strain of virus and bacterial superinfection. CAV-2 may be transmitted by aerosol, whereas CAV-1 is spread by other direct means such as contact with urine or saliva from infected animals. CAV-1 and CAV-2 are oncogenic in experimentally infected hamsters (Sarma et al., 1967; Dulcac et al., 1970).

Immunization. Dogs that recover from natural CAV-1 infection are immune for a long period. The first CAV-1 vaccines were produced by formalin inactivation of tissue homogenates from infected dogs.

CAV-1 was first adapted to tissue culture by Cabasso et al. (1954) and by Fieldsteel and Emery (1954). The latter modified the virus by serial passage in porcine and canine tissue cultures; the resulting vaccine immunized dogs and did not produce clinical signs of infection except for occasional corneal opacity similar to that caused by natural infection. Dogs immunized with CAV-1 vaccines are also protected against CAV-2 (Appel et al., 1973). The immunity produced by the attenuated live-virus CAV-1 vaccines is long lasting and has drastically reduced the incidence of the canine disease.

Although CAV-2 is closely related to CAV-1, when it is inoculated parenterally into dogs, it does not cause disease, although the virus is shed from the respiratory tract (Appel et al., 1973). Such dogs become immune to both CAV-1 and CAV-2. An attenuated live-virus vaccine containing CAV-2 is now being widely used in place of older CAV-1 vaccines (Bass *et al.*, 1980); this has resulted in a much lower incidence of corneal opacity in recipients. However, because of the oncogenicity of adenoviruses in other hosts, the respiratory shedding of CAV-2 virus should be a concern.

2. Human Adenovirus

In man, adenoviruses mainly produce disease of the respiratory tract which varies in severity depending on the virus and the age of infected individuals. The viruses cause acute pharyngitis in infants and children, pharyngitis and conjunctivitis in children, and acute respiratory disease (ARD) in military recruits and institutionalized young adults. Pneumonia may also occur, expecially following ARD.

Immunization.   A vaccine consisting of adenovirus types 3, 4, and 7, grown in monkey kidney cell culture and inactivated with formalin, was introduced in 1958 for use in U.S. military recruits. The vaccine was effective in reducing ARD in this population (Sherwood *et al.*, 1961). However, the vaccine was withdrawn from use in 1963 because of concern for possible oncogenicity of the adenoviruses, and of the SV_{40} virus present in the monkey kidney cell culture.

A subsequent adenovirus, type 4, was passed in human tissue and was, therefore, devoid of SV_{40} genomic material. This virus, encapsulated in enteric-coated capsules, proved to be a safe and effective vaccine (Chanock *et al.*, 1966; Edmonson *et al.*, 1966). An adenovirus 7 vaccine, prepared in the same way and given simultaneously with adenovirus 4 vaccine, was equally effective (Top *et al.*, 1971). The administration of a vaccine with only one of these viruses was not effective in controlling ARD caused by any of several different adenoviruses, but formulation of a vaccine with both viruses proved to be broadly cross-protective and have had a major influence in controlling ARD in U.S. military recruits.

C. HERPESVIRIDAE

Over 70 herpesviruses produce disease in man and animals. These viruses have an affinity for epithelial tissues and nervous system tissues. These tropisms lead to specific disease syndromes involving the respiratory and urogenital tracts, and the central and peripheral nervous systems. The viruses often cause persistent infections, which can be latent and can be reactivated. Herpesvirus disease are generally much more severe in young humans and animals. Some herpesviruses, including Epstein–Barr virus (EBV) in humans and Marek's disease virus in fowl, are associated with malignancies.

The presence of specific antibodies may prevent or modify the clinical disease but does not prevent infection. Vaccines have been developed for those herpesviruses causing major diseases in animals; however, despite the seriousness of human herpesvirus diseases, including those caused by herpes simplex virus, EBV virus, cytomegalovirus, and varicella virus, progress has been slow in developing vaccines for humans. This stems from concern over possible persistence and oncogenicity of vaccine viruses. In the past few years, several attenuated live-virus varicella vaccines have been tested and found safe and efficacious (Takahashi *et al.*, 1974; Asano *et al.*, 1977; Arbeter *et al.*, 1983).

1. Infectious Bovine Rhinotracheitis Virus

Since the initial recognition of infectious bovine rhinotracheitis (IBR) in the early 1950s and the later recognition of another manifestation of the disease, infectious pustular vulvovaginitis, this bovine herpesvirus has been acknowledged as a major problem in livestock. The respiratory disease varies from mild to severe, and herd mortality can be as high as 10% in an acute outbreak. The virus may cause abortions in pregnant cattle, and the genital disease results in a chronic vulvovaginitis but not abortions, apparently due to a lack of viremia.

Immunization. Attenuated live-virus vaccines were developed by serial passage of field isolates in bovine kidney cell cultures. Such vaccine viruses have reduced virulence when administered intranasally and do not produce disease when administered parenterally (Schwarz *et al.*, 1957; York *et al.*, 1957). Vaccine virus does not spread from vaccinated to unvaccinated contact animals. The widescale use of such vaccines has controlled this disease effectively. When administered by the intranasal route (Todd *et al.*, 1971), these vaccines had the advantage of producing more rapid protection, but long-term protection was no greater than with perenterally administered vaccines (McKercher and Crenshaw, 1971). Because of the possibility that the attenuated live-virus vaccines given parenterally might cause abortion, their use has been restricted to nonpregnant animals. A formalin-inactivated vaccine has also been developed, but requires multiple inoculations, and the serum neutralizing (SN) antibody response is low (Matsuaba *et al.*, 1972). However, inactivated vaccines are used especially in dairy cattle because of concern that the attenuated live-virus vaccines may cause abortion.

2. Equine Rhinopneumonitis Virus

Four herpesviruses affect horses: equine rhinopneumonitis virus (EHV-1) causes abortion which may be epizootic, and also, occasionally, rhinopneumonitis; EHV-2 is cytomegalovirus found in buffy coat cells of most horses, but its role in causing disease is unknown; EHV-3 causes equine coital exanthema, a urogenital tract disease; and EHV-4 is the main cause of equine rhinopneumonitis. EHV-1 and -4 are related antigenically, whereas types 2 and 3 are distinct (Sabine *et al.*, 1981; Studdert and Blackney, 1979).

Immunization. The first vaccine for equine rhinopneumonitis was developed by Doll and Bryans (1963), who adapted an EHV-1 isolate to suckling hamsters. This vaccine produced a mild disease, but induced protective immunity against the more serious respiratory disease and abortion that occurs in older animals. However, this vaccine sometimes caused abortions, and the virus was known to spread from vaccinated to unvaccinated horses.

A more attenuated strain of EHV-1 has been used widely and is considered to be reasonably effective (Mayr, 1970). This strain was attenuated by passage in hamsters and in pig kidney cell culture before adaptation to an equine cell line (Gerber *et al.*, 1977). This vaccine induces low levels of SN antibodies, and protects against respiratory disease but not against abortion.

A formalin-inactivated vaccine, emulsified in an oil adjuvant, has also been found safe and effective in preventing respiratory disease. This vaccine, in controlled field trials, lowered the abortion rate significantly (Bryans, 1980; Bryans and Allen, 1981). The attenuated live-virus and the inactivated vaccines contain only EHV-1, but apparently there is enough cross-protection induced by repeated vaccinations to protect against the EHV-4 respiratory disease.

3. Pseudorabies Virus

This herpesvirus is unusual in that it occurs naturally in many species—cattle, sheep, goats, swine, dogs, cats, rats, and mice. It produces a fatal disease in all of these species except adult swine, in which the disease is mild. In each species except swine the primary sign is intense puritis resulting in the animal biting the affected area. Infection rapidly spreads to the central nervous system, leading to paralysis and death. In adult swine, the signs of infection are mild, usually of a respiratory nature, but abortions follow in approximately 50% of pregnant sows. In young pigs, especially neonates, the infection may be fatal.

Immunization. Since the disease is prevalent only in swine, this is the only animal for which a vaccine has been developed. In examining a virulent strain of pseudorabies virus, Bartha and Kojnok (1963) found two plaque sizes. The small plaque size variant, called K, occurred naturally and had reduced virulence for rabbits. Further studies with this strain passaged in chick embryo or calf testicle cell culture produced a safe vaccine for swine. One dose induced partial immunity and a second dose yielded good immune responses in all recipients.

McFerran and Dow (1975) adapted the K strain to Vero cells and showed that one dose of a vaccine prepared from this passage material was protective. Pigs vaccinated with this vaccine did not shed the virus. Although the vaccine did not prevent infection, it prevented clinical disease. This attenuated live-virus vaccine is used widely.

4. Feline Rhinotracheitis Virus

Feline rhinotracheititis virus, which was first isolated in 1957, produces a widespread respiratory disease in cats (Crandell and Maurer, 1958). The virus may also cause fetal death.

Immunization. An attenuated live-virus vaccine was developed by passage of a field isolate in feline kidney cells (Bittle and Rubic, 1975). The vaccine is given parenterally and is safe and effective (Scott, 1977). Low levels of SN antibodies persist for at least 6 months. Vaccinated cats are resistant to intranasal instillation of virulent virus; they may be reinfected, but do not develop clinical disease (Bittle and Rubic, 1976; Kahn *et al.,* 1975). The vaccine has controlled this important respiratory pathogen and, when combined with a feline calicivirus vaccine, has drastically reduced the incidence of respiratory disease in this species.

5. Avian Infectious Laryngotracheitis Virus (LTV)

This herpesvirus is highly contagious and causes lesions in the larynx, trachea, and bronchi of infected fowl. The infection causes the formation of an exudate that produces the characteristic respiratory distress and rattling in severely affected birds. Birds that recover from this disease are immune for a long period, but may remain as carriers and a source of virus for reinfection of flocks.

Immunization. The earliest method of immunization was developed by Beaudette and Hudson (1933), who applied virulent virus from tracheal exudate to the mucosa of the bursa of Fabricius and the cloaca with a stiff brush. This produced a local infection and a solid systemic immunity. The use of fully virulent virus caused occasional outbreaks of disease, particularly when the scarification was not properly done or insufficient virus was present, and birds did not become immune. The virus was propagated on the chorioallantoic membrane of embryonated eggs by Burnet (1934), and this became a source of vaccine material. Other methods of vaccination involved intranasal instillation (Benton et al., 1958) and feeding in drinking water (Zamberg et al., 1971). Attenuated strains of LTV have been developed by serial passage in cell culture (Gelenczei and Marty, 1964) and by feather follicle passage (Molgard and Cavett, 1947). Attenuated strains isolated from outbreaks or selected from passage are now used in preference to virulent virus.

6. Marek's Disease Virus

Marek's disease virus causes lymphoproliferative disease in chickens, occurring in three forms: neural, ocular, and visceral (the latter mainly in young birds) (Sevoian and Chamberlain, 1962; Biggs and Payne, 1963). Sevoian was the first to provide evidence that Marek's tumors were caused by a virus and were transmissible. The virus has been established as a gamma herpesvirus (Churchill and Biggs, 1967; Nazerian and Burmeister, 1968; Soloman et. al., 1968).

Immunization. Fatalities from Marek's disease caused major economic losses in the poultry industry until a vaccine was developed for its control. This was accomplished by Churchill et al. (1969), who attenuated by serial passage a virus isolated from chickens that is parenterally administered at 1 day of age. Thereafter, Okazaki et al. (1970) selected a herpesvirus from turkeys (HVT) that was relatively avirulent in chickens, and Zander et al. (1972) and Schat and Calnek (1978), selected a natural avirulent strain from chickens.

These three vaccines are effective, but the HVT strain has been more widely used because it can be obtained from infected cells and can be lyophilized (Calnek et al., 1970). The vaccines are given parenterally to chicks at hatching and produce good protection (80–100%) against virulent virus challenge (Purchase et al., 1972).

D. Poxviridae

Viruses of the family Poxviridae infect most domestic animals and man. From the standpoint of immunoprophylaxis, the most important poxviruses are: *Orthopoxvirus,* smallpox (variola), mousepox (ectromelia); *Avipoxvirus,* fowlpox, pigeonpox; *Capripoxvirus,* sheeppox, goatpox; *Leporipoxvirus,* myxomatosis virus; *Parapoxvirus,* contagious pustular dermatitis virus. All these poxviruses cause serious disease in their primary host species and some may infect other species. Each of the poxviruses causes characteristic vesicular lesions on the skin and mucous membranes, with the exception of myxomatosis virus which produces hyperplastic lesions in the form of myxomas and fibromas.

Ectromelia (mousepox) is caused by a virus closely related to vaccinia virus and produces a serious disease of laboratory mice. Vaccination with vaccinia apparently will reduce the morbidity and mortality of mousepox in a colony, but it will not prevent infection and may act to maintain a silent reservoir of virus (Buller and Wallace, 1985).

Sheeppox is one of the most serious pox diseases, occurring in Europe, the Middle East, and Africa, but it is controlled by vaccination (Aygun, 1955; Sabban, 1955). Goatpox occurs mainly in the Middle East and Africa; a goatpox vaccine has been reported to also immunize against sheeppox (Rafyi and Ramyar, 1959).

Contageous pustular dermatitis virus is unrelated to sheeppox, but causes a pox-like disease in young lambs in which vesicles form around the skin of lips, nostrils, and eyes. Boughton and Hardy (1935) showed that animals could be protected by scarification with dried contageous pustullar dermatitis virus material similar to that use with vaccinia.

Myxomatosis virus causes a fatal disease of domestic rabbits and may be spread by direct contact or by blood meals of insects such as mosquitos and fleas (Myers *et. al.,* 1954). McKercher and Saito (1964) developed a safe and efficacious attenuated live-virus vaccine by passage of the virus in rabbit kidney cell culture.

1. Smallpox (Variola) Virus

This virus, once the cause of epidemics that decimated entire cities, has now been eradicated. The control was brought about by world-wide vaccination and isolation of infected persons. Another factor in the control of smallpox was that variola virus had no other host except man.

Immunization. Material from lesions of smallpox-infected individuals had been used for centuries to infect susceptible persons so they would develop a mild form of the disease and become resistant. This variolation was dangerous but much safer than natural exposure to the smallpox virus. Jenner (1798) practiced an improved form of this method by using cowpox virus (vaccinia) to inoculate susceptible persons, as described in Chapter 6.

Most vaccinia vaccines were produced by scarifying the skin of a calf with infected material and harvesting the lymph from the crusted lesions as aseptically as possible. This was stored in 40% glycerol to stabilize the virus and preservatives were added to destroy bacteria. Sheep and rabbits were also used similarly for vaccine production. Vaccinia virus was also adapted to grow in embryonated eggs (Goodpasture *et al.*, 1935). Vaccinia virus is very stable, can be produced at a low cost, and is simple to administer. These factors played a major role in allowing the wide-scale use of vaccinia for the eradication of smallpox.

2. Fowlpox Virus

Fowlpox virus occurs mainly in chickens and produces pox lesions on the wattles, comb, mouth, nostrils, and eyes. The disease is spread mainly by direct contact with infected birds and blood-sucking parasites such as mosquitoes. Although it is a fairly resistant virus, it is not otherwise very transmissible.

Immunization. Fowlpox vaccine was originally made by scarifying cockrel combs with virulent virus and harvesting the exudate. Johnson (1929) demonstrated that dried exudate would produce immunity when scarified in the wing web or applied to the thigh skin free of feathers. Fowlpox virus was later cultivated on the chorio allontoic membrane by Goodpasture *et al.* (1931) and used as a source of vaccine material. Later the virus was adapted to tissue culture. An attenuated live-virus fowlpox vaccine produced in cell culture may be used in 1-day-old chicks (Siccardi, 1975). Another vaccine, an attenuated strain (HP-1) developed by Mayr *et al.* (1976), is given orally to 5-day-old chicks, then repeated after 3 to 4 months.

E. HEPADNAVIRIDAE

Hepadnaviridae is a new-found family of viruses containing hepatitis B virus of man as well as three similar but distinct viruses that infect woodchucks, beechey ground squirrels, and Pekin ducks. These viruses have many of the same ultrastructural, molecular, and biological features and their surface antigens cross-react to a small, variable degree. The host range appears to be specific for each virus. Hepatitis B infects man and certain higher primates, including the chimpanzee and gibbon. Infection with these hepadnaviruses results in subacute hepatitis, which often becomes progressive and chronic.

Hepatitis B Virus

The most important of these viruses is hepatitis B virus, which produces a chronic disease in man (Blumberg *et al.*, 1967; Prince, 1968). Hepatitis B virus is transmitted by blood, saliva, and semen, but also from mother to offspring, the latter route accounting for as much as one-third of persistent infections. The disease is usually self-limiting, but in 5–10% of patients the infection becomes chronic, with the virus persisting in a carrier state. There are over 200 million chronic carriers of this virus worldwide. A late sequela in chronic carriers is hepatocellular carcinoma. It is estimated that 40–60% of malignancies in Africa are the result of hepatitis B-induced onco-genesis.

Immunization. The development of a vaccine for hepatitis B was hampered by the difficulty of growing the virus in cell culture. Krugman *et al.* (1970) was the first to show that hepatitis B virus-infected serum could be heat-inactivated and retain its antigenicity. They also showed that this inactivated serum given parenterally could protect subjects exposed to virulent hepatitis B virus. This led to the use of plasma from infected but healthy virus carriers as the source of antigen. Carriers produce large quantities of the hepatitis B virus, along with its outer coat protein. By purifying and inactivating the coat protein, a safe and effective vaccine was developed (Hilleman *et al.*, 1978). The coat protein, naturally formed into 22-nm particles, was purified by ammonium sulfate concentration, isopycnic banding, rate zonal separation and enzymatic digestion. The purified protein parti-cles were then inactivated with 1 : 4000 formalin. The particles induce good levels of protective antibody when given in a series of three injections (Symuness *et al.*, 1980). However, the high cost of this vaccine has limited its use. Newer vaccines produced by recombinant DNA methods are now being used, as described in other chapters.

II. Vaccines for RNA Viruses

A. Picornaviridae
 1. Foot-and-Mouth Disease (FMD) Virus
 2. Poliomyelitis Virus
 3. Avian Encephalomyelitis (AE) Virus

B. Caliciviridae
 Feline Calcivirus

C. Reoviridae
 1. Reoviruses
 Avian Reovirus
 2. Rotaviruses
 a. Bovine Rotavirus
 b. Porcine Rotavirus

 3. Orbiviruses
 a. Bluetongue Virus
 b. African Horse Sickness Virus

D. Birnaviridae
 Infectious Bursal Disease (IBD) Virus

E. Togaviridae
 1. *Alphavirus*
 2. *Pestivirus*
 a. Hog Cholera (HC) Virus
 b. Bovine Virus Diarrhea (BVD) Virus
 3. *Rubivirus*
 Rubella Virus
 4. *Arterivirus*
 Equine Arteritis Virus

F. Flaviviridae (Yellow Fever Virus)

G. Orthomyxoviridae
   1. Human Influenza Virus
   2. Equine Influenza Virus

H. Paramyxoviridae
   1. Parainfluenza Virus
      a. Sendai Virus
      b. Canine Parainfluenza Virus
      c. Bovine Parainfluenza Virus
   2. Mumps Virus
   3. Newcastle Disease Virus
   4. Measles Virus
   5. Canine Distemper Virus

6. Rinderpest Virus
7. Bovine Respiratory Syncytial Virus (RSV)

I. Rhabdoviridae
   Rabies Virus

J. Retroviridae
   Feline Leukemia Virus (FeLV)

K. Coronaviridae
   1. Avian Infectious Bronchitis Virus (IBV)
   2. Transmissible Gastroenteritis Virus (TGE)

A. PICORNAVIRIDAE

The four genera in the family Picornaviridae are: *Aphthovirus, Rhinovirus, Enterovirus,* and *Cardiovirus.* Viruses in the first three genera cause important diseases in domestic animals and man, whereas viruses in the fourth infect rodents. The picornaviruses in general have a primary affinity for superficial tissues especially of the digestive and respiratory tracts. Viruses in the first three genera also have an ability to mutate, thus yielding many serotypes.

Rhinoviruses cause clinical disease in man, horses, and cattle. No vaccines have been developed for the infections of humans because of the multiplicity of viral serotypes. The number of serotypes in horses (three) and cattle (two) is fewer; nevertheless, no vaccines are available.

Over 100 enteroviruses exist; of these, vaccines have been developed only for poliomyelitis viruses, avian encephalomyelitis, and duck hepatitis viruses. Other viruses in this group either are of low pathogenicity or the number of serotypes is so large as to preclude the development of vaccines. The exception is human hepatitis A virus, which causes a serious disease and has one serotype; the development of both inactivated virus and attenuated live-virus vaccines is in progress (Hilleman *et al.,* 1982; Provost *et al.,* 1983).

1. Foot-and-Mouth Disease (FMD) Virus

FMD was the first animal disease shown to be caused by a virus (Loeffler and Frosch, 1898). FMD viruses cause one of the most economically important diseases of animals and its control is critical to the world's supply of animal protein. The viruses are widespread and occur in many cattle producing regions of the world. The viruses also affect other cloven-footed animals including sheep, swine, and goats. FMD virus infection produces vesicles on oral mucous membranes, including the tongue, gums, and dental pads, but also on the skin including the interdigital spaces and teats. These vesicles on the mucous membranes coalesce and erupt, leaving large denuded areas. The mucous membrane and skin lesions can incapacitate an animal for weeks, thus severely disrupting its productivity. The viruses are highly contagious and persist for long periods in infected animals. Animals that recover from natural infection are immune for approximately one year. Vallee and Carre (1922) showed that there was more than one FMD virus; seven serotypes with over 60 subtypes have now been identified, making the development of effective vaccines difficult.

Immunization. The first FMD vaccine for cattle was reported in 1925 and consisted of a formalinized emulsion of vesicular epithelium (Vallee *et al.,* 1925). A similar but improved version called the Schmidt–Waldmann vaccine followed and contained vesicle material from the tongue epithelium of infected cattle. This material was treated with formalin and used with aluminum hydroxide (Schmidt, 1936; Waldmann and Klobe, 1938). Another advance was described by Frenkel (1947), who infected superficial layers of bovine tongue epithelium in culture and inactivated the newly replicated virus with formalin to produce a more uniform product. Although this method is used today in some areas of the world, most FMD vaccines are now produced by growing the virus in baby hampster kidney cells (MacPherson and Stoker, 1952; Mowat and Chapman, 1962; Capstick *et al.,* 1962).

The imines replaced formalin as an inactivant in most FMD vaccines after Brown *et al.* (1963) showed that viral inactivation was more complete, and safer vaccines could be produced by this process. All inactivated FMD vaccines contain more than one serotype, including the serotypes most common in the area in which the vaccines are to be used. Although inactivated vaccines that are produced and used properly can effectively lead to the control FMD, their stability could be improved, thereby lowering their cost. This is discussed further in the chapter by Brown.

Attenuated live-virus FMD vaccines have been developed (Henderson, 1978) but are not used because of the fear that the virus might persist in animals and in meat and milk products from animals (Hyslop, 1966-1967).

2. *Poliomyelitis Virus*

There are three polio viruses and minor variants of each. The viruses infect man by entry into the upper alimentary tract, infecting cells, and spreading via the blood to the central nervous system, producing neuronal destruction in the medulla and spinal cord. The degree of paralysis that follows infection depends on such factors as virus strain and virus tropism. The vast majority of persons infected with wild polioviruses show no apparent clinical disease. Paralysis occurs only in an estimated 1% of infected individuals; polio 1 virus is responsible for at least 85% of cases.

Immunization.   Early attempts to develop inactivated poliovirus vaccines were hampered by not knowing that there are three distinct viruses. The differentiation of the three viruses by Bodian (1949) and Kessel and Pait (1949) was a major step toward controlling the disease. Enders *et al.* (1949) found that poliovirus would grow in extraneural tissues of human origin and thus laid the groundwork for the development of poliovirus vaccines. The first vaccine (Salk) contained all three polio viruses grown in monkey kidney cell culture and inactivated with formalin (Salk *et al.*, 1954). This vaccine, introduced in 1953, reduced the incidence of paralytic poliomyelitis 80–90% where it was used; however, multiple doses were required and intestinal tract infection was not prevented, thus allowing the virus to continue to spread.

There was an intense effort in the 1950s to develop an attenuated live-virus vaccine that could be administered orally, and could protect the intestinal tract, thus breaking the chain of transmission. Koprowski, Sabin, and Cox each developed vaccine strains of reduced neurovirulence that underwent extensive laboratory and field studies (Koprowski *et al.*, 1956; Sabin, 1955; Cox *et al.*, 1959). The strains developed by Sabin were finally licensed in the United States; they produced rapid immunity as well as protection of the intestinal tract while preventing spread to unvaccinated, susceptible persons in contact with vaccinees. This improved the overall level of immunity in communities. With the widescale use of oral poliomyelitis vaccine, the incidence of paralytic disease in the United States has dropped to less than 10 cases per year. The occasional reaction to the attenuated vaccine is discussed in the chapter by Hogle and Filman.

3. Avian Encephalomyelitis (AE) Virus

Avian encephalomyelitis was first discribed and shown to have a viral etiology by Jones (1932, 1934). The virus is widespread and affects young chickens (1–3 weeks old). Characteristic clinical signs are ataxia and tremors of the head and neck. Extensive neuronal degeneration occurs in the anterior horn of the cord and in the medulla and pons. The virus may affect older laying birds, causing a drop in egg production.

Immunization. Flocks that have survived an outbreak or subclinical infection during the growing period are resistant to further infection (Schaaf and Lamoreux, 1955). Moreover, infected chickens 16–20 weeks of age undergo only mild disease, providing an opportunity for vaccination (Schaff, 1958).

Calnek and Taylor (1960) successfully immunized immature birds with an attentuated live-virus vaccine delivered in drinking water. A number of vaccines have been developed including the 1143 strain (Calnek, 1961), the NSW-1 strain (Westbury and Senkovic, 1978), the Philips Duphar strain (Folkers *et al.,* 1976), and a strain grown in chicken pancreas cell culture (Miyamae, 1978). Inactivated AE virus vaccines have been developed for use in susceptible breeding flocks that are in production (Schaaf, 1959; Calnek and Taylor, 1960; Butterfield *et al.,* 1961; MacLeod, 1965).

B. Caliciviridae

Two viruses in the family Caliciviridae cause significant disease in animals, vesicular exanthema virus in swine and sea lions and feline calicivirus. Caliciviruses have also been isolated from humans, calves, reptiles, nonhuman primates, birds, dogs, and fish, but do not produce significant disease in these animals.

Vesicular exanthema virus caused a disease in swine closely resembling FMD (Traum, 1933). Eradication of this disease followed the discovery that the main source of contagion was uncooked infected meat in garbage fed to swine, and the consequent enforcement of garbage cooking laws.

Feline Calicivirus

Fastier (1957) first isolated a calicivirus from a domestic cat and showed that it produced an upper respiratory tract infection. A large number of viral isolates, with different neutralization patterns, were made from clinically ill cats (Crandell *et al.,* 1960; Bittle *et al.,* 1960). These serotypes were later shown to have a common antigen and are now considered a single serotype (Povey and Ingersoll, 1975). This virus is widespread, having been isolated from cats in many countries. The virus produces a disease that is generally mild, but, if allowed to progress, the lesions may extend from the upper respiratory tract into the lung causing pneumonia and death (Kahn and Gillespie, 1971).

Immunization. Cats that recover from natural infection and have neutralizing antibodies can be reinfected, but they do not have recurrent clinical disease. An attenuated live-virus calicivirus vaccine has been prepared by serial passage at low temperature; this

vaccine virus produces only mild clinical signs in recipients (Bittle and
Rubic, 1976). This attenuated live-virus vaccine is administered parenterally; it induces high levels of neutralizing antibody and protects
vaccinated cats challenged intranasally with both homologous and
heterologous strains (Kahn *et al.,* 1975; Scott, 1977). Immunity from
vaccination persists for at least 6 months and probably longer. The
calicivirus is combined with feline rhinotracheitis and feline panleukopenia to make a multivalent vaccine that is routinely used in
domestic cats (Bittle and Rubic, 1975). Inactivated vaccines have also
been licensed and are used in multivalent vaccines.

C. REOVIRIDAE

The family Reoviridae is divided into three genera: *Reovirus, Rotavirus,* and *Orbivirus.* Infections cause by member viruses are common in mammals and birds.

1. *Reoviruses*

Reoviruses are commonly isolated from dogs, cats, sheep, cattle,
horses, mice, rats, rabbits, birds, and man. Only in birds is the disease
serious enough to warrant control with vaccines. The reoviruses are
commonly found in sewage, and the mode of transmission is thought to
be the fecal–oral route.

Avian Reovirus.   In chickens and turkeys, reoviruses produce a
widespread disease called viral arthritis (tenosynovitis). This disease
of the synovial membranes, tendon sheaths, and myocardium was first
recognized by Dalton (1967) and by Olsen and Solomon (1968). Viral
arthritis occurs primarily in meat-producing birds, and in acutely
affected flocks there is a high rate of condemnation. There are at least
five avian reovirus serotypes, but they are antigenically unrelated to
the mammalian reoviruses.

Immunization.   Vaccination of breeding stock is an effective way to
control viral arthritis. Van der Heide *et al.* (1976) used an attenuated
live-virus vaccine and Cessi and Lombardini (1975) used an inactivated vaccine in laying hens to protect chicks with maternal antibody.
This eliminated transmission and protected susceptible day-old chicks.

2. *Rotaviruses*

Rotaviruses produce acute gastroenteritis in many species, especially in newborns, including newborn calves, foals, lambs, piglets,
puppies, monkeys, and humans. The clinical signs are similar in all
species; in each there is acute diarrhea followed by dehydration and

rapid loss of weight. Secondary bacterial infection may exaggerate the symptoms and also cause pneumonia. The viruses infect epithelial cells of villi, causing desquamation and loss of absorptive function, resulting in diarrhea, rapid dehydration, and emaciation. Secretory antibody is very important in protecting the epithelial surface of the small intestine (Snodgrass and Wells, 1976); antibody contained in colostrum is protective when in high titer.

a. *Bovine Rotavirus.* Bovine rotovirus causes a rapidly spreading disease in neonatal calves (Mebus, 1969). The antigenic relationship of the bovine rotavirus and other rotaviruses isolated from children, calves, piglets, mice, and foals is very close (Woode *et al.*, 1976).

Immunization. An attenuated live-virus vaccine developed by Mebus *et al.* (1976) is administered in two doses to cows prior to calving. This is meant to stimulate colostral antibody, which is passed on to the nursing calves. This vaccine has also been combined with an attenuated live-virus coronavirus vaccine and entero-toxigenic *E. coli* vaccine to prevent calf scours.

b. *Porcine Rotavirus.* Leece *et al.* (1976) isolated a rotavirus from piglets with fatal diarrhea. Additional reports of this disease showed that it was widespread and warranted the development of a vaccine for its control.

Immunization. Early attempts to immunize pigs by oral administration of a bovine attenuated live-virus rotavirus vaccine were unsuccessful (Leece and King, 1979). Presently an attenuated porcine rotavirus vaccine containing two serotypes, A^1 and A^2, is licensed in the United States and is being used in combination with a transmissible gastroenteritis (TGE) vaccine. The vaccines are administered to pregnant sows by both parenteral and oral routes. At least two doses of vaccine are given orally, 5 and 3 weeks before farrowing, and one dose is given parenterally 1 week before farrowing. This induces antiviral colostral antibody for the protection of suckling piglets.

3. Orbiviruses

The member viruses of this genus replicate in arthropods as well as in vertebrates. The most important viruses are the bluetongue viruses, and African horse sickness viruses. Colorado tick fever virus, the only virus in this genus that infects man, is transmitted by the bite of infected ticks. The disease is usually benign, and infection produces long-lasting immunity.

a. *Bluetongue Virus.* Bluetongue viruses infect ruminants and are transmitted by *Culicoides* gnats. The most serious disease is in sheep, which develop fever, depression, oral lesions, pneumonia, and lameness. Mortality can be high, especially in lambs. Ewes infected early in gestation may produce lambs with hydrocephalus and other congenital deformities. Although cattle rarely have clinical bluetongue disease, *in utero* transmission can occur, resulting in congenital deformities.

Of the 24 distinct bluetongue viruses, 5 occur in the United States. Infection with one bluetongue virus confers resistance to reinfection with that same virus for several months, but cross-protection against infection with other viruses is minimal.

Immunization. A multivalent attenuated live-virus vaccine developed in South Africa by serial passage of several different viruses in sheep proved difficult to standardize. A more uniform vaccine was later developed by Alexander *et al.* (1947); it contained strains of at least five viruses, attenuated by passage in chick embryos, and gave broad protection against the multiple viruses seen in the field. A similar vaccine was developed by McKercher *et al.* (1953), who isolated bluetongue virus in the United States and also attenuated a strain of serotype 10 by serial passage in chick embryos (McKercher *et al.*, 1957). Recently McConnell and Livingston (1982) have been attempting to incorporate more bluetongue virus strains into multivalent attenuated live-virus vaccines.

Inactivated vaccines for bluetongue would have the advantage of greater safety than attenuated live-virus vaccines. They would eliminate the possible chance of reversion to virulence, and the chance of vaccine-associated abortion and birth defects. Such vaccines are under development (Stott *et al.*, 1979).

b. African Horse Sickness Virus. African horse sickness virus causes an acute disease in equine animals in Africa, the Middle East, and Asia. It was shown to be caused by a virus (McFadyean, 1900) and has been more thoroughly characterized by Breeze *et al.* (1969). The viruses are transmitted to horses by *Culicoides* species and affect principally the vasculature of the respiratory tract causing edema of the lungs, head, and neck. The viruses also cause cardiac lesions.

Immunization. Some animals that recover from natural infection may be reinfected, so immunity is not permanent. A spleen pulp vaccine inactivated with formalin was made by DuToit *et al.* (1933) and administered in multiple doses. Later, an attenuated live-virus vaccine was developed by serial intracerebral passage of a field isolate in mice (Alexander and DuToit, 1934). However, because there are nine African horse sickness viruses, it has been necessary to adapt each to mice and to combine them in a polyvalent vaccine. Such vaccine has been effective in protecting horses.

D. BIRNAVIRIDAE

Infectious Bursal Disease (IBD) Virus

The virus that causes IBD was first isolated by Winterfield and Hitchner (1962) using embroyonated eggs. It causes a disease of chickens in commercial poultry-producing areas. The virus affects mainly young birds 3–6 weeks of age, with clinical signs of diarrhea and dehydration. The lesions arise in lymphoid tissues such as the bursa of Fabricius, thymus, and spleen, producing immunosupression with the associated opportunistic infections.

Immunization. Both attenuated live-virus and inactivated vaccines have been developed to control IBD. The vaccines are used mainly for immunizing breeder flocks to confer passive immunity through the yolk sac of the egg. Maternal antibody protects chicks for 1–3 weeks. If breeder flocks are boosted with oil–adjuvant-inactivated vaccines, maternal antibody may last longer. There are several types of attenuated live-virus vaccines with varying degrees of virulence. These vaccines are administered in water, etc., to chicks from 1 day to 2–3 weeks of age in broiler-breeder flocks, followed by vaccination with an inactivated product at approximately 16–18 weeks of age (Lukert and Hitchner, 1984).

E. TOGAVIRIDAE

The four genera in the family Togaviraidae are: *Alphavirus, Pestivirus, Rubivirus,* and *Arterivirus.* Each of these genera contain important pathogens.

1. Alphavirus

The *Alphavirus* genera include:

1. Western equine encephalomyelitis (WEE) virus
2. Eastern equine encephalomyelitis (EEE)
3. Venezuelan equine encephalomyelitis (VEE) virus

All cause encephalitis in horses and humans. In horses, the mortality rate of EEE in over 80%, and that from WEE is about 20–30%. The main mode of transmission is by culicine mosquitoes; however, VEE has been transmitted from horse to horse by contact with body fluids.

Immunization. Infections with togaviruses produce viremia, long-term humoral antibody responses, and immunity. Early vaccines were made from formalin-inactivated infected animal brain tissue. The cultivation of both WEE and EEE in the chick embryo by Higbee and Howitt (1935) made possible the development of successful inactivated vaccines (Beard *et al.*, 1938). More recent vaccines for WEE and EEE are produced in tissue culture. An attenuated live-virus VEE vaccine, first developed for humans, is also used for horses in endemic areas (Berge *et al.*, 1961; McKinney *et al.*, 1963). The vaccine virus is grown in primary chick embryo cell cultures; it induces long-lasting immunity. An inactivated VEE vaccine has also been developed and is combined with WEE and EEE vaccines in a trivalent formulation.

2. *Pestivirus*

a. Hog Cholera (HC) Virus. Hog cholera virus and bovine virus diarrhea (BVD) virus antigenically are closely related pestiviruses, but are specific in the diseases they cause in swine and cattle, respectively.

HC virus produces an acute febrile disease marked by multiple hemorrhages, necrosis, and infarcts in internal organs. Lethargy, vomiting, and encephalomyelitis are seen in a high percentage of infected animals during an outbreak and mortality is high.

Immunization. Passive protection with convalescent swine serum from swine has been used effectively for short-term control of outbreaks for many years (Dorset *et al.*, 1908). Antiserum and either virulent or partially attenuated virus strains were also used to establish active immunity. Although there is only one antigenic type of HC virus, variant biotypes have arisen that are more difficult to protect against with standard vaccines. The presence of neutralizing antibody correlated well with protection.

An inactivated virus vaccine prepared from defibrinated swine blood taken during the acute phase of the disease and treated with crystal violet or phenol was safe, but required multiple doses (McBryde and Cole, 1936).

Attenuation of HC virus was first accomplished by passage in rabbits (Baker, 1946; Koprowski *et al.*, 1946). Tissue culture attenuated live-virus vaccines eventually replaced the rabbit vaccine; the latter produced a rapid and long-lasting immunity.

A large number of different attenuated live-virus HC vaccines with different characteristics have been used over the years, but residual pathogenicity, shedding, and spread of vaccine viruses have remained problems. A vaccine containing BVD virus was tested in swine, based on evidence that this virus could block replication of HC virus (Sheffy *et al.*, 1961). However, the BVD vaccine did not protect against all strains of HC virus (Tamoglia *et al.*, 1966).

Formerly, control of HC was difficult because HC virus persists in infected meat scraps fed to swine in uncooked garbage. However, since 1969 no vaccines have been used in the United States. By controlling the transport of swine and cooking all garbage used as feed, the disease has been eradicated from the United States, and several European countries.

b. *Bovine Virus Diarrhea (BVD) Virus.* BVD virus causes a widespread disease of cattle, especially in young stock. Clinical signs, which vary in severity, include scouring, ulcerations of the oral cavity, and abortion. Young animals that recover often remain stunted and unproductive for long periods. BVD viral strains differ in their cytopathic effects in tissue culture; cattle infected with noncytopathogenic strains during the first 3 months of gestation can transmit the virus to the fetus, which may be born viremic and immunologically tolerant. Later exposure to cytopathogenic strains, naturally or by vaccination, can cause offspring to develop the more severe form of the disease (Bolin *et al.,* 1985).

Immunization. A cytopathogenic strain of virus isolated from a calf and designated Oregon (C24V) strain (Gillespie *et al.,* 1960) became less pathogenic for calves after 32 passages in bovine kidney tissue culture (Coggins *et al.,* 1961). This has been the standard vaccine strain and has been used widely for many years. For cattle never exposed to BVD antigen, this vaccine strain is safe and effective; however, persistently infected cattle may react strongly to vaccination with the cytopathic strain of BVD virus, causing a mucosal disease syndrome. It is important to identify and eliminate persistently infected cattle from herds.

3. Rubivirus

Rubella Virus. In man, rubella virus causes a generally mild exanthematous disease, with malaise and respiratory symptoms. Complications include arthritis, thrombocytopenia purpura, and encephalitis. Gregg's observation (1941) that rubella virus produces fetal abnormalities if infection occurs early in pregnancy emphasized the destructive effects of this virus and the need to develop a means to protect against infection.

Immunization. Natural exposure to rubella virus evokes nasopharyngeal antibody, which is important in preventing reinfection. Antibody, especially IgG antibody in mother's plasma, is important in preventing fetal infection.

Two groups isolated rubella virus in tissue culture (Parkman *et al.,* 1962; Weller and Nova, 1962), allowing the first attempts to develop vaccines. Both inactivated and attenuated live-virus vaccines were tried before the latter evolved as superior products. The attenuated live-virus vaccines were developed using different cell culture systems, including monkey kidney (Parkman et al., 1966), duck embryo (Buynak, 1968), rabbit kidney (Peetermans and Huygelen, 1967), canine kidney (Musser and Hilsabeck, 1969), and human diploid cells (Plotkin, 1967). The vaccines now being used are more than 95% effective in inducing protective levels of antibody that persist for at least 9 years. The annual incidence of rubella in the United States has dropped from 56,000 reported cases in 1970 to less than 700 in 1985.

4. Arterivirus

Equine Arteritis Virus. Equine arteritis virus was first isolated by Doll et al. (1957). The disease caused by this virus is characterized by edema of limbs, stiffness, and swelling in the tissues surrounding the eye, and abortion.

Immunization. Horses that recover from infection develop long-lasting immunity. An effective attenuated live-virus vaccine was developed by serial passage of Bucyrus field strain virus in primary equine and rabbit kidney cell culture and an equine dermal cell line (Doll et al., 1968; Wilson et al., 1962; McCollum, 1986). The vaccine has been shown in challenge trials to protect recipients for as long as 24 months (McCollum, 1986); it does not cause any clinical manifestations and it is not spread to susceptible horses in contact with vaccinated recipients.

F. FLAVIVIRIDAE (YELLOW FEVER VIRUS)

Yellow fever virus causes acute hepatitis and hemorrhagic fever in man, characterized by jaundice, shock, and renal damage. Transmission is by mosquitoes belonging to the *Aedes* genus throughout tropical areas of South America and Africa. The virus is maintained in a transmission cycle between mosquitoes and monkeys, with man being infected when he enters a territory in which the monkey–mosquito cycle exists.

Immunization. An attenuated live-virus yellow fever vaccine was developed by passage of the virulent Asibi strain in mouse brain and cell culture until it had lost its pathogenicity for monkeys and man (Theiler, 1951). The vaccine virus, termed 17D, is propagated in embryonated eggs. The vaccine, given as a single dose, is extremely safe and efficacious, providing immunity for at least 10 years.

G. ORTHOMYXOVIRIDAE

The family Orthomyxovirus comprises the influenza viruses, the cause of acute, highly contagious respiratory disease in man, horses, swine, and birds. Two structural viral proteins (NF and M) divide this family into three distinct genera: A, B, and C.

The viruses, especially influenza A virus, undergo genetic reassortment, which allows variant viruses to emerge. Two viral proteins, the hemagglutinin and neuraminidase, both located on the surface of virions, are important in inducing immunity.

Vaccines have been widely used for controlling influenza with reasonably good success. Since immunity is more closely related to local secretory IgA antibody than to serum antibody, it is difficult to stimulate and maintain protection with the presently used inactivated vaccines. With human infections, the type A viruses undergo occasional antigenic shifts and drifts, after which the antigens in the vaccine may not be representative of those viruses found in the field. This potential antigenic variability, as well as animal reservoirs for this virus, are responsible for the pandemics associated with this virus. As an example, the acute respiratory disease of swine caused by a type A strain of virus was first recognized in 1918 during the human influenza epidemic and is believed to have been transmitted from swine from humans. Both swine and humans are susceptible to the swine virus. However, the disease in swine occurs sporadically and has not been enough of a problem to warrant the use of vaccines in that species.

1. Human Influenza Virus

Influenza is a respiratory infection with systemic manifestations that include fever, chills, muscular aches, etc. The severity of the disease depends on the virus strain and the susceptibility of the population.

Persons that have recovered from an influenza infection are usually immune to rechallenge with the homologous virus. However, the change of a few amino acids in hemagglutinin may give rise to antigenic drift and reinfection of populations.

Immunization. Because of the epidemic threat of influenza viruses, careful surveillance for new strains is carried out in many parts of the world. The strains that public health officials predict will be the cause of the next winter's epidemics are then scheduled for vaccine production. For vaccine production, virus is grown in the allantoic cavity of embryonated eggs and is purified and concentrated by zonal centrifugation. The virus is inactivated with formalin, β-propiolactone, or irradiation. The quantity of viral antigen per dose is standardized before use. The vaccine usually contains several type A viruses and a type B virus. These inactivated whole virus vaccines produce protective levels of antibody in approximately 85% of primed recipients and in 60% of the unprimed recipients. Antibody levels are maintained for approximately 1 year in primed individuals. Attenuated live-virus influenza vaccines have been used extensively in the USSR with varying results. Problems of adverse reactions, inconsistent potency, and questionable appropriateness of strains make it difficult to evaluate the effectiveness of these vaccines.

More recent attempts to develop attenuated live-virus vaccines involve genetic reassortment, a method that offers considerable promise (reviewed by Wright and Karzon, 1987).

2. Equine Influenza Virus

Influenza in horses resembles the disease in man and swine. The two type A influenza viruses of importance in the horse are: A/Equi 1/Prague/56 type 1 and A/Equi 2/Miami/63 type 2. The disease spreads rapidly through susceptible horses, and those that recover are protected for only a short time. Recovery from infection with one virus type does not provide immunity against the other.

Immunization. Vaccines for equine influenza are produced in essentially the same manner as human influenza vaccines. Formal-inactivated vaccines contain both equine type 1 and 2 viruses and one of several adjuvants, as described by Bryans *et al.* (1973). Vaccines of this type are widely used and effectively control equine influenza.

H. PARAMYXOVIRIDAE

The family Paramyxoviridae contains several viruses that cause significant disease in animals. The family is composed of three genera that include the following viruses for which vaccines have been developed.

Paramyxovirus   (parainfluenza virus, mumps virus, and Newcastle's disease virus)
Morbillivirus   (measles virus, canine distemper virus, and rinderpest virus)
Pneumovirus   (bovine respiratory syncytial virus)

These viruses are transmitted by the respiratory route and are antigenically rather stable.

1. Parainfluenza Virus

Parainfluenza viruses infect humans, rodents, swine, dogs, and cattle. These viruses, by themselves, cause mild upper respiratory tract disease, but when combined with other viral and bacterial pathogens may cause a more severe syndrome. Parainfluenza types 1, 2, 3, and 4a/4b infect humans, especially young children. Type 3 is considered the most pathogenic, causing a bronchitis and pneumonitis.

Vaccines for parainfluenza of rodents (Sendai virus infection), dogs (canine parainfluenza), and cattle (bovine parainfluenza) have been developed. There is no licensed parainfluenza vaccine for man.

a. *Sendai Virus.* Sendai virus, first isolated during attempts to recover human respiratory viruses in mice (Kuroya *et al.*, 1953), is a parainfluenza type 1 virus that causes respiratory disease in mice, rats, hamsters, and swine. The disease occurs either in an acute-short duration form or a chronic-persistent, clinically inapparent form. Spread is by either direct contact or by aerosol. In mouse colonies, this disease is difficult to control because the virus is so highly infective.

Immunization. Formalin-inactivated vaccines have been effective in controlling the disease in mice and rats (Fukumi and Takeuchi, 1975; Eaton *et al.*, 1982; Tsukui *et al.*, 1982). Additionally, a temperature-sensitive mutant strain of Sendai virus has been used as an aerosol-delivered vaccine in mice. It suppresses virus replication, but the vaccine virus spreads throughout the colony and makes it difficult to monitor for wild virus strains (Kimura *et al.*, 1979).

b. *Canine Parainfluenza Virus.* Outbreaks of mild respiratory disease in laboratory dogs have been attributed to parainfluenza type 2 virus (Binn *et al.*, 1968; Crandell *et al.*, 1968). When other respiratory agents such as mycoplasma and *Bordetella bronchiseptica* were given intranasally after exposure to this parainfluenza virus, more severe respiratory signs occurred (Appel and Percy, 1970). This encouraged efforts to develop a vaccine for canine parainfluenza virus.

Immunization. An attenuated live-virus parainfluenza vaccine has been shown to protect dogs against aerosol challenge with virulent virus (Emery *et al.*, 1976). The vaccine produces no untoward effects and has been combined with canine distemper and canine adenovirus vaccines in multivalent formulations.

c. *Bovine Parainfluenza Virus.* A parainfluenza type 3 virus isolated from cattle can also cause mild respiratory disease (Reisinger *et al.*, 1959). The virus, when combined with other respiratory pathogens including *Pasteurella* and infectious bovine rhinotracheitis virus, causes the severe pneumonia syndrome, called "shipping fever."

Immunization.   An attenuated live-virus parainfluenza type 3 vaccine administered parenterally induces good levels of antibodies and affords protection against experimental challenge (Mohanty and Lillie, 1964; Thorsen *et al.*, 1969). This vaccine has been combined with infectious bovine rhinotracheitis virus and bovine virus diarrhea vaccines in multivalent formulations. An inactivated vaccine, requiring two inoculations, induces high hemagglutination-inhibition titers and lessens the severity of the disease in cattle challenged with the same virus (Gale *et al.*, 1963).

2. *Mumps Virus*

Mumps virus causes an acute infection in man with parotitis as the main clinical manifestation, although the central nervous system and other organs including the testes and ovaries can be affected. Mumps virus has a limited host range; in addition to man, only certain monkey species and laboratory rodents can be infected.

Immunization.   Recovery from natural infection with mumps virus confers long-term immunity. Early experiments with formalin-inactivated virus derived from infected parotid glands of monkeys showed that monkeys and humans could be immunized (Enders *et al.*, 1945; Stokes *et al.*, 1946). Habel (1946) found that chick embryo grown virus could be inactivated with ultraviolet light or formalin and would induce protection in monkeys. A similar vaccine was later shown to induce protection in man (Habel, 1951; Henle *et al.*, 1951). Poor antibody responses to multiple inoculations of this type of vaccine encouraged the search for a more effective vaccine.

A mumps virus strain (Jeryl Lynn) has been attenuated by passage in chick embryos (Weibel *et al.*, 1980). The vaccine is immunogenic in 93–98% of subjects, and neutralizing antibodies persist for at least 10 years. The annual incidence of mumps in the United States has been reduced from 160,000 cases in 1968 to less then 3,000 in 1985 by application of this vaccine. As presently used, mumps vaccine is combined with measles and rubella vaccines in a pediatric formulation called MMR.

3. *Newcastle Disease Virus*

Newcastle disease is one of the most serious widespread diseases affecting poultry. The disease was first described by Kranevelt (1926) and shortly thereafter by Doyle (1927), who named it after the area in England where an outbreak occurred and showed that its cause was a filterable virus. The disease has several forms causing mainly respiratory, enteric, and central nervous system manifestations. The morbidity and mortality vary depending on the virus strain. Burnet (1942) described the hemagglutinating property of the virus, which has been very helpful in its quantitation and immunodiagnosis.

Immunization. A number of attenuated live-virus vaccines have been developed which are widely used to control the disease. The B1 strain (Hitchner and Johnson, 1948), the LaSota strain (Winterfield *et al.*, 1957), and the F strain (Asplin, 1952) are used to immunize birds of all ages by different routes, including by addition to drinking water and by spraying.

Vaccines containing inactivated virus do not produce long-lasting immunity but may be used in certain situations when only short-term immunity is needed, such as when boosting immunity is needed in laying flocks. Increasing the antigen content and using oil–emulsion adjuvants improves the quality of these inactivated vaccines (Stone *et al.*, 1980; Zanella and Marchi, 1982).

4. Measles Virus

Measles is a highly contagious disease of humans, occurring mostly in children, causing exanthemata and sometimes more serious manifestations including encephalomyelitis. The virus has two principal immunogens, the hemagglutinin and the fusion protein (Norrby *et al.*, 1975). The immunity produced by natural infection is long lasting.

Immunization. The growth of measles virus in chick embryo fibroblasts by Enders and Peebles (1954) paved the way for the development of vaccines. A formalin-inactivated measles virus vaccine was shown to induce partial immunity. However, some vaccinated children later exposed to measles virus, either naturally or as attenuated live-virus measles vaccine, developed atypical measles (atypical rashes, edema of hands and feet, and respiratory disease). It was later found that formalin-inactivated vaccine failed to stimulate antibody to the fusion protein: consequently the virus could spread from cell to cell, causing the atypical manifestations of disease (Norrby *et al.*, 1975).

An attenuated live-virus vaccine was developed from the *Edmonston* strain of measles virus by passage first in human cell culture, then in the amnionic sac of embryonated hen's eggs, and finally in chick embryo cells (Milovanovic *et al.*, 1957). This vaccine (Enders Passage Level B) was effective in inducing immunity but produced some adverse effects (Katz and Enders, 1959; Stokes *et al.*, 1962). Further attenuation by growth at lower temperature yielded an equally effective vaccine that produced fewer side effects (Schwarz, 1964; Hilleman *et al.*, 1968). Attenuated live-virus measles vaccine has been combined with mumps and rubella vaccines. Measles vaccine usage has reduced the incidence of measles in the United States from 440,000 cases in 1960 to 3,000 in 1985.

5. Canine Distemper Virus

Canine distemper virus affects most carnivores, causing respiratory, gastrointestinal, and central nervous system disease. The mortality rate in dogs is about 20%. Dunkin and Laidlaw (1926) first described the disease in detail and confirmed the viral etiology proposed earlier by Carre (1905).

Immunization. Laidlaw and Dunkin (1926, 1928a,b) prepared a vaccine by treating virus derived from spleens of infected dogs with formalin. Initial administration of this vaccine, followed 2 weeks later with a small dose of virulent virus, usually produced only a mild disease with solid immunity. This approach was replaced with inactivated virus vaccines, given in multiple doses, which served as the main means of controlling the disease from 1930 to 1950. Green (1945) serially passaged canine distemper virus in ferrets and produced the first attenuated live-virus vaccine; however, this vaccine caused disease in some dogs.

The adaptation of canine distemper virus to the chorioallantoic membrane of embryonated eggs by Haig (1948) was a major step in developing an attenuated live-virus vaccine. Cabasso and Cox (1949) applied this method and after 28 passages showed that the virus lost virulence for ferrets but retained its immunizing property for dogs. Rockborn (1958) adapted a strain of canine distemper virus to cell culture, and this method is now widely used to produce attenuated live-virus vaccines.

6. Rinderpest Virus

Rinderpest is an acute highly contagious disease of ruminants characterized by erosions and necrosis of the intestinal mucosa. The disease is epizootic in parts of Africa and Asia, causing great losses of cattle and buffalo.

Immunization. Koch in 1897 developed one of the first means of immunizing cattle against rinderpest by administering bile from infected cattle. Animals that survived were permanently immune. Formalin- and chloroform-inactivated vaccines were developed using tissues from infected animals. These vaccines were safe, but required two or three doses and protection lasted less than a year (Walker *et al.*, 1946). Rinderpest virus has been adapted to several foreign hosts, including goats (Daubney, 1949) and rabbits (Nakamura *et al.*, 1938) and has been attenuated by passage in these animals. Tissues of these animals have been used to produce vaccines in many countries. However, on continued passage, the seed strains tend to lose their immunogenicity, and vaccines become contaminated with adventitious agents from the foreign host.

The Kabete strain of rinderpest virus was adapted to grow on the chorioallantoic membrane of embryonated eggs, becoming attenuated for cattle after 19 passages (Shope *et al.*, 1946). This vaccine and another containing a lapinized strain of virus adapted to embryonated eggs have been used widely in Africa (Nakamura and Miyamoto, 1953). More recently, the Kabete strain was adapted to bovine kidney cell culture and after 70 passages became avirulent for cattle. This vaccine strain is safe and efficacious in most cattle breeds (Plowright and Ferris, 1962). Protection persists for at least 4 years. Over 150 million doses of this vaccine have been used in Africa, with good success (Maurer, 1980).

7. Bovine Respiratory Syncytial Virus (RSV)

Bovine RSV produces a rhinitis and catarrhal bronchiolitis in cattle (Mohanty *et al.*, 1975; Jacobs and Edington, 1975; Paccaud and Jacquier, 1970). The virus appears to be widespread having been isolated in Europe, the United States, and Asia. Human and bovine virus are related antigenically (Paccaud and Jacquier, 1970); however, the cattle virus is not known to infect man.

Immunization. Nasal secretory antibody is protective but the disease may occur in the presence of serum antibody. An inactivated bovine RSV vaccine is combined with vaccines for infectious bovine rhinotracheitis, bovine virus diarrhea, and bovine parainfluenza components in a multivalent formulation. The efficacy of the RSV component in this formulation is unclear.

I. Rhabdoviridae

Of the viruses in the family Rhabdoviridae that cause disease in man and domestic animals, the most important is rabies virus. Others include vesicular stomatitis viruses (VSV) and bovine emphemeral fever virus (BEFV). VSV occurs sporadically and epizootically, affecting horses, cattle and swine in the United States. There is a formalin-inactivated vaccine (Gearhart *et al.*, 1987), but it is used rarely. BEFV is an arthropod-transmitted disease of cattle occurring mainly in Africa, but also in Asia and Australia; it is controlled by immunization with attenuated live-virus vaccines (Van der Westhuizen, 1967; Inaba *et al.*, 1973; Spradbrow, 1977; Theodoridis *et al.*, 1973).

Rabies Virus

Rabies is an infection of the central nervous system; the disease can occur in most mammals and is usually fatal. There are only a few documented cases of human survivors. After isolating the virus, Pasteur (1881) developed a vaccine for its control. Historically rabies virus has been considered as a single serotype. But now shared antigens have been found in other viruses in Africa of which two, Mokola and Duvenhage, may be associated with human disease (Shope *et al.,* 1970). Mokola virus causes a rabies-like disease in dogs and cats in Zimbabwe (Foggin, 1983).

Immunization. Protection against rabies correlates with SN antibody, which can be assessed by a number of tests. Pasteur's classical vaccine, developed from infected spinal cord tissue dried at room temprerature for 3–14 days, was given in a series of 21–28 inoculations beginning with material dried the longest and progressing through material dried for only 3 days (Pasteur 1881). Even though the last inoculum was virulent enough to cause rabies, the earlier inoculations conferred sufficient immunity to protect the recipients. This method of producing a vaccine was successful in most instances but caused the disease occasionally and was eventually replaced by chemically inactivated vaccines prepared from infected brain tissue. Although effective, these vaccines gave rise to undesirable side-effects because they contained a myelin-related encephalitogen present in brains from mature animals. Substitution of brain tissue from immature animals such as suckling mice, rats, and rabbits with their lesser myelin antigenic content greatly reduced these post-vaccination reactions.

The adaptation of the Flury strain of rabies virus to growth in chick embryos led to the development of attenuated live-virus vaccines produced in this tissue (Leach and Johnson, 1940; Koprowski and Cox, 1948; Koprowski and Black, 1950, 1954).

The growth of rabies virus in tissue culture has further improved rabies vaccines (Kissling, 1958; Cabasso *et al.,* 1965; Emery *et al.,* 1968; Brown *et al.,* 1967; Fenje, 1960; Abelseth, 1964). Yet, despite their benefits, the attenuated rabies vaccines occasionally caused rabies, particularly in cats. Therefore, suckling mouse brain and tissue culture again became the substrates of choice to produce inactivated rabies virus vaccines for animals. In humans the requirement for a safe substrate is more exacting than in animals. For this reason, duck embryos proved better than brain tissue to produce rabies virus (Peck *et al.,* 1956). After inactivation with β-propriolactone (BPL), this virus was an improved product for humans, although the allergenic effects from duck embryo tissue still present a problem. Therefore the adaptation of the PM rabies virus strain to human diploid cells and inactivation with BPL (Wiktor *et al.*, 1964) was a further improvement. This vaccine is less reactive and more effective for pre- and post-exposure use in humans than any other yet made (Bahmanyar *et al.*, 1976). A similar vaccine produced in BHK cells is also beneficial in animals.

J. Retroviridae

Retroviruses have an RNA genome, a portion of which encodes the unique enzyme reverse transcriptase. This enzyme imparts to retroviruses the ability to make RNA-directed DNA copies of their genome, which can then act as a transposable element and can be integrated into the host cell DNA. Thus, once a cell is infected, it may escape immune surveillance and destruction and the host animal may be infected for life. The retroviruses thus constitute a considerable challenge to traditional vaccine approaches, as discussed further in the chapters by Arlinghaus and by Nathanson and Gonzalez-Scarano.

Many retroviruses infect mammalian species, from mouse to man. Most notable are the C-type retroviruses, including the primate, murine, and feline leukemia viruses, as well as human T-cell leukemia viruses types I and II; the B-type retroviruses, particularly mouse mammary tumor virus; and the lentiviruses, including caprine infectious anemia virus, Visna virus, equine infectious anemia virus, feline immunodeficiency virus, bovine immunodeficiency virus, and human immunodeficiency viruses (HIV-1 and HIV-2).

In recent years, as HIV has become a major threat, massive efforts have been directed to developing an efficacious vaccine. So far, all attempts have met with failure. In fact, there are only two retrovirus vaccines that have been proven effective: a formalin-inactivated whole virus preparation of the primate SAIDS type D retrovirus, which is capable of protecting monkeys from a lethal challenge (Marx *et al.*, 1986), and the commercially available vaccine for feline leukemia.

Feline Leukemia Virus (FeLV)

FeLV commonly infects cats in urban areas, usually by the oral–nasal route. Kittens under 6 months of age are particularly susceptible. About 1% of infected cats develop persistent anemia from which myeloproliferative disease and hypoplastic anemia may follow. The immunosuppression caused by FeLV infection may predispose to severe chronic opportunistic infections. Because cats that develop neutralizing antibody are usually immune to infection, vaccines have been developed and tested with that goal in mind.

Immunization. The problem in developing a vaccine for feline leukemia was to find immunogens that could be used without exposing animals to oncogenic materials. Early studies with inactivated whole virus were unsuccessful (Yohn *et al.*, 1976). Although attenuated live-virus vaccines induce sufficiently high levels of neutralizing antibodies to be protective (Jarrett *et al.*, 1974; Pedersen *et al.*, 1979), their oncogenic potential makes them unacceptable. Efforts to develop vaccines containing only viral proteins, such as envelope protein, have had variable results. However, cultivation of FeLV in FL 74-transformed cells, followed by treatment to release viral and cell proteins, yields a vaccine that stimulates antibodies to both viral and cell membrane components. A commercial vaccine using this method of antigen production has been approved for use in the United States; it is based on studies done by Olsen and Lewis (1981). Subsequently, the efficacy of this vaccine has been disputed (Pederson and Ott, 1985).

K. CORONAVIRIDAE

Viruses in the family Coronaviridae cause important diseases including avian infectious bronchitis, transmissible gastroenteritis of swine (TGE), feline infectious peritonitis (FIP), and human coronavirus infections. Other coronaviruses may cause disease in calves, dogs, mice, rats, turkeys, horses, and parrots, but the diseases are of less importance. Coronavirus diseases usually follow a similar pattern, except for FIP. FIP is a chronic debilitating disease manifested as fibrinous peritonitis and pleuritis. The infection may be inapparent, but is fatal in a small proportion of infected cats. The immune response to FIP virus seems to mediate the disease; the immune response is not protective and antibody levels are higher in diseased animals. Immune complexes have also been demonstrated in renal glomeruli of cats with FIP.

Bovine coronavirus causes acute diarrheal disease in neonatal calves (Mebus *et al.*, 1973). An attenuated live-virus vaccine is being used in combination with an attenuated live-virus rotavirus vaccine to control calf diarrhea. The vaccine is administered to pregnant cows near the end of gestation and stimulates colostral antibodies that offer protection to nursing calves.

With the exception of avian infectious bronchitis, most coronavirus infections have been difficult to control with vaccines. Perhaps this is because primary lesions are in mucous membranes of the respiratory and gastrointestinal tracts, sequestered from immune reactivity. Coronaviruses produce about 15% of common colds in man, second only to rhinoviruses. There are two groups of human coronaviruses that are antigenically distinct.

1. Avian Infectious Bronchitis Virus (IBV)

IBV is a highly contagious respiratory infection of young chickens. The virus may also infect older birds, causing a decrease in egg production. The disease was first shown to be caused by a virus by Bushnell and Brandley (1933). Beaudette and Hudson (1937) propagated the virus in chick embryos, making possible the quantification of the virus and the means for attenuation. There are a number of serotypes of IBV, making the development of an effective vaccine difficult.

Immunization. Immunity following natural infection may last up to 1 year, depending on the serotype and the severity of challenge. Van Roekel *et al.* (1950) first developed an immunization procedure; he used a field strain of virus to infect 7- to 15-week-old birds before they start to lay, inoculating a few of the birds and allowing infection to spread naturally through the flock. Today, there are a number of attenuated live-virus vaccines licensed in the United States. There is good protection (90–100%) against homologous virus strains and about 40% against heterologous strains (Hofstad, 1981). Reduced pathogenicity may be associated with reduced immunogenicity, so a balance must be maintained. The attenuated live-virus vaccines are administered by the usual labor-saving devices of spraying, dusting, or placing the vaccine in drinking water. The wide-scale use of IBV vaccines has significantly reduced the economic loss caused by this disease.

2. Transmissible Gastroenteritis Virus (TGE)

TGE is an often fatal disease of pigs under 2 weeks of age. The main lesion is enteritis, resulting in malabsorption, diarrhea, and dehydration. TGE virus is serologically related to FIP virus, but the diseases have entirely different characteristics. There is one serotype of TGE virus and one serotype of FIP virus.

High levels of maternal TGE antibody in sows' colostrum protect piglets if fed continuously. Immunity of this type has been produced by feeding sows tissues containing virulent TGE virus several weeks prior to gestation. The effects of this virus are relatively mild in older animals.

Immunization. Attenuated live-virus vaccines administered parenterally to pregnant swine in the latter part of the gestation period produce colostral antibodies. Apparently, in sows previously exposed to TGE, this vaccine produces sufficient immune responsiveness to be of value. The vaccine is also used orally in pigs 1–3 days old to induce local immunity. The effectiveness of this use of the vaccine has not been thoroughly demonstrated.

III. Vaccines for Gram-Positive Bacteria

A. *Corynebacterium*
   1. *C. pseudotuberculosis*
   2. *C. diphtheriae*

B. *Bacillus*

C. *Erysipelothrix*

D. *Clostridium*
   1. *C. perfringens*
   2. *C. tetani*

   3. *C. novyi*
   4. *C. chauvoei*
   5. *C. septicum*

E. *Mycobacterium*

F. *Streptococcus*
   1. *S. agalactiae*
   2. *S. pneumoniae*

A. *Corynebacterium*

The genus *Corynebacterium* is a heterogeneous grouping with its species placed together largely on the basis of similar cell wall components (Goodfellow and Minnikin, 1981). These species share a basic cell wall chemistry (Barksdale, 1981) of which the mycolic acids (Silva and Ioneda, 1977), especially trehalose dimycolate, are frequently used as potent adjuvants in immunization protocols.

Two corynebacteria—*C. pyogenes* and *C. pseudotuberculosis*—are important in veterinary medicine. The former is frequently associated with ruminate suppurative conditions and abscesses, but it rarely affects man. Infections with this organism are sporadic, because it is an opportunist that gains entry through wounds and abrasions. It may also be seen as a secondary invader in devitalized tissues; e.g., vaccination site abscesses. The efficacy of vaccines, toxoids, and antisera against *C. pyogenes* is equivocal; little is known about immunity to the bacterium.

1. Corynebacterium pseudotuberculosis

Corynebacterium pseudotuberculosis causes caseous lymphadenitis of goats and sheep. It is recognized as a worldwide problem and a serious cause of economic loss to the goat industry (Burrell, 1981; Ashfaq and Campbell, 1980). As with *C. pyogenes,* the responsible bacterium, *C. pseudotuberculosis,* is primarily an opportunist entering wounds or abrasions, where it causes local inflammation before settling in the regional lymph nodes.

Immunization. Cell-mediated immunity is necessary for acquired resistance and protection against *C. pseudotuberculosis* (Jolly, 1965; Tashjian and Campbell, 1983; Irwin and Knight, 1975). Killed and autogenous vaccines and a toxoid vaccine have been used in attempts to immunize against the bacterium (Cameron, 1972; Brogden *et al.,* 1984; Nairn *et al.,* 1977; Burrell, 1978; Anderson and Nairn, 1984; Brown *et al.,* 1986); however no one vaccine has proven highly efficacious.

2. Corynebacterium diphtheriae

Diphtheria, characterized by the formation of a tightly adherent pseudomembrane on the pharyngeal mucous membranes of the throat and trachea, is a highly contagious disease of man caused by the bacterium *C. diphtheriae.* The bacterium can also be isolated from the pharyngeal mucosa of normal individuals. The organism produces a lethal protein exotoxin (Gill and Pappenheimer, 1971; Collier and Kandel, 1971).

Immunization. Successful immunization against *C. diphtheriae* actually protects against the diphtherial exotoxin. Because diphtheria toxin is produced in high yield by the Park-Williams Number 8 strain (PW8), PW8 is used to make diphtherial toxoid for vaccines. As a source of toxin it is rendered nontoxic by incubation with formalin under alkaline conditions. The product's retention of antigenicity, enabling it to induce antitoxin antibodies, makes it an excellent pediatric vaccine. It is commonly utilized in combination with antigens from *C. tetani* and *B. pertussis.*

B. Bacillus

The most important species of the *Bacillus* genus, *B. anthracis,* is the organism responsible for the disease anthrax in both man and animals. Anthrax was the first bacterial disease ever to be reported, being described by Davaine in 1863. Koch in 1876 reproduced the disease via animal inoculation and in 1881 Pasteur successfully vaccinated against anthrax. In animals, natural infection usually occurs by ingestion of spores that germinate in the mucosa of the esophagus or the intestinal tract. Herbivorous animals, especially cattle, horses, sheep, and goats, are highly susceptible to the disease, usually the result of grazing in infected pastures or consuming infected foods.

In man, anthrax is manifested in three forms: cutaneous (malignant carbuncle), pulmonary (woolsorter's disease), and gastrointestinal with cutaneous being the most common. Death results from the combined effects of an extracellular toxic protein complex (Vodkin and Leppla, 1983) comprised of three components: edema factor, protective antigen, and lethal factor (Leppla, 1982; Stephen, 1981). Effective vaccines require all three components.

Immunization. The attenuated Pasteur vaccine has been supplanted in veterinary medicine by stable spore vaccines, carbo-zoo vaccine, or Stern vaccine (Jackson *et al.,* 1957) prepared from avirulent, nonencapsulated variants of *B. anthracis.* The viable bacterial spores are suspended in 10% saponin. Immunity is attributed to the development of antibodies to the toxins released from growing bacteria. Vaccines of killed bacteria provide little immunity, since no bacterial toxins are produced; hence, no antitoxin antibodies are generated. Purified protective antigen (complex toxin) is both antigenic and immunogenic and has been used as a vaccine for humans. It is prepared by aluminum potassium sulfate precipitation of sterile *B. anthracis* culture filtrates and has proven highly efficacious.

C. *Erysipelothrix*

Erysipelothrix is found in soil, water, and decaying vegetative material and carcasses. The major species of interest is *E. rhusiopathiae,* which has 20 serotypes (Norrung, 1979). The bacterium, most notable for causing swine erysipelas, is capable of invading the tissues of both man and animal. Fatally affected animals develop welt-like, discolored cutaneous lesions, and numerous hemorrhagic lesions in thoracic and abominal viscera; chronic debilitating arthritis predominates in surviving animals.

Immunization. The principal vaccines used to control erysipelas are formalin-killed, alum-adsorbed, whole-cell culture vaccines. These combinations of soluble bacterial glycoprotein and whole killed bacterial cells are usually produced from strains of serotype 2, which possess highly antigenic soluble cell wall glycoproteins. Animals immunized with cell-free culture fluids develop agglutinins to the whole bacteria (White and Verway, 1970). Such vaccines are highly effective in controlling swine erysipelas.

D. *Clostridium*

The pathogenic clostridia invade both man and many animal species of veterinary interest, in which they cause such diseases as tetanus (*C. tetani*), gas gangrene (*C. perfringens, C. septicum, C. oedematous*), botulism (*C. botulinum*), enterotoxemia, and dysentery (*C. perfringens*). The clostridia are widely distributed in soil and water and are common inhabitants of the intestinal tracts of animals and humans. Additionally, the bacteria can often be isolated from infected wounds. Vaccination is not routinely practiced against all clostridial organisms, notably *C. botulinum*. The toxins of *C. botulinum*, which exert their effects upon the nervous system (Schantz and Sugiyama, 1974), are as potent as those of *C. tetani*. The lethal dose of the toxin, however, is less than that required to induce an antibody response.

1. *Clostridium perfringens*

Clostridium perfringens has five serotypes, A–E, classified according to the production of lethal exotoxins. Types A and C are pathogenic for man, whereas all five serotypes can affect animals (see Table I).

Immunization. The exotoxins of *C. perfringens* are antigenic proteins that can be detoxified for use in vaccines. The existence of common capsular antigens, which elicit cross-reactions between the serotypes, demonstrates the considerable heterogeneity of this group. Ewes and lambs are frequently vaccinated against *C. perfringens* enterotoxemias. Effective vaccines employ type-specific alum-

TABLE I

DISEASES CAUSED BY AND THE MAJOR SOLUBLE ANTIGENS OF *C. perfringens* SEROTYPES A, B, C, D, AND E

Type	Host	Disease	Toxins			
A	Man Sheep Horses	Gas gangrene, food poisoning Yellow lamb disease	α			
B	Sheep	Lamb dysentery	α,	β,	ε	
C	Man Sheep Cattle Piglets	Enteritis necroticans "Struck," toxemia Hemorrhagic enteritis	α,	β,	γ,	σ
D	Sheep	Enterotoxemia	α,	σ,	ε	
E	Sheep, cattle	Enterotoxemia	α,	ι		

precipitation or formalinized toxoids (Smith and Matsuoka, 1959; Kennedy *et al.*, 1977).

2. *Clostridium tetani*

Clostridium tetani elaborates potent neurotropic exotoxins (tetanospasmin and tetanolysin) that may be lethal for susceptible species such as man, horses, mules, swine, cattle, and sheep. Birds are not naturally susceptible to the bacterium. Tetanus toxin is one of the most poisonous toxins known. It acts only on the nervous system and its effect characteristically causes spastic paralysis and generalized convulsions.

Immunization. Protective antitoxin blood levels are obtained by immunizing both humans and susceptible animals with alum-precipitated or absorbed tetanus toxoid (Chodnik *et al.*, 1959). Ramon and Lemetayer (1931) first introduced the concept of active immunization against tetanus when they used formalinized tetanus toxoid precipitated with alum to vaccinate horses. *Clostridium tetani* vaccines are very effective at inducing long-lasting immunity in both man and domestic animal species. A serious, often fatal disease has been successfully controlled with these vaccines.

3. *Clostridium novyi*

Clostridium novyi possesses four antigenic types, A, B, C, and D; type A is the most common clinical pathogen. Types A and B are responsible for gas gangrene both in man and animals (Elder and Miles, 1957). In areas where sheep simultaneously carry a heavy liver-fluke infestation, exposure to *C. novyi* is often associated wtih hepatic necrosis and subcutaneous edema. Migrating flukes produce foci of hepatic necrosis suitable for the germination of spores and the subsequent elaboration of lethal toxins (Williams, 1962).

Immunization. Effective vaccinations for *C. novyi* in animals employ chemically inactivated, detoxified, and adjuvanted suspensions of alum-precipitated formalinized whole broth cultures.

4. *Clostridium chauvoei*

Clostridium chauvoei, which is the etiologic agent for the disease "blackleg" and is pathogenic for animals only, occurs primarily in ruminant species. Protective antigens and toxins with hemolytic and necrotizing activity are formed in susceptible animals (Jayaraman *et al.*, 1962). The necrotizing toxin may effect fatal toxemia with degenerative foci of myonecrosis.

Immunization. Immunity to *C. chauvoei* can be produced via vaccination with its alum-precipitated formalinized cultures (Chandler and Gulasekhuram, 1970).

5. Clostridium septicum

Clostridium septicum, in contrast to *C. chauvoei,* is pathogenic for both man and animal. In man, it is associated with gas gangrene and in affected animals, primarily ruminants, it is the agent most closely identified with the diseases malignant edema and braxy. The organism produces four lethal necrotizing, hemolyzing toxins that cause an increase in capillary permeability and myonecrosis.

Immunization. Immunity to *C. septicum* is induced with injection of formalinized bacterial cultures. The antitoxin provides homologous protection and additionally protects against *C. chauvoei.* Animals are often vaccinated with mixtures of Clostridial species; i.e., *novyi, chauvoei, septicum, perfringens,* and *sordelli* in one combination vaccine. These are highly efficacious vaccines and are routinely used in veterinary medicine.

E. Mycobacterium

Although infections with *Mycobacterium tuberculosis* primarily occur through inhalation of the tubercle bacillus, ingestion of large numbers of the bacilli in contaminated milk or infectious sputum can readily produce disease in susceptible species. The bacterium is pathogenic in man, but can also cause disease in monkeys, pigs, and occasionally in cattle, dogs, and parrots. The disease may be asymptomatic or produce severe, debilitating pulmonary lesions. If infection is not restricted by the immune system, the disease may be fatal (Comstock, 1982; Bloom and Godal, 1983). Since bacteriocidal mechanisms of the normal macrophage prevent *M. tuberculosis* from multiplying intercellularly (Goren, 1977; Goren *et al.,* 1976), protective immunity depends on cell-mediated immunity (Lagrange, 1984).

Mycobacterium bovis, closely related to *M. tuberculosis,* and *M. avium* causes disease primarily in cattle and birds. They can, however, be contagious to man, sheep, and pigs.

Immunization. Immunoprophylaxis for tuberculosis is based on vaccination with an attenuated, relatively avirulent strain of *M. bovis* that does not produce lesions. The strain is known as BCG or the bacillus of Calmette and Guérin (1924, 1926). Worldwide, this is one of the most widely used human vaccines, as it has proven efficacious in controlling a severe disease. Additionally, BCG has been used for nonspecific enhancement of resistance against tumors and other infections. The cell wall of *M. tuberculosis* is a potent immunostimulant when used in Freund's adjuvant.

F. *Streptococcus*

Although streptococci may be normal inhabitants of the gastrointestinal tract, they may also be pathogenic for both man and animals. On the basis of characteristic cell wall components, the streptococci are traditionally divided into Lancefield groupings (Lancefield, 1934).

1. *Streptococcus agalactiae*

Streptococcus agalactiae, a streptococcus group B organism, causes severe mastitis in the bovine species and has been identified as a major cause of serious neonatal infections in man (Eickoff *et al.,* 1964). Capsular antigens form the four major type-specific antigens (Ia, Ib, II, and III), with type III organisms being most commonly associated with neonatal meningitis. In infants, early-onset disease occurs within the first days of life and is characterized by sepsis and pneumonia. The mortality rate is high. Late-onset disease occurs around 1 month of age and is characterized by meningitis (Einstein *et al.,* 1982).

Immunization. There is a direct correlation between the absence of maternal IgG antibody to type III antigen and the incidence of neonatal infection. Thus, susceptibility to the bacterium is related to the absence of significant levels of maternal serum antibody being transferred transplacentally to the fetus. Current vaccine developments are directed toward maternal immunization with type III antigen (Einstein *et al.,* 1982).

2. *Streptococcus pneumoniae*

Streptococcus pneumoniae, the etiologic agent of pneumococcal pneumonia in human infants and adults, may cause septicemia, meningitis, and inner ear infections. Aerosol transmission of the bacterium, often in association with viral upper respiratory infections, is the major mode of transmitting *S. pneumoniae* infections. *Streptococcus pneumoniae* possesses a capsular polysaccharide capable of deterring phagocytosis, thus enhancing the virulence of the bacterium. Of over 80 types of the bacterium identified, 10 serotypes are most frequently associated with the disease.

Immunization. A polyvalent pneumococcal vaccine prepared from soluble purified capsular polysaccharides of the 23 most predominant *S. pneumoniae* serotypes has proven effective in adults. The capsular polysaccharides are well-tolerated and highly immunogenic; significant rises in protective serum antibody titers are achieved following vaccination (Kasper *et al.*, 1982). However, vaccination of infants has not proven beneficial, because they develop no higher antibody titers to the bacteria than do unvaccinated infants (Ginsburg, 1986).

IV. Vaccines for Gram-Negative Bacteria

A. Entobacteria
  1. *Escherichia coli*
  2. *Salmonella* spp.
  3. *Yersinia pestis*

B. *Pasteurella*
  1. *P. multocida*
  2. *P. haemolytica*

C. *Hemophilus*
  1. *H. pleuropneumoniae*
  2. *H. somnus*

D. *Bordetella*
  1. *B. pertussis*
  2. *B. bronchiseptica*

E. *Brucella*
  1. *B. abortus*
  2. *B. melitensis*
  3. *B. ovis*

F. *Campylobacter*
  1. *C. fetus venerealis*
  2. *C. fetus intestinalis*

G. *Vibrio*
  V. cholera

H. *Leptospira* spp.

I. *Neisseria*
  N. meningitidis

J. *Rickettsia*

A. Enterobacteria

Many members of this family are indigenous to the gastrointestinal tract with the fecal–oral route, often the most important mode of transmission in animals. Established carriers may intermittently shed bacteria.

1. Escherichia coli

Enterotoxigenic pathogenic strains of *Escherichia coli* may cause severe, potentially fatal, diarrheal disease in both man and domestic species, particularly neonatal cattle and swine. The capsular (K) antigens are cell-surface proteins and/or polysaccharides associated with virulence. The K88 antigen mediates adhesion to the microvillus of intestinal epithelial cells; production and release of enterotoxin follow (Bywater, 1970; Lonroth *et al.*, 1979). *Escherichia coli* neonatal enteritis of newborn calves is also a serotype-specific disease (Myers and Guinee, 1976). All important colostral antibodies in both swine and cattle are anti-K antibodies (usually K99) (Myers and Guinee, 1976; Moon et al., 1978).

Immunization. Vaccination of gilts, sows, heifers, and cows with vaccines prepared from the K88 or other pilus-associated antigens has reduced morbidity and mortality from *E. coli* nec natal enteritis of newborn piglets and calves (Nagy et al., 1978; Rutter, 1975; Kohler et al., 1975; Childrow and Porter, 1979; Myers and Guinee, 1976). To prepare the porcine vaccines, bacterial strains specific for the herds to be vaccinated are used to immunize animals 3 weeks prior to parturition, thereby generating specific, protective colostral antibodies. Recombinant DNA technology, discussed in the chapter by Collett has introduced the potential to construct *E. coli* vaccine strains that would afford considerably better protection than those currently available.

2. Salmonella spp.

Salmonella species are a major cause of invasive enteric infections in humans and domestic animals, with domestic poultry constituting the largest reservoir of *Salmonella* organisms in nature. Normally, infection occurs through the oral route. *Salmonella* is a facultative intracellular pathogen; therefore, cell-mediated immunity is more important than humoral immunity in resistance to the disease, salmonellosis (Fields et al., 1986a,b; Dougan et al., 1987; Woolcock, 1973).

Salmonella typhi, the only *Salmonella* species that has a capsular polysaccharide (Vi antigen), is the etiologic agent of typhoid fever, a serious and common disease in underdeveloped areas (Edelman and Levine, 1986). This pathogen infects humans only; there is no suitable animal model for typhoid fever.

Immunization. Few vaccines have been developed for *Salmonella,* and most are of low efficacy with undesirable side-effects. Live vaccines are more effective than killed ones in promoting better immunity (Levine et al., 1983; Dougan et al., 1987; Roantree, 1967). With respect to *S. typhi,* vaccines containing the inactivated bacteria offer only limited and transient protection with undesirable side-effects (Levine, et al., 1983). The attenuated strain of *S. typhi,* Ty-21a, requires multiple doses to achieve 60–70% protection (Hirschel et al., 1985). Consequently, typhoid fever has not been controlled by immunization, although the Vi antigen has recently been hailed as the agent of a preventative vaccine (Robbins and Robbins, 1984) without adverse side-effects (Acharya et al., 1987).

3. Yersinia pestis

Yersinia pestis is the etiologic agent of plague or "black death" in man, a highly fatal disease with fever and purulent lymphadenopathy. Although not a disease of domestic animals, rats, ground squirrels, and other rodents may be affected. The bacterium is spread by the rat flea, *Xenopsylla cheopis,* from rat to rat and from rat to man.

Immunization. The most widely used vaccine for the prevention of *Y. pestis* infection is Haffkine's vaccine, first developed in 1897. This vaccine is prepared from heat and phenol-killed virulent cultures. Formalin-killed virulent bacteria are also successful, as are living avirulent strains (Grasset, 1946). The is no evidence that any vaccine protects against pneumonic plague, the most contagious and fatal form of the disease. Furthermore, vaccine protection is only recommended for plague research workers. Disease control is primarily dependent upon eradication of rodent carriers of *Y. pestis.*

B. Pasteurella

Pasteurella multocida and *P. haemolytica* are common commensals of the mucous membranes of the respiratory tract and oropharynx of healthy cattle, sheep, swine, dogs, and cats. When the bacteria multiply unchecked, they can penetrate the oral and/or respiratory mucosa, where they quickly grow and overpower the host's defense systems.

1. Pasteurella multocida

Pasteur first described this bacterium as the etiologic agent of fowl cholera; it is also associated with bovine pneumonia, swine plague, and an epizootic hemorrhagic septicemia in ungulates. The bacterium's heat-stable antigens have been used as serologic indicators in the gel diffusion precipitin test to define its 16 serotypes (Brogden *et al.,* 1978).

Immunization. Pasteur's successful bacterial vaccine to fowl cholera, and the first vaccine ever used, consisted of avirulent cultures of the *P. multocida* attenuated by prolonged growth on artificial medium. Killed *P. multocida* vaccines are prepared from virulent immunogenic strains of the bacterium. The organisms are suspended in formalinized saline, incorporated into an adjuvant, and injected subcutaneously (Heddleston *et al.,* 1974). These vaccines induce substantial immunity to fowl cholera. Additionally, live vaccines for oral administration have been developed for use in the poultry industry (Dougherty *et al.*, 1955; Heddleston *et al.*, 1974; Olson, 1977; Bierer and Derieux, 1972).

Pasteurella multocida is usually mixed with modified live or killed bovine rhinotracheitis virus, parainfluenza 3 virus, bovine viral diarrhea virus, and *P. hemolytica* bacteria in combination vaccines to protect against *Pasteurella* pneumonia in cattle.

2. *Pasteurella haemolytica*

Bovine pneumonic pasteurellosis (shipping fever) is a severe fibrinous pneumonia of feedlot cattle usually associated with biotype A, serotype 1 infections with this organism.

Immunization. Administration of either killed or live vaccines has been of limited efficacy in controlling shipping fever. Partial protection from experimental disease follows immunization of cattle with either live *P. haemolytica* by aerosol or parenteral routes (Panciera *et al.*, 1984; Confer *et al.*, 1984) or lyophilized *P. haemolytica* vaccines consisting of chemically altered, streptomycin-dependent, or modified live organisms given intramuscularly or intradermally (Confer *et al.*, 1986). Humoral antibody responses appear to correlate strongly with protection against experimental disease (Confer *et al.*, 1985; McKinney *et al.*, 1985). For example, purified *P. haemolytica* lipopolysaccharide stimulates specific antibody formation and has protected calves challenged with the bacterium from developing the disease (Hilwig *et al.*, 1985).

C. *Hemophilus*

These obligate parasites, restricted to respiratory and pharyngeal mucous membranes, cause important diseases in porcine (*H. pleuropneumonia, H. suis,* and *H. parasuis*), equine (*H. equigenitalis*), bovine (*H. somnus*), and avian (*H. gallinarum, H. paragallinarum*) hosts. Most *Hemophilus* species require two factors, hemin (X) and nicotinamide adenine dinucleotide (V), for growth.

Antigens associated with protection and virulence have been described for *H. paragallinarum* (Yamamoto, 1984), the etiologic agent of infectious coryza in chickens. Birds that have recovered from natural infection possess varying degrees of immunity to re-exposure (Page *et al.*, 1963); immunity is serotype-specific. Adjuvanted vaccines containing multiple bacterial serotypes are prepared from chicken embryos or formalinized bacterial broth cultures and are effective vaccines in preventing infectious coryza in chickens.

1. *Hemophilus pleuropneumoniae*

This bacterium is the etiologic agent of the porcine disease, contagious pleuropneumonia, which is characterized by severe multifocal, necrotizing pneumonia with venous thrombosis and associated serofibrinous pleuritis (Didier *et al.*, 1984). The disease is of considerable economic importance to the swine industry, being most prevalent in situations where swine are raised under intensive management conditions. *Hemophilus pleuropneumoniae* possesses major and minor antigens that are both common and serotype specific (Gunnarson *et al.*, 1978; Gunnarson, 1979; Mittal *et al.*, 1982). Since high antibody titer apparently provides little protection from the disease, cell-mediated immunity may be important in protection from infection (Rapp and Ross, 1984; Rosendal *et al.*, 1981).

Immunization. No adequate immunoprophylaxis against contagious pleuropneumonia is currently available, although many vaccines have been tried (Nielsen, 1976; Henry and Marstellar, 1982; Christensen, 1982; Masson *et al.*, 1982). Prior infection with one serotype provides protection from heterologous serotypes (Nielsen, 1976). The bacterial strains used in vaccines are serotype specific and, while not preventing the disease, can reduce its severity (Christensen, 1982).

2. *Hemophilus somnus*

Hemophilus somnus is the cause of infectious meningoencephalitis, a disease with low morbidity but high mortality in cattle. Whole or sonicated bacterial cells and bacterial protein are immunogenic (Noyer *et al.*, 1976) and efficacious bacterins foster protective immunity in calves (Williams *et al.*, 1978). The bacterins of *H. somnus*, adjuvanted with aluminum hydroxide, are prepared from highly immunogenic strains of the bacterium and grown in serum-free media for use as vaccines.

D. *Bordetella*

The species in this genera, *B. pertussis, B. bronchiseptica,* and *B. parapertussis,* can be either parasites or, as in swine and dogs, common inhabitants of the upper respiratory tract. These small, serologically related bacilli produce a dermonecrotic toxin. Infection is by aerosol transmission with bacteria adherent to tracheal cilia (Bemis *et al.*, 1977). Local, not serum, antibody concentration is important in clearance of the infection.

1. Bordetella pertussis

The etiologic agent of whooping cough, *B. pertussis*, produces two distinct hemagglutinins, leukocytosis-promoting factor-hemagglutinin (LPF-HA) and filamentous hemagglutinin (FHA), and various toxins (pertussis toxin [PT] and dermonecrotic toxin). FHA is involved in bacterial adherence to the respiratory mucosa, whereas PT is believed to be the major protective (Sato and Sato, 1984) and pathogenic antigen (Steinman *et al.*, 1985).

Immunization.   Although efficacious, the safety of the human vaccines currently in use, suspensions of killed whole cells containing protective antigens, is open to question (Robinson *et al.*, 1985). Undesirable side-effects such as screaming, collapse, encephalopathy, and other serious neurological complications have been reported in association with *B. pertussis* vaccinations (Dick, 1978). The potencies of whole cell vaccines correlate with the antigenic content of PT (Reiser and Germanier, 1986).

2. Bordetella bronchiseptica

Bordetella bronchiseptica is an obligate parasite of the upper respiratory tract of both dogs and pigs. In dogs the bacterium frequently invades the lungs as a sequela to canine distemper (caused by a morbillivirus), causing an often fatal bronchopneumonia. The bacterium is also associated with mild to severe tracheobronchitis, "kennel cough," in dogs (Bemis *et al.*, 1977). In pigs, a deformation of the bony structures of the nasal area (atrophic rhinitis) and reduction of the total volume of nasal turbinates commonly follow the bacterial infection (Ross *et al.*, 1963). Degenerative changes in the osteoblasts and osteocytes may be caused by elaboration of a dermonecrotic toxin (DNT), which is released from *B. bronchiseptica* after colonization or multiplication of the organisms on the nasal mucosa (Nakai *et al.*, 1985). The release of DNT from *P. multocida* type D is thought to exacerbate the disease.

Immunization.   Vaccines to control canine *B. bronchiseptica* infections are commonly incorporated into combination packages containing attenuated live-virus canine distemper, and canine adeno and parainfluenza viruses. To control atrophic rhinitis, avirulent live, or inactivated organisms alone or in combination with *P. multocida, Erysipelothrix rhusiopathiae* and *E. coli* have been utilized in vaccines.

E. Brucella

The organisms in this group, *B. abortus, B. suis, B. melitensis, B. canis,* and *B. ovis,* cause the disease brucellosis in domestic animals and man. The bacterium may localize in the reproductive tract which, in the female, can lead to fetal death with subsequent abortion. Brucellosis, due to *B. abortus* or *B. melitensis,* is a zoonotic disease, readily transmitted from animal to man.

1. Brucella abortus

The potentially severe consequences of brucellosis, fetal death and abortion, in the pregnant cow and epididymitis and sterility in the bull result in significant economic loss to the cattle industry. The primary source of infection is infected animals, whose mammary and/or genital secretions may contain the bacterium. Calves can become infected *in utero;* however, the main portals of infection are oral mucosa, nasopharynx, and conjuctiva of exposed animals. Immunity to *B. abortus* is dependent upon cell-mediated immunity, as the presence of serum antibodies, although a significant indicator of infection, does not correlate with the immune status of the host (Fitzgeorge *et al.,* 1967; Kaneene, *et al.,* 1978; Swiderska *et al.,* 1971; Montaraz and Winter, 1986).

2. Brucella melitensis

Most humans who contract brucellosis have been exposed either to *B. melitensis,* the etiologic agent of Malta or Mediterranean fever, or *B. abortus. Brucella melitensis,* found in the milk of infected sheep and goats, may produce fatal disease when ingested by humans. Brucellosis of sheep and goats mimics the disease as it is seen in cattle, with fetal death and abortion occurring in ewes and does and epididymitis in rams and billies.

3. Brucella ovis

Brucella ovis infects sheep, causing late fetal death and abortion in pregnant ewes and epididymitis in rams, such as *B. abortus* does in cattle.

Immunization. Brucella abortus (Strain 19) is currently used as the vaccine of choice for control of brucellosis of cattle in the United States. This is a viable, smooth strain that, while posing virtually no threat for cattle, may cause disease in man. The major objections to the vaccine are this pathogenicity for humans and the difficulty of differentiating vaccinated from naturally infected animals since persistent serum antibodies are induced by the vaccine. Killed *B. melitensis* in adjuvant or live avirulent strains have been used for vaccines to induce a high degree of immunity in sheep and goats. *Brucella ovis* bacterins in adjuvant, as well as *B. melitensis* vaccines, have been used to protect animals from the disease *B. ovis* causes, since the antigens of these two pathogens are cross-protective (Diaz *et al.*, 1967).

F. *Campylobacter*

Pathogenic members of this genus are associated with venereal disease, fetal death, and abortion in cattle.

1. *Campylobacter fetus venerealis*

This bacterium is transmitted to uninfected cattle by coitus or artificial insemination and is an obligate parasite of the genital tract.

Immunization. Stimulation of opsonizing antibodies of the IgG class by systemic vaccination with adjuvanted vaccines is effective in preventing natural infection in bulls (Bouters *et al.*, 1973) and infertility in cows (Corbeil *et al.*, 1974; Hoerlin and Kramer, 1964), and prevents the carrier state (Wilkie and Winter, 1971).

2. *Campylobacter fetus intestinalis*

Unlike *C. fetus venerealis,* this bacterium is contracted by ingestion and is not transmitted venereally. Both sheep and cattle can be infected; however, the disease is most severe in pregnant ewes, which undergo a high percentage of abortions or premature births within a flock.

Immunization. In sheep, vaccination with polyvalent adjuvanted vaccines is efficacious in preventing disease (Thompson and Gilmour, 1978).

G. *Vibrio*

The most important organism of this genus, *V. cholera,* causes severe, acute enteritis in humans and nonhuman primates.

Virbrio cholera

The etiologic agent of cholera in humans, *V. cholera,* causes a potentially fatal diarrheal disease. Infection results in the production of a powerful enterotoxin in the small intestine, which stimulates an increase in cyclic AMP in intestinal epithelial cells and causes a profuse outpouring of isotonic fluids. *Vibrio* possesses immunogenic heat-labile flagellar (H) protein and heat-stable (O) lipopolysaccharide somatic antigens. The cholera toxin is immunologically and functionally similar to the heat-labile enterotoxin of *E. coli* (Yamamoto *et al.,* 1984). It consists of six light subunits (L) that assist in toxin adherence to intestinal cell receptors and one heavy subunit (H), which is the toxic entity.

Immunization. Present cholera vaccines are administered by parenteral or oral routes. Parenteral vaccines consist of formalin/phenol-inactivated bacteria, whereas oral vaccines employ killed or live bacteria. Vaccines given by either route provide protection for approximately 3–9 months. The predominant immune mechanism is antibacterial rather than antitoxic (Levine *et al.,* 1979); antibacterial antibodies prevent attachment of the bacterium, whereas antitoxic antibodies inhibit toxin adherence to cell receptors. Because current vaccines often produce adverse side-effects (Feeley, 1970), synthetic and semi-synthetic vaccines are currently under investigation. For the latter, a nonpyrogenic, bivalent cell-surface protein–polysaccharide conjugate is being investigated (Kabir, 1986).

H. *Leptospira* spp.

The pathogenic genera of this family can penetrate the gastrointestinal mucosa and abraded epidermis. Leptospires are transmitted through contact with the urine of animal carriers, either directly or in contaminated water or soil. Rodents are the primary reservoir of the bacteria which, due to its ability to synthesize urease, colonizes the renal nephron and subsequently is shed into the urine. Leptospirosis causes economically serious disease in cattle and swine by causing fetal death, abortion, and infertility. Recovery from infection with one serotype lends immunity only to that serotype. This immunity is predominantly humoral, since agglutinins (IgM) are responsible for the initial clearance of the bacteria; neutralizing antibodies (IgG) are also protective (Hanson, 1974; Negi *et al.,* 1971). Canine leptospirosis infections may be severe, occurring more commonly in male dogs than in females. Man is a dead-end host for leptospires; infection in man is accidental and usually related to occupational exposure.

Immunization. Killed, multivalent, leprospira vaccines protect against clinical disease in cattle and swine; however, in pigs, immunity does not protect against renal colonization (Stalheim, 1968). Dogs can be vaccinated successfully with formalin or phenol-killed vaccines that contain antigens from the two most common infecting serotypes, *L. canicola* and *L. icterohemorrhagica* (Kerr and Marshall, 1974). Vaccines for humans, prepared from chemically inactivated cells of leptospires, have been used extensively in certain areas of the world.

I. *Neisseria*

Neisseria meningitidis

Neisseria meningitidis is a frequent cause of endemic purulent meningitis in human infants and adults, although the incidence of the disease is substantially higher in young infants (Hoffman, 1986). Bacterial invasion of the meninges is usually hematogenous from the upper respiratory tract and is a life-threatening affliction. *Neisseria meningitidis* has been classified into at least nine groups (A, B, C, W-135, X, Y, Z, L, 29-E) on the basis of its capsular polysaccharides (Morse, 1986).

Immunization. Protection against meningococcus meningitis results primarily from the presence of antibodies against the capsular polysaccharide of *N. meningitidis* (Frasch *et al.*, 1982). Group A and C polysaccharide vaccines are especially effective against disease in children over two years of age and in adults.

J. *Rickettsia*

Epidemic typhus fever has afflicted mankind since ancient times. It is an acute highly infectious disease with the potential for explosive epidemics in man. Significant outbreaks of the disease have been intimately associated with war and famine. The disease is characterized by sustained high fevers, headache, panencephalitis, a diffuse maculopapular skin rash, and toxic vascular damage. The fatality rate may be high. The etiologic agent, *R. prowazeki,* is transmitted from person to person by the human body louse *Pediculus humanus corporis*. Infection is established by inoculating infected louse feces into the skin by scratching.

Immunization. Although no etiologic relationship has been demonstrated between *R. prowazeki* and the bacterial strain *Proteus* OX19, these two species share a common polysaccharide antigen (Castaneda, 1934). The sera of infected typhus patients agglutinates *Proteus* OX19 and this test is now standard (Weil–Felix reaction) for diagnosis of the acute disease. Additionally, *R. prowazeki* has two major antigenic components—one heat labile and the other heat stable (Craigie *et al.*, 1946; Topping *et al.*, 1945). Typhus fever vaccine contains killed organisms propagated in the yolk-sac membranes of developing chick embryos (Cox, 1948). This vaccine not only diminishes the symptoms of typhus in immunized persons, but it also greatly reduces the mortality rate (Gilliam, 1946). The usefulness of the attenuated (Madrid E strain) vaccine is hampered because, under appropriate conditions, the strain may revert to virulence (Brezina, 1982).

ACKNOWLEDGMENTS

The authors wish to acknowledge Drs. Frederick Murphy, Fred Brown, Erling Norrby, John Elder, Donald McCarthy, and Ms. Phyllis Minick for their advice. Hagan and Bruner's *Infectious Diseases of Domestic Animals* and Braude's *Infectious Diseases and Medical Microbiology* were useful references in writing this chapter.

REFERENCES

Abelseth, M. K. (1964). *Can. Vet. J.* **5**, 279–286.

Acharya, I. L., Lowe, C. U., Thapa, R., and Gurubacharya, V. L. (1987). *N. Engl. J. Med.* **317**, 1101–1104.

Alexander, R. A., and DuToit, R. M. (1934). *Onderstepoort J. Vet. Sci. Anim. Ind.* **2**, 357.

Alexander, R. A., Haig, D. A., and Adelaar, T. F. (1947). *Onderstepoort J. Vet. Sci. Anim. Ind.* **21**, 231–241.

Anderson, M. J., and Pattison, J. R. (1984). *Arch. Virol.* **82**, 137–148.

Anderson, V. M., and Nairn, M. E. (1984). *Colloq. INRA* **28**, 601–609.

Appel, M. J. G., and Percy, D. H. (1970). *Am. Vet. Med. Assoc.* **156**, 1778–1785.

Appel, M. J. G., Bistner, S. I., Menegus, M., Albert, D. A., and Carmichael, L. E. (1973). *Am. J. Vet. Res.* **34**, 543–550.

Appel, M. J. G., Cooper, G. J., Greisen, H., Scott, F., and Carmichael, L. E. (1979). *Cornell Vet.* **69**, 123–133.

Appel, M. J. G., Scott, F. W., and Carmichael L. E. (1979b). *Vet. Rec.* **105**, 156–159.

Arbeter, A. M., Starr, S. E., Weibel, R. E., Neff, B. J., and Plotkin, S. A. (1983). *Pediatrics* **71**, 307–312.

Asano, Y., Hirose, S., Tsuzuki, K., Ito, S., Isomura, S., Takahashi, M., Nakayama, H., Yazaki, T., and Nato, R. (1977). *Pediatrics* **59**, 3–7.

Ashfaq, M. K., and Campbell, S. G. (1980). *Am. J. Vet. Res.* **41**, 1789–1192.

Asplin, F. D. (1952). *Vet. Rec.* **64**, 245–249.

Aygun (1955). *Arch. Exp. Vet. Med.* **9**, 145.

Bahmanyar, M., Fayaz, A., Nour-Saiebi, S., Mohammadi, M., and Koprowski, H. (1976). *J. Am. Med. Assoc.* **36**, 2751–2754.

Baker, J. A. (1946). *Proc. Soc. Exp. Biol. Med.* **63**, 183–185.

Barksdale, L. (1981). *In* "The Prokaryotes" (M. P. Starr, H. Stolp, H. G. Truper, and A. Barlows, and H. G. Schlegel, eds.), Vol. 2. Springer-Verlag, New York.

Bartha, A., and Kojnok, J. (1963). *Proc. World Vet. Congress, 17th* Vol. 1, p. 53.

Bass, E. P., Gill, M. A., and Beckenhauer, W. H. (1980). *J. Am. Vet. Med. Assoc.* **177**, 234–242.

Beard, J. W., Finkelstein, H., Sealy, W. C., and Wyckoff, R. W. G. (1938). *Science* **87**, 490.

Beaudette, F. R., and Hudson, C. B. (1933). *J. Am. Vet. Med. Assoc.* **82**, 460.

Beaudette, F. R., and Hudson, C. B. (1937). *J. Am. Vet. Med. Assoc.* **90**, 51–60.

Bemis, D. A., Greiser, H. A., and Appel, M. J. G. (1977). *J. Infect. Dis.* **135**, 753–762.

Benton, W. J., Cover, M. S., and Greene, L. M. (1958). *Avian Dis.* **2**, 383–396.

Berge, T. O., Banks, I. S., and Tigertt, W. D. (1961). *Am. J. Hyg.* **73**, 209–218.

Bierer, B. W., and Derieux, W. T. (1972). *Poult. Sci.* **51**, 408–416.

Biggs, P. M., and Payne, L. N. (1963). *Vet. Rec.* **75**, 177–179.

Binn, L. N., Lazar, E. C., Rogul, M., Shepler, V. M., Swango, L. J., Claypool, T., Hubbard, D. W., Asbill, S. G., and Alexander, A. D. (1968). *Am. J. Vet. Res.* **29**, 1809–1815.

Bittle, J. L., and Rubic, W. (1975). *Am. J. Vet. Res.* **36**, 89–91.

Bittle, J. L., and Rubic, W. (1976). *Am. J. Vet. Res.* **37**, 275–278.

Bittle, J. L., York, C. J., Newberne, J. W., and Martin, M. (1960). *Am. J. Vet. Res.* **21,** 547–550.

Bittle, J. L., Emrick, S. A., and Garber, F. B. (1970). *J. Am. Vet. Med. Assoc.* **12,** 2052–2056.

Bloom, B. R., and Godal, T. (1983). *Rev. Infect. Dis.* **5,** 765–780.

Blumberg, B. S., Gerstley, B. J., Hungerford, D. A., London, W. T., and Sutnick, A. I. (1967). *Ann. Intern. Med.* **66,** 924–931.

Bodian, D. (1949). *Am. J. Hyg.* **49,** 200–224.

Bolin, S. R., McClurken, A. W., Cutlip, R. C., and Coria, M. F. (1985). *Am. J. Vet. Res.* **46,** 573–576.

Boughton, I. B., and Hardy, W. T. (1935). *Tex. Agric. Exp. Stn. [Bull.]* **504.**

Bouters, R. B., De Keyser, J., Vandeplassche, M., Van Aert, A., Brone, E., and Bonte, P. (1973). *Br. Vet. J.* **129,** 52–57.

Breeze, S. S., Ozawa, Y., and Dardiri, A. H. (1969). *Am. J. Vet. Med. Assoc.* **155,** 391–400.

Brezina, R. (1982). *In* "Infectious Diseases and Medical Microbiology" (A. I. Braude, C. E. Davis, and J. Fierer, eds.), pp. 1231–1234. Saunders, Philadelphia, Pennsylvania.

Brogden, K. A., Roades, K. R., and Heddleston, K. L. (1978). *Avian Dis.* **22,** 185–190.

Brogden, K. A., Cutlip, R. C., and Lehmkuhl, H. D. (1984). *Am. J. Vet. Res.* **45,** 2393–2395.

Brown, A. L., Davis, E. V., Merry, D. L., and Beckenhauer, W. H. (1967). *Am. J. Vet. Res.* **28,** 751–759.

Brown, F., Hyslop, N. St. G., Crick, J., and Morrow, W. W. (1963). *J. Hyg.* **61,** 337–344.

Brown, C. C., Olander, H. J., Biberstein, E. L., and Morse, S. M. (1986). *Am. J. Vet. Res.* **47,** 1116–1119.

Bryans, J. T. (1973). *Immunobiol. Stand.* **20,** 311.

Bryans, J. T. (1980). *Am. J. Vet. Res.* **41,** 1743–1746.

Bryans, J. T., and Allen, G. P. (1981). *Dev. Biol. Stand.* **52,** 493–498.

Buller, R. M. L., and Wallace, G. D. (1985). *Lab. Anim. Sci.* **35,** 473–476.

Burnet, F. M. (1934). *Br. J. Exp. Pathol.* **15,** 52–55.

Burnet, F. M. (1942). *Aust. J. Exp. Biol. Med. Sci.* **20,** 81–88.

Burrell, D. H. (1978). *Proc. Annu. Conf. Aust. Vet. Assoc.* **55,** 79–81.

Burrell, D. H. (1981). *Aust. Vet. J.* **57,** 105–110.

Bushnell, L. D., and Brandley, C. A. (1933). *Poult. Sci.* **12,** 55–60.

Butterfield, W. K., Luginbuhl, R. E., Helmboldt, C. F., and Sumner, F. W. (1961). *Avian Dis.* **5,** 445–450.

Buynak, E. B. (1968). *JAMA, J. Am. Med. Assoc.* **204,** 195–200.

Bywater, R. J. (1970). *J. Comp. Pathol.* **80,** 565–573.

Cabasso, V. J., and Cox, H. R. (1949). *Proc. Soc. Exp. Biol. Med.* **71,** 246–250.

Cabasso, V. J., Stebbins, M. R., Norton, T. W., and Cox, H. R. (1954). *Proc. Soc. Exp. Biol. Med.* **85,** 239.

Cabasso, V. J., Stebbins, M. R., Douglas, A., and Sharpless, G. R. (1965). *Am. J. Vet. Res.* **26,** 24–32.

Calmette, A., and Guérin, C. (1924). *Ann. Inst. Pasteur, Paris* **38,** 371–398.

Calmette, A., and Guérin, C. (1926). *Ann. Inst. Pasteur, Paris* **40,** 574–581.

Calnek, B. W. (1961). *J. Am. Vet. Med. Assoc.* **139,** 1323.

Calnek, B. W., and Taylor, P. J. (1960). *Avian Dis.* **4,** 116–122.

Calnek, B. W., Hitchner, S. B., and Aldinger, H. S. (1970). *Appl. Microbiol.* **20,** 723–726.

Cameron, C. M. (1972). *J. S. Afr. Vet. Med. Assoc.* **43,** 343–349.

Capstick, P. B., Telling, R. C., Chapman, W. G., and Stewart, D. L. (1962). *Nature (London)* **195,** 1163–1164.

Carmichael, L. E., Medic, B. L. S., Bistner, S. I., and Aguirre, G. D. (1975). *Cornell Vet.* **65,** 331–351.

Carré, H. (1905). *C. R. Hebd. Seances Acad. Sci.* **140,** 689 and 1489.

Castaneda, M. R. (1934). *J. Exp. Med.* **60,** 119–125.

Cessi, D., and Lombardini, F. (1975). *Clin. Vet.* **98,** 426–430.

Chandler, H. M., and Gulasekhuram, J. (1970). *Aust. J. Exp. Biol. Med. Sci.* **48,** 187–197.

Chanock, R. M., Ludwig, W., Huebner, R. J., Cate, T. R., and Chu, L. W. (1966). *JAMA J. Am. Med. Assoc.* **195,** 445–452.

Childrow, J. W., and Porter, P. (1979). *Vet. Rec.* **104,** 496–499.

Chodnik, K. S., Watson, R. A., and Hepple, J. R. (1959). *Vet. Rec.* **71,** 904- 908.

Christensen, G. (1982). *Nord. Veterinaer Med.* **34,** 113–123.

Churchill, A. E., and Biggs, P. M. (1967). *Nature (London)* **215,** 528–530.

Churchill, A. E., Chubb, R. C., and Baxendale, W. (1969). *J. Gen. Virol.* **4,** 557–564.

Coggins, L., Gillespie, J., Robson, D. S., Thompson, J. D., Phillips, W. W., Wagner, W. C., and Baker, J. A. (1961). *Cornell Vet.* **51,** 539–545.

Collier, R. J., and Kandel, J. (1971). *J. Biol. Chem.* **246,** 1496–1503.

Comstock, G. W. (1982). *In* "Tuberculosis in Bacterial Infections in Humans: Epidemiology and Control" (A. S. Evans and H. A. Feldman, eds.), pp. 605–632. Plenum, New York.

Confer, A. W., Panciera, R. J., Corstvet, R. E., Rummage, J. A., and Fulton, R. W. (1984). *Am. J. Vet. Res.* **45,** 2543–2545.

Confer, A. W., Lessley, B. A., Panciera, R. J., Fulton, R. W., and Kreps, J. A. (1985). *Vet. Immunol. Immunopathol.* **10,** 265–278.

Confer, A. W., Panciera, R. J., Gentry, M. J., and Fulton, R. W. (1986). *Am. J. Vet. Res.* **47,** 1853–1857.

Corbeil, L. B., Schurig, D. D., Duncan, J. R., Corbeil, R. R., and Winter, A. J. (1974). *Infect. Immun.* **10,** 422–429.

Cox, H. R. (1948). *In* "Symposium on Rickettsial Diseases, 1946." Am. Assoc. Adv. Sci., Boston, Massachusetts.

Cox, H. R., Cabasso, V. J., Markam, F. S., Moses, M. J., Mayer, A. W., Roca-Garcia, M., and Ruegsegger, J. M. (1959). *Br. Med. J.* **2,** 591–597.

Craigie, J., Watson, D. W., Clark, E. M., and Malcomson, M. E. (1946). *Can. J. Res., Sect. E* **24,** 84–103.

Crandell, R. A., and Maurer, F. D. (1958). *Proc. Soc. Exp. Biol. Med.* **97,** 487–490.

Crandell, R. A., Niemann, W. H., Ganaway, J. R., and Mauer, F. D. (1960). *Virology* **10,** 283–285.

Crandell, R. A., Brumlow, W. B., and Davison, V. E. (1968). *Am. J. Vet. Res.* **29,** 2141–2147.

Dalton, P. J. (1967). *Vet. Rec.* **80,** 107–109.

Daubney, R. (1949). *FAO Agric. Stud.* **8,** 6–23.

Davis, E. V., Gregory, G. G., and Beckenour, W. H. (1970). *VM/SAC, Vet. Med. Small Anim. Clin.* March, pp. 237–242.

Diaz, R., Jones, L. N., and Wilson, N. J. B. (1967). *J. Bacteriol.* **93**(2) 1262–1268.

Dick, G. (1978). *In* "New Trends and Developments in Vaccines" (A. Voller and H. Friedman, eds.), pp. 29–54. University Park Press, Baltimore, Maryland.

Didier, P. J., Perino, L., and Urbance, J. (1984). *J. Am. Vet. Med. Assoc.* **184,** 716–719.

Doll, E. R., and Bryans, J. T. (1963). *J. Am. Vet. Med. Assoc.* **139,** 1324–1330.

Doll, E. R., Bryans, J. T., McCallum, W. H., and Crowe, M. E. W. (1957). *Cornell Vet.* **47,** 3–41.

Doll, E. R., Bryans, J. T., and Wilson, J. C. (1968). *Cornell Vet.* **58,** 497–524.

Dorset, M., McBryde, C. N., and Niles, W. B. (1908). *U.S. Bur. Anim. Ind. Bull.* **102.**

Dougan, G., Maskell, D., Sweeney, K., O'Callighan, D. O., Fairweather, N., Brown, A., and Hormaeche, C. (1987). *In* "Vaccines '87: Modern Approaches to New Vaccines" (R. M. Chanock, R. A. Lerner, F. Brown, and A. Ginsberg, eds.), pp. 279–282. Cold Spring Harbor Lab., Cold Spring Harbor, New York.

Dougherty, E., Sanders, L. Z., and Parsons, E. H. (1955). *Am. J. Pathol.* **31,** 475–487.

Doyle, T. M. (1927). *J. Comp. Pathol. Ther.* **40,** 144–169.

Dulcac, G. C., Swango, L. J., and Bernstein, T. (1970). *Can. J. Microbiol.* **16,** 391–394.

Dunkin, G. W., and Laidlaw, P. P. (1926). *J. Comp. Pathol. Ther.* **39,** 201.

DuToit, R. M., Alexander, R. A., and Neitz, W. O. (1933). *Ondersteport J. Vet. Sci. Anim. Ind.* **1,** 25.

Eaton, G., Lerro, A., and Custer, R. (1982). *Lab. Anim. Sci.* **32,** 384–386.

Edelman, R., and Levine, M. M. (1986). *Rev. Infect. Dis.* **8,** 329–349.

Edmonson, W. P., Purcell, R. H., Gundelfinger, B. F., Love, J. W. P., Ludwig, W., and Chanock, R. M. (1966). *J. Am. Med. Assoc.* **195,** 453–459.

Eickoff, T. C., Klein, J. O., and Daly, A. K. (1964). *N. Engl. J. Med.* **271,** 1221–1228.

Einstein, T. K., Carey, R. B., Schockman, G. D., Smith, S. M., and Swenson, R. M. (1982). *Semin. Infect. Dis.* **4,** 279–284.

Elder, W. G., and Miles, D. A. (1957). *J. Pathol. Bacteriol.* **74,** 133–139.

Emery, J. B., Elliot, A. Y., Bordt, D. E., Burch, G. R., and Kugal, B. S. (1968). *J. Am. Vet. Med. Assoc.* **152(5),** 476–482.

Emery, J. B., House, J. A., Bittle, J. L., and Spotts, A. M. (1976). *Am. J. Vet. Res.* **37,** 1323–1327.

Enders, J. F., and Hammond, W. D. (1940). *Proc. Soc. Exp. Biol. Med.* **43,** 194–200.

Enders, J. F., and Peebles, T. C. (1954). *Proc. Soc. Exp. Biol. Med.* **86,** 277–286.

Enders, J. F., Kane, L. W., Cohen, S., and Levens, J. H. (1945). *J. Exp. Med.* **81,** 93–117.

Enders, J. F., Weller, T. H., and Robbins, F. C. (1949). *Science* **109,** 85–87.

Eugester, A. K. (1978). *Tex. Vet. Med. J.* **40,** 19–78.

Fastier, L. B. (1957). *Am. J. Vet. Res.* **18,** 382–389.

Feeley, J. C. (1970). *In* "Principles and Practice of Cholera Control," p. 87. World Health Organ., Geneva.

Fenje, P. (1960). *Can. J. Microbiol.* **6,** 605–609.

Fields, P. I., Haidaris, C. G., Swanson, R. V., Parsons, R. L., and Heffron, F. (1986a). *In* "Vaccines '86" (F. Brown, R. M. Chanock, and R. A. Lerner, eds.), pp. 205–212, Cold Spring Harbor Lab., Cold Spring Harbor, New York.

Fields, P. I., Swanson, R. V., Haidaris, C. G., and Heffron, F. (1986b) *Proc. Natl. Acad. Sci. U.S.A.* **83,** 5189–5193.

Fieldsteel, A. H., and Emery, J. B. (1954). *Proc. Soc. Exp. Biol. Med.* **86,** 819.

Fitzgeorge, R. B., Solotorovsky, M., and Smith, H. (1967). *Br. J. Exp. Pathol.* **48(2),** 522–528.

Foggin, C. M. (1983). *Vet. Rec.* **113,** 115.

Folkers, C. D., Jaspers, M. E., Stumpel, E. N., and Willebrongel, E. A. C. (1976). *Dev. Biol. Stand.* **33,** 364–369.

Frasch, C. E., Peppler, M. S., Cate, T. R., and Zahradnik, J. M. (1982). *Semin. Infect. Dis.* **4,** 263–267.

Frenkel, H. S. (1947). *Bull. Off. Int. Epizoot.* **28,** 155.

Fujisaki, Y., Watanabe, Y., and Kodama, K. (1978). *Natl. Inst. Anim. Health Q.* **18,** 184–185.

Fukumi, H., and Takeuchi, Y. (1975). *Dev. Biol. Stand.* **28,** 477–481.

Gale, C., Hamdy, A. H., and Trapp, A. L. (1963). *J. Am. Vet. Med. Assoc.* **142**, 884–887.
Gearhart, M. A., Webb, P. A., Knight, A. P., Salman, M. D., Smith, J. A., and Erickson, G. D. (1987). *J. Am. Vet. Med. Assoc.* **191**, 7, 819–822.
Gelenczei, E. F., and Marty, E. W. (1964). *Avian Dis.* **8**, 105–122.
Gerber, J. D., Marron, A. E., Bass, E. P., and Beckenhauer, W. H. (1977). *Can. J. Comp. Med.* **41**, 471–478.
Gill, D. M., and Pappenheimer, A. M. (1971). *J. Biol. Chem.* **246**, 654–658.
Gillespie, J. H., Baker, J. A., and McEntee, K. (1960). *Cornell Vet.* **50**, 73–79.
Gilliam, A. G. (1946). *Am. J. Hyg.* **44**, 401–410.
Ginsburg, I. (1986). *In* "Infectious Diseases and Medical Microbiology" (A. I. Braude, C. E. Davis, and J. Fierer, eds.), 2nd ed., pp. 242–253. Saunders, Philadelphia, Pennsylvania.
Goodfellow, M., and Minnikin, D. E. (1981). *In* "The Prokaryotes" (M. P. Starr, H. Stolp, H. G. Truper, A. Barlows, and H. G. Schlegel, eds.), Vol. 2. Springer-Verlag, New York.
Goodpasture, E. W., Woodruff, A. M., and Buddingh, G. J. (1931). *Science* **74**, 371–372.
Goodpasture, E. W., Buddringh, G. J., Richardson, L., and Anderson, K. (1935). *Am. J. Hyg.* **21**, 319–360.
Goren, M. B. (1977). *Annu. Rev. Microbiol.* **31**, 507–533.
Goren, M. B., D'Arcy Hart, P., Young, M. R., and Armstrong, J. A. (1976). *Proc. Natl. Acad. Sci. U.S.A.* **73**, 2510–2514.
Grasset, E. (1946). *Trans. R. Soc. Med. Hyg.* **40**, 275–294.
Green, R. G. (1945). *Am. J. Hyg.* **41**, 7.
Gregg, N. M. (1941). *Trans. Ophthalmol. Soc. Aust.* **3**, 35–46.
Gunnarson, A. (1979). *Am. J. Vet. Res.* **40**, 469–472.
Gunnarson, A., Hurvell, B., and Biberstein, E. L. (1978). *Am. J. Vet. Res.* **39**, 1286–1292.
Habel, K. (1946). *Public Health Rep.* **61**, 1655–1664.
Habel, K. (1951). *Am. J. Hyg.* **54**, 295–311.
Haig, D. A. (1948). *Onderstepoort J. Vet. Sci. Anim. Ind.* **23**, 149–155.
Hanson, L. E. (1974). *J. Dairy Sci.* **59**, 1166–1170.
Heddleston, K. L., Rebers, P. A., and Wessman, G. (1974). *Poult. Sci.* **54**, 217–221.
Henderson, W. M. (1978). *Br. Vet. J.* **134**, 3–9.
Henle, G., Bishe, W. J., Burgoon, J. S., Burgoon, C. F., Hunt, G. R., and Henle, W. (1951). *J. Immunol.* **66**, 561–577.
Henry, S., and Marstellar, T. A. (1982). *Int. Pigm. Vet. Soc.* Congr. p. 114.
Higbee, E., and Howitt, B. (1935). *J. Bacteriol.* **29**, 399–406.
Hilleman, M. R., Buynak, E. B., Weibel, R. E., Stoes, J., Whitman, J. E., and Leagus, M. B. (1968). *JAMA, J. Am. Med. Assoc.* **206**, 587–590.
Hilleman, M. R., Bertland, A. V., and Buynak, E. B. (1978). *In* "Viral Hepatitis" (G. Vyas, S. N. Cohen, and R. Schmid, eds.), pp. 525–537. Franklin Inst. Press, Philadelphia, Pennsylvania.
Hilleman, M. R., Buynak, E. B., McAleer, W. J., McLean, A. A., Provost, P. J., and Lytell, A. A. (1982). *In* "Viral Hepatitis," (W. Szmuness, H. J. Alter, and J. E. Maynard, eds.), pp. 385–397. Franklin Inst. Press, Philadelphia, Pennsylvania.
Hilwig, R. W., Songer, J. G., Joens, L. A., and Cubberley, J. (1985). *Proc. West. States Food Anim. Conf.*
Hirschel, B., Wuthrich, R., Somaini, B., and Steffen, R. (1985). *Eur. J. Clin. Microbiol.* **4**, 295–298.
Hitchner, S. B., and Johnson, E. P. (1948). *Vet. Med. (Kansas City, Mo.)* **43**, 525–532.
Hoerlin, A. B., and Kramer, T. K. (1964). *Am. J. Vet. Res.* **25**, 371–379.

Hoffman, T. A. (1986). In "Infectious Diseases and Medical Microbiology" (A. I. Braude, C. E. Davis, and J. Fierer, eds.), 2nd ed., pp. 1060–1065. Saunders, Philadelphia, Pennsylvania.

Hofstad, M. S. (1981). Avian Dis. 25, 650–654.

Hyslop, N. St. G. (1966–1967). "Vaccination against Foot and Mouth Disease," Vet. Annu., p. 140. John Wright & Sons, Bristol, England.

Inaba, Y., Kurogi, H., Sato, K., Goto, Y., Omori, T., and Matsumoto, M. (1973). Arch. Gesamte. Virusforsch. 42, 42–53.

Irwin, M. R., and Knight, H. D. (1975). Infect. Immun. 12(5), 1098–1103.

Jackson, F. C., Wright, G. G., and Armstrong, J. (1957). Am. J. Vet. Res. 18, 771–777.

Jacobs, J. W., and Edington, N. N. (1975). Res. Vet. Sci. 18(3), 299–306.

Jarrett, W., Mackey, L., Jarrett, O., Laird, H. M., and Hood, C. (1974). Nature (London) 248, 230–232.

Jayaraman, M. S., Lal, R., and Dhanda, M. R. (1962). Indian Vet. J. 39, 481–487.

Jenner, E. (1798). "An Inquiry into the Cause and Effects of the Vanidae Vaccinae." Sampson Low, London.

Johnson, R. H. (1967a). Res. Vet. Sci. 8, 256–264.

Johnson, R. H. (1967b). J. Small Anim. Pract. 8, 319–324.

Johnson, R. H., Margolis, G., and Kilham, L. (1967). Nature (London) 214, 175–177.

Johnson, W. T. (1929). J. Am. Vet. Med. Assoc. 75, 629.

Jolly, R. D. (1965). N. Z. Vet. J. 13, 148–153.

Jones, E. E. (1932). Science 76, 331–332.

Jones, E. E. (1934). J. Exp. Med. 59, 781–798.

Joo, H. S., and Johnson, R. H. (1977). Aust. J. Vet. 53, 550–552.

Kabir, S. (1986). In "Vaccines '86" (F. Brown, R. M. Chanock, and R. A. Lerner, eds.), pp. 231–234. Cold Spring Harbor Lab., Cold Spring Harbor, New York.

Kahn, D. E., and Gillespie, J. A. (1971). Am. J. Vet. Res. 32, 521–533.

Kann, D. E., Hoover, E. A., and Bittle, J. L. (1975). Infect. Immun. 11, 1003–1009.

Kaneene, J. M., Johnson, D. W., Anderson, R. K., Agnes, R. D., Pietz, D. E., and Muscoplat, C. C. (1978). Am. J. Vet. Res. 39, 585–589.

Kasper, D. L., Baker, C. J., Edwards, M. S., Nicholson-Weller, A., and Jennings, H. J. (1982). Semin. Infect. Dis. 4, 275–278.

Katz, S. L., and Enders, J. F. (1959). Am. J. Dis. Child. 98, 605–607.

Kennedy, K. K., Norris, S. J., Bechenhauer, W. H., and White, R. G. (1977). Am. J. Vet. Res. 38, 1515–1517.

Kerr, D. D., and Marshall, V. (1974). VM/SAC, Vet. Med. Small Anim. Clin. 69, 1157–1160.

Kessel, J. F., and Pait, C. F. (1949). Proc. Soc. Exp. Biol. Med. 70, 315–316.

Kilham, L., and Margolis, G. M. (1966). Am. J. Pathol. 48, 991–1011.

Kimura, Y., Aoki, H., Shimokata, K., Ito, Y., Takano, M., Kurabayashi, N., and Norrby, E. (1979). Arch. Virol. 61, 297–304.

Kissling, R. E. (1958). Proc. Soc. Exp. Biol. Med. 98, 223–225.

Koch, R. (1897). Cited by Todd, C. (1930). In "A System of Bacteriology" (P. Filders and J. C. G. Ledingham, eds.), Vol. 7, p. 284. H. M. Stationery Office, London.

Kohler, B. M., Cross, R. F., and Bohl, E. H. (1975). Am. J. Vet. Res. 36, 757–764.

Koprowski, H., and Black, J. (1950). J. Immunol. 64, 185–196.

Koprowski, H., and Black, J. (1954). J. Immunol. 72, 503–510.

Koprowski, H., and Cox, H. (1948). J. Immunol. 60, 533–554.

Koprowski, H., James, T. R., and Cox, H. R. (1946). Proc. Soc. Exp. Biol. Med. 63, 178–183.

Koprowski, H., Norton, T. U., Jervis, G. A., and Nelson, T. L. (1956). *JAMA, J. Am. Med. Assoc.* **160**, 954–966.

Kranevelt, F. C. (1926). *Ned. Indisch. Bl. Diergeneeskd.* **38**, 448–450.

Krugman, S., Giles, J. P., and Hammond, J. (1970). *J. Infect. Dis.* **122**, 432–436.

Kuroya, M., Ishida, N., Shiratori, T., and Yakoham. (1953). *Med. Bull.* **4**, 217–233.

Lagrange, P. H. (1984). *In* "The Mycobacteria: A Source Book, Part B" (G. P. Kubica and G. W. Lawrence, eds.). Dekker, New York.

Laidlaw, P. P., and Dunkin, G. W. (1926). *J. Comp. Pathol. Ther.* **39**, 222–230.

Laidlaw, P. P., and Dunkin, G. W. (1928a). *J. Comp. Pathol. Ther.* **41**, 1–17.

Laidlaw, P. P., and Dunkin, G. W. (1928b). *J. Comp. Pathol. Ther.* **41**, 209–227.

Lancefield, R. C. (1934). *J. Exp. Med.* **57**, 441–459.

Leach, C. N., and Johnson, H. N. (1940). *Am. J. Trop. Med.* **20**, 335–340.

Leasure, F. E., Lienhardt, H. F., and Taberner, F. R. (1934). *North Am. Vet.* **15**, 30–44.

Leece, J. G., and King, M. W. (1979). *Can. J. Comp. Med.* **43**, 90–93.

Leece, J. G., King, M. W., and Mock, R. (1976). *Infect. Immun.* **14**, 816–885.

Leppla, S. H. (1982). *Proc. Natl. Acad. Sci. U.S.A.* **79**, 3162–3166.

Levine, M. M., Nalin, D. R., Craig, J. P., Hoover, D., Berquist, E. J., and Waterman, D. (1979). *Trans. R. Soc. Trop. Med. Hyg.* **73**, 3–9.

Levine, M. M., Kaper, J. B., Black, R. E., and Clements, M. L. (1983). *Microbiol. Rev.* **47**, 510–550.

Loeffler, F., and Frosch, P. (1898). *Zentralbl. Bakteriol. Parasitenkd. Infektionskr., Abt. 1* **23**, 371–391.

Lonroth, I., Andren, B., Lange, S., Martinsson, K., and Holmgren, J. (1979). *Infect. Immun.* **24**, 900–905.

Lukert, P. D., and Hitchner, S. B. (1984). "Diseases of Poultry," 8th ed. Iowa State Univ. Press, Ames.

McBryde, C. N., and Cole, C. G. (1936). *J. Am. Vet. Med. Assoc.* **89**, 652–663.

McCollum, W. H. (1986). *Am. J. Vet. Res.* **47(9)**, 1931–1934.

McConnell, S., and Livingston, C. W. (1982). *Proc. U. S. Anim. Health Assoc.* **86**, 103–113.

McFadyean, J. (1900). *J. Comp. Pathol. Ther.* **13**, 1–30.

McFerran, J. B., and Dow, C. (1975). *Res. Vet. Sci.* **19**, 17–22.

McKercher, D. G., and Crenshaw, G. L. (1971). *J. Am. Vet. Med. Assoc.* **159**, 1362–1369.

McKercher, D. G., and Saito, J. (1964). *Nature (London)* **202**, 933–934.

McKercher, D. G., McGowan, B., Howarth, J. A., and Saito, J. K. (1953). *J. Am. Vet. Med. Assoc.* **122**, 300–301.

McKercher, D. G., McGowan, B., Cabasso, V. J., Roberts, G. I., and Saito, J. K. (1957). *Am. J. Vet. Res.* **18**, 310–316.

McKinney, K. L., Confer, A. W., Rummage, J. A., Gentry, M. J., and Durham, J. A. (1985). *Vet. Microbiol.* **10**, 465–480.

McKinney, R. W., Berge, T. O., Sawyer, W. D., Tigertt, W. D., and Crozier, D. (1963). *Am. J. Trop. Med. Hyg.* **12**, 597–603.

MacLeod, A. J. (1965). *Vet. Rec.* **77**, 335–338.

MacPherson, I. A., and Stoker, M. (1952). *Virology* **16**, 147–151.

Marx, P. A., Pedersen, N. C., Lerche, N. W., Osborn, K. G., Lowenstine, L. J., Lackner, A. A., and Maul, D. H. (1986). *J. Virol.* **60**, 431–435.

Masson, R. W., McKay, R. W., and Corbould, A. (1982). *Aust. Vet. J.* **58**, 108–110.

Matsuaba, T., Folkerts, T. M., and Gale, C. (1972). *JAMA, J. Am. Med. Assoc.* **160**, 333–337.

Maurer, F. D. (1980). "Bovine Medicine and Surgery," 2nd ed. pp. 142–153. Am. Vet. Publ., Santa Barbara, California.

Mayr, A. (1970). *Proc. Int. Conf. Equine Infect. Dis., 2nd, 1969* pp. 41–45.

Mayr, A., and Danner, K. (1976). *Dev. Biol. Stand.* **33,** 249–259.

Mebus, C. A. (1969). *Res. Bull.—Nebr. Agric. Exp. Stn.* **233,** 1.

Mebus, C. A., White, R. G., Bass, E. P., and Twiehaus, M. J. (1973). *J. Am. Vet. Med. Assoc.* **163,** 880–883.

Mebus, C. A., Wyatt, R. G., Sharpee, R. L., Sereno, M. M., Kalica, A. R., Kapakian, A. Z., and Tweihaus, M. J. (1976). *Infect. Immun.* **14,** 471–474.

Mengeling, W. I., Brown, T. T., and Paul, P. S. (1979). *Am. J. Vet. Res.* **40,** 204–207.

Milovanovic, M. V., Enders, J. F., and Mitus, A. (1957). *Proc. Soc. Exp. Biol. Med.* **95,** 120–127.

Mittal, K. R., Higgins, R., and Lariviere, S. (1982). *J. Clin. Microbiol.* **15,** 1019–1023.

Miyamae, T. (1978). *Am. J. Vet. Res.* **39,** 503–504.

Mohanty, S. B., and Lillie, M. G. (1964). *Am. J. Vet. Res.* **25,** 1653–1657.

Mohanty, S. B., Ingling, A. L., and Lillie, M. G. (1975). *Am. J. Vet. Res.* **36,** 417–419.

Molgard, P. C., and Cavett, J. W. (1947). *Poult. Sci.* **26,** 563–567.

Montaraz, J. A., and Winter, A. J. (1986). *Infect. Immun.* **53,** 245–251.

Moon, H. W., McClurkin, A. N., Isaacson, R. E., Problenz, J., Skartvedt, S. M., Gillette, K. G., and Baetz, N. A. L. (1978). *J. Am. Vet. Med. Assoc.* **173,** 577–583.

Morse, S. A. (1986). *In* "Infectious Diseases and Medical Microbiology" (A. I. Braude, C. E. Davis, and J. Fierer, eds.), 2nd ed., pp. 278–286. Saunders, Philadelphia, Pennsylvania.

Mowat, C. N., and Chapman, W. E. (1962). *Nature (London)* **194,** 253–255.

Musser, S. J., and Hilsabeck, L. J. (1969). *Am. J. Dis. Child.* **118,** 355–361.

Myers, K., Marshall, I. D., and Fenner, F. (1954). *J. Hyg.* **52,** 337–360.

Myers, L. L., and Guinee, P. A. (1976). *Infect. Immun.* **13,** 1117–1119.

Nagy, E., Moon, H. W., Isaacson, R. E., To, C. C., and Brinton, C. C. (1978). *Infect. Immun.* **21,** 269–274.

Nairn, M. E., Robertson, J. P., and McQuade, N. C. (1977). *Proc. Annu. Conf. Aust. Vet. Assoc.* **54,** 159–161.

Nakai, T., Sawata, A., and Kume, K. (1985). *Am. J. Vet. Res.* **46,** 870–874.

Nakamura, J., and Miyamoto, T. (1953). *Am. J. Vet. Res.* **14,** 307–317.

Nakamura, J., Wayatsuma, S., and Fukusko, K. (1938). *J. Jpn. Soc. Vet. Sci.* **17,** 185.

Nazerian, K., and Burmeister, B. R. (1968). *Cancer Res.* **28,** 2454–2462.

Negi, S. K., Myers, W. L., and Segré, D. (1971). *Am. J. Vet. Res.* **32,** 1915–1927.

Nielsen, R. (1976). *Nord. Veterinaer med.* **28,** 337–348.

Norrby, E., Enders-Ruekle, G., and TerMeulen, V. (1975). *J. Infect. Dis.* **132,** 262–269.

Norrung, V. (1979). *Nord. Veterinaer med.* **31,** 462–465.

Noyer, P. S. G., Ward, G. F., Saunders, J. R., and MacWilliams, P. (1976). *Can. Vet. J.* **18,** 159–163.

Olsen, N. O., and Solomon, D. P. (1968). *Avian Dis.* **12,** 311–316.

Olsen, R. G., and Lewis, M. G. (1981). *In* "Feline Leukemia" (R. G. Olsen, ed.), pp. 135–148. CRC Press, Boca Raton, Florida.

Olson, L. D. (1977). *Avian Dis.* **21,** 178–184.

Okazaki, W., Purchase, H. G., and Burmeister, B. R. (1970). *Avian Dis.* **14,** 413–429.

Paccaud, M. F., and Jacquier, C. (1970). *Arch. Gesamte Virusforsch.* **30,** 327–342.

Page, L. A., Rosenwald, A. S., and Price, F. C. (1963). *Avian Dis.* **7,** 239–565.

Panciera, R. J., Corstvet, R. E., Confer, A. W., and Gresham, C. N. (1984). *Am. J. Vet. Res.* **45,** 2538–2542.

Parkman, P. D., Buescher, R. S., and Arnstein, M. S. (1962). *Proc. Soc. Exp. Biol. Med.* **111**, 225–230.

Parkman, P. D., Meyer, H. M., Jr., Kirschstein, R. L., and Hopps, H. E. (1966). *N. Engl. J. Med.* **275**, 569–574.

Pasteur, L. (1881). *C. R. Hebd. Seances Acad. Sci.* **86**.

Paul, P. S., and Mengeling, W. L. (1980). *Am. J. Vet. Res.* **41**, 2007–2011.

Peck, F. B., Powell, H. M., and Culbertson, C. G. (1956). *JAMA, J. Am. Med. Assoc.* **162**, 1373–1376.

Pederson, N. C., and Ott, R. L. (1985). *Feline Pract.* **15(6)**, 7–20.

Pedersen, N. C., Theilen, G. H., and Werner, L. L. (1979). *Am. J. Vet. Res.* **40**, 1120–1126.

Peetermans, J., and Huygelen, C. (1967). *Arch. Gesamte Virusforsch.* **21**, 133–143.

Plotkin, S. A. (1967). *Am. J. Epidemiol.* **86**, 468–477.

Plowright, W., and Ferris, R. D. (1962). *Res. Vet. Sci.* **3**, 172–182.

Pollack, R. U. H., and Carmichael, L. E. (1983). *Am. J. Vet. Res.* **44(2)**, 169–175.

Povey, C., and Ingersoll, J. (1975). *Infect. Immun.* **11**, 877–885.

Prince, A. M. (1968). *Proc. Natl. Acad. Sci. U.S.A.* **60**, 814–821.

Provost, P. J., Conti, P. A., Giesa, P. A., Banker, F. S., Buynak, E. B., McAleer, W. G., and Hilleman, M. R. (1983). *Proc. Soc. Exp. Biol. Med.* **172**, 357–363.

Purchase, H. G., Okazaki, W., and Burmeister, B. R. (1972). *Avian Dis.* **16**, 57–71.

Rafyi, A., and Ramyar, H. (1959). *J. Comp. Pathol. Ther.* **69**, 141–147.

Ramon, G., and Lemetayer, E. (1932). *C. R. Seances Soc. Biol. Ses. Fil.* **109**, 827.

Rapp, V. J., and Ross, R. F. (1984). *Proc. Conf. Res. Work. Anim. Dis.* p. 169.

Reiser, J., and Germanier, R. (1986). *In* "Vaccines '86" (F. Brown, R. M. Chanock, and R. A. Lerner, eds.), pp. 235–238. Cold Spring Harbor Lab., Cold Spring Harbor, New York.

Reisinger, R. C., Heddleston, K. L., and Manthei, C. A. (1959). *J. Am. Vet. Med. Assoc.* **135**, 147–152.

Roantree, R. J. (1967). *Annu. Rev. Microbiol.* **21**, 443–466.

Robbins, J. D., and Robbins, J. B. (1984). *J. Infect. Dis.* **150**, 436–449.

Robinson, A., Irons, L. I., and Ashworth, L. A. E. (1985). *Vaccine* **3**, 11–22.

Rockborn, G. (1958). *Arch. Gesamte/Virusforsch.* **8**, 485–492.

Rosendal, S., Carpenter, D. S., Mitchell, W. R., and Wilson, M. R. (1981). *Can. Vet. J.* **22**, 34–35.

Ross, R. F., Duncan, J. R., and Switzer, W. T. (1963). *Vet. Med.* **58**, 566–569.

Rutter, J. M. (1975). *Vet. Rec.* **96**, 171–175.

Sabban, M. S. (1955). *Am. J. Vet. Res.* **16**, 209–213.

Sabin, A. B. (1955). *Ann. N.Y. Acad. Sci.* **61**, 924–938.

Sabine, M., Robertson, G. R., and Whalley, J. M. (1981). *Aust. Vet. J.* **57**, 148–149.

Salk, J., Krech, V., Youngner, J. S., Bennett, B. L., Lewis, L. J., and Blazeley, P. L. (1954). *An. J. Public Health* **44**, 563–570.

Sarma, P. S., Voss, W., Heubner, R. J., Igel, H., Lane, W. T., and Turner, H. C. (1967). *Nature (London)* **215**, 293–294.

Sato, H., and Sato, Y. (1984). *Infect. Immun.* **46**, 422–428.

Schaaf, K. (1958). *Avian Dis.* **2**, 279–289.

Schaaf, K. (1959). *Avian Dis.* **3**, 245–256.

Schaaf, K., and Lamoreux, W. F. (1955). *Am. J. Vet. Res.* **16**, 627–633.

Schantz, E. J., and Sugiyama, H. (1974). *Agric. Food. Chem.* **22**, 26–30.

Schat, K. A., and Calnek, B. W. (1978). *J. Natl. Cancer Inst. (U.S.)* **60**, 1075–1082.

Schmidt, S. (1936). *Z. Immunitaetsforsch.* **88**, 91–103.

Schultz, R. D., Mendel, H., and Scott, F. W. (1973). *Infect. Immun.* **7(4)**, 547–549.
Schwarz, A. J. F. (1964). *Ann. Paediatr.* **202**, 241–252.
Schwarz, A. J. F., York, C. J., Zirbel, L. W., and Estella, L. A. (1957). *Proc. Soc. Exp. Biol. Med.* **96**, 453–458.
Scott, F. W. (1977). *Am. J. Vet. Res.* **38**, 229–234.
Scott, F. W., and Glauberg, A. F. (1975). *J. Am. Vet. Med. Assoc.* **166**, 147–149.
Sevoian, M., and Chamberlain, D. M. (1962). *Vet. Med. (Kansas City, Mo.)* **57**, 608–609.
Sheffy, B. E., Coggins, L., and Baker, J. A. (1961). *Proc. 65th Annu. Meet. U.S. Livestock Sanit. Assoc.* p. 347.
Sherwood, R. W., Buescher, E. L., Nitz, R. E., and Cooch, J. W. (1961). *JAMA, J. Am. Med. Assoc.* **178**, 1125–1127.
Shope, R. E., Griffiths, H. J., and Jenkins, D. L. (1946). *Am. J. Vet. Res.* **7**, 135–141.
Shope, R. E., Murphy, F. A., Harrison, A. K., Causey, O. R., Kemp, G. E., Simpson, D. I. H., and Moore, D. L. (1970). *J. Virol.* **6**, 690–692.
Siccardi, F. J. (1975). *Avian Dis.* **19**, 362–365.
Silva, L., and Ioneda, T. (1977). *Chem. Phys. Lipids* **20**, 217–233.
Slater, E. A., and Kucera, C. J. (1966). U.S. Patent 3,293,130.
Snodgrass, D. R., and Wells, P. W. (1976). *Arch. Virol.* **52**, 201–205.
Soloman, J. J., Witter, R. L., Nazerian, K. I., and Burmeister, B. R. (1968). *Proc. Soc. Exp. Biol. Med.* **127**, 173–177.
Spradbrow, P. B. (1977). *Aust. Vet. J.* **53**, 351–352.
Stahlheim, O. H. V. (1968). *Am. J. Vet. Res.* **29(2)**, 1463–1468.
Steinman, L. A., Weiss, N., Adelman, M., Lim, R., Zuniga, J., Oehlert, J., Henlett, E., and Falkow, S. (1985). *Proc. Natl. Acad. Sci. U.S.A.* **82**, 8733–8736.
Stephen, J. (1981). *Pharmacol. Ther.* **12**, 501.
Stokes, J., Enders, J. F., Maris, E. P., and Kane, L. W. (1946). *J. Exp. Med.* **84**, 407–428.
Stokes, J., Weibel, R., Halenda, R., Reilly, C. M. and Hilleman, M. R. (1962). *Am. J. Dis. Child.* **103**, 366–372.
Stone, H., Brugh, M., Erickson, G. A., and Beard, C. W. (1980). *Avian Dis.* **24**, 99–111.
Stott, J. L., Osburn, B. I., and Barker, T. L. (1979). *Proc. U. S. Anim. Health Assoc.* **83**, 55–62.
Studdert, M. J., and Blackney, M. H. (1979). *Aust. Vet. J.* **55**, 488–492.
Suzuki, H., and Fujisaki, F. (1976). *Bull. Natl. Inst. Anim. Health* **72**, 17–23.
Swiderska, H., Osuch, T., and Brzoska, W. J. (1971). *Exp. Med. Microbiol* **23B**, 133–138.
Symuness, M. D., Stevens, C. E., Harley, E. J., Zang, E. A., and Oleszko, W. R. (1980). *N. Eng. J. Med.* **303**, 834–841.
Takahashi, M., Otsuka, T., and Okuno, Y. (1974). *Lancet* **2**, 1288–1290.
Tamoglia, T. W., Tellejohn, A. L., Phillips, C. E., and Wilkinson, F. B. (1966). *Proc. 69th Annu. Meet. U.S. Livestock Sanit. Assoc.* p. 385.
Tashjian, J. J., and Campbell, S. G. (1983). *Am. J. Vet. Res.* **44(4)**, 690–693.
Theiler, G. (1951). *In* "The Virus in Yellow Fever" (G.K. Strode, ed.), pp. 39–136. McGraw-Hill, New York.
Theodoridis, A., Giesecke, W. H., and DuToit, I. J. (1973). *Onderstepoort J. Vet. Res.* **40(3)**, 83–92.
Thompson, D. A., and Gilmour, J. L. (1978). *Vet. Rec.* **102**, 530.
Thorsen, J., Sanderson, R., and Bittle, J. (1969). *Can. J. Comp. Med.* **33(2)**, 105–107.
Todd, J. D., Volenec, F. J., and Paton, I. M. (1971). *J. Am. Vet. Med. Assoc.* **159**, 1370–1374.
Top, F. H., Grossman, R. A., Bartelloni, P. J., Segal, H. E., Dudding, B. A., Russel, P. K., and Buescher, E. L. (1971). *J. Infect. Dis.* **124(2)**, 148–154.

Topping, N. H., Bengtson, I. A., Henderson, R. G., Shephard, C. C., and Sitear, M. J. (1945). *Nat. Inst. Health Bull.* No. 183.

Traum, J. (1933). *Proc. Int. Vet. Congr.* pp. 87–98.

Tsukui, M., Ito, H., Tada, M., Nakata, M., Miyajima, H., and Fujiwara, K. (1982). *Lab. Anim. Sci.* **32**, 143–146.

Vallee, H., and Carré, H. (1922). *C. R. Hebd. Seances Acad. Sci.* **174**, 1498.

Vallee, H., Carré, H., and Rinjard, P. (1925). *Recl. Med. Vet.* **101**, 297.

Van der Heide, L. M., Kalbac, L. M., and Hall, W. C. (1976). *Avian Dis.* **20**, 647–648.

Van der Westhuizen, B. (1967). *Ondersteport. J. Vet. Res.* **34**, 29–40.

Van Roekel, H., Bullis, K. L., and Clark, M. K., Olesink, O. M., and Sperling, F. G. (1950). *Mass., Agric. Exp. Stn., Bull.* **460**, 1–47.

Verge, J., and Christoforoni, N. (1928). *C. R. Seances Soc. Biol. Ses. Fil.* **99**, 312.

Vodkin, M. H., and Leppla, S. H. (1983). *Cell* **34**, 693–697.

Waldmann, O., and Kobe, K. (1938). *Berl. Tieraerztl. Wochenschr.* **22**, 317–320.

Walker, R. V. L., Griffiths, H. J., Shope, R. E., Maurer, F. D., and Jenkins, D. L. (1946). *Am. J. Vet. Res.* **7**, 145–151.

Warren, K. S. (1985). *In* "Vaccines '85" (R. Lerner. R. M. Chanock, and F. Brown, eds.), pp. 373–378. Cold Spring Harbor Lab., Cold Spring Harbor, New York.

Weibel, R. E., Buynak, E. B., McLean, A. A., Roehm, R. R., and Hilleman, M. R. (1980). *Proc. Soc. Exp. Biol. Med.* **165**, 260–263.

Weller, T. H., and Nova, F. A. (1962). *Proc. Soc. Exp. Biol. Med.* **111**, 215–225.

Westbury, H. A., and Senkovic, B. (1978). *Aust. Vet. J.* **54**, 68–71.

White, R. R., and Verway, W. F. (1970). *Infect. Immun.* **1**, 380–386.

Wiktor, T. J., Fernandes, M. V., and Koprowski, H. (1964). *J. Immunol.* **93**, 353–366.

Wilkie, B. N., and Winter, A. J. (1971). *Can. J. Comp. Med.* **35**, 301–312.

Williams, B. M. (1962). *Vet. Rec.* **74**, 1536–1542.

Williams, J. M., Smith, G. L., and Murdock, F. M. (1978). *Am. J. Vet. Res.* **39**, 1756–1762.

Wilson, J. C., Doll, E. R., and McCollum, W. H. (1962). *Cornell Vet.* **2**, 205–208.

Winterfield, R. W., and Hitchner, S. B. (1962). *Am. J. Vet. Res.* **23**, 1273–1279.

Winterfield, R. W., Goldman, C. L., and Seadale, E. H. (1957). *Poult. Sci.* **36**, 1076–1088.

Woode, G. N., Bridger, J. C., Jones, J. M., Bryden, A. S., Davies, H. A., White, G. B. B., and Flewett, A. S. (1976). *Infect. Immun.* **14**, 804–810.

Woolcock, J. B. (1973). *Aust. Vet. J.* **49**, 307–317.

Wratthal, A. E., Wells, D. E., and Cartwright, S. T. (1984). *Res. Vet. Sci.* **36**, 136–143.

Wright, P. F., and Karzon, D. T. (1987). *Prog. Med. Virol.* **34**, 70–88.

Yamamoto, R. (1984). *In* "Diseases of Poultry," 8th ed., pp. 178–186. Iowa State Univ. Press, Ames.

Yamamoto, T., Tamura, T., and Yokota, T. (1984). *J. Biol. Chem.* **259**, 5037–5044.

Yohn, D. S., Olsen, R. G., Schaller, J. P., Hoover, E. A., Mathes, L. E., and Heding, L. (1976). *Cancer Res.* **36**, 382–387.

York, C. J., Schwarz, A. J. F., and Estella, L. A. (1957). *Proc. Soc. Exp. Biol. Med.* **94**, 740–744.

Zamberg, E. E., Cuperstein, V., Bendheim, V., and Aronovia, C. (1971). *Avian Dis.* **15**, 413–417.

Zander, D. V., Hill, R. W., Raymond, R. E., Balch, R. K., Mitchell, R. W., and Bunsong, J. W. (1972). *Avian Dis.* **16**, 163–178.

Zanella, A., and Marchi, R. (1982). *Dev. Biol. Stand.* **51**, 19–32.

Poliovirus: Three-dimensional Structure of a Viral Antigen

JAMES M. HOGLE AND DAVID J. FILMAN

*Department of Molecular Biology, Research Institute of Scripps Clinic,
La Jolla, California*

I. Introduction

An understanding of the nature of the interactions between viral antigens and the immune system is crucial to understanding the mechanisms utilized by vertebrates to clear viral infection and to the development of effective immunization strategies for protection against viral diseases. The development of rapid genome sequencing methods, the introduction of methods for preparing monoclonal antibodies (and more recently cloned T-cell lines), and the demonstration that short synthetic peptides can serve as useful probes of the immune response to protein antigens have allowed the important B- and T-cell epitopes of a number of viruses to be mapped onto the linear sequence of their constituent proteins. In several instances the three-dimensional structures of the viral antigens have also been determined by X-ray crystallographic methods, allowing the antigenic sites to be understood in the context of a complete three-dimensional structure.

65

In the first such study, Wilson, Wiley, and Skehel described the three-dimensional structure of the hemagglutinin of influenza virus A/Hong Kong (Wilson et al., 1981). In a companion paper they analyzed the three-dimensional distribution of sequence differences between natural isolates of influenza virus and the location of mutations selected by neutralizing antibodies (Wiley et al., 1981). They observed that the sequence changes that accompanied escape from immune recognition were located in exposed loops on the outer surface of the hemagglutinin molecule and were clustered in three to four distinct regions on the molecule that were separated by regions of more strict sequence conservation. From this observation, and by analysis of sequence changes that accumulate during the natural antigenic drift of the virus, the authors concluded first that the hemagglutinin has three to four distinct neutralizing antigenic sites, and second that the influenza virus requires at least one mutation in each of these sites to escape immune surveillance and cause significant disease in a previously exposed population.

In a similar study, Colman et al. (1983; Varghese et al., 1983) determined the structure of the other surface glycoprotein of influenza virus, the neuraminidase, and mapped its antigenic sites. These authors also found that mutations that accumulated under immune selection were located in exposed loops on the surface of the protein and were clustered in three to four discrete sites on the protein surface. Recently, Colman et al. (1987) have also determined the structure of the neuraminidase in complex with a Fab fragment. The structure of the complex showed that the interaction between the neuraminidase and the Fab involved an extensive area on the surface of both contributing proteins. The observed interactions included several exposed loops of the neuraminidase that had previously been identified as components of an antigenic site, as well as all four complementarity-determining loops of the Fab molecule. A similar conclusion concerning the extent of the contacts between an antibody and its cognate antigen had been drawn from studies of complexes between hen egg white lysozyme and Fab fragments from antilysozyme monoclonal antibodies (Amit et al., 1986; Sheriff et al., 1987). In contrast to the lysozyme–Fab complexes, wherein three were little or no indications of conformational changes in either the lysozyme molecule or the Fab, the formation of the neuraminidase–Fab complex resulted in substantial local conformational changes in the vicinity of the interaction sites in both the neuraminidase and the Fab.

Both of these structural studies of viral antigenic sites have focused on the sites recognized by neutralizing antibodies (that is, on the sites recognized by the humoral or B-cell response). More recently, several workers have begun to describe the sequences of the hemagglutinin and neuraminidase (Hurwitz *et al.,* 1984; Katz *et al.,* 1985) [as well as non-external proteins such as the matrix and nucleocapsid proteins (Yewdell *et al.,* 1985)], which are recognized by T cells. The present uncertainty as to the nature of the antigens that are presented to T cells, however, clouds the significance of mapping these sites on the three-dimensional structures of the viral proteins. Indeed, recent evidence suggests that the presentation of antigens to helper T cells by class II MHC antigens and, by analogy, the presentation of antigens to cytotoxic T cells by class I MHC antigens involve processed peptides approximately 10–20 amino acids in length (Babbit *et al.,* 1985; Buus *et al.,* 1986). This suggests that T-cell epitopes might be better analyzed as free peptides or as peptides complexed to the appropriate MHC antigen. In this regard it is interesting to note that in the recently described structure of a class I MHC protein (HLA A2) there is a clear indication in the electron density map for a peptide or mixture of peptides in the probable antigen presenting site of the molecule (Bjorkman *et al.,* 1987a,b).

In addition to the earlier structural studies on the isolated surface glycoproteins of influenza virus, three-dimensional structures now have also been determined for the complete virions of several members of the picornavirus family including the Mahoney strain of type 1 poliovirus (Hogle *et al.,* 1985) the Sabin strain of type 3 poliovirus (Filman *et al.,* 1988), rhinovirus 14 (Rossmann *et al.,* 1985), and Mengo virus (Luo *et al.,* 1987). In the cases of poliovirus and rhinovirus 14, the structure determinations were preceded or accompanied by sequence analyses of a number of mutants selected by panels of neutralizing monoclonal antibodies (Minor *et al.,* 1983, 1985, 1986; Diamond *et al.,* 1985; Blondel *et al.,* 1986; Page *et al.,* 1988; Sherry *et al.,* 1986), thus allowing the three-dimensional structure of the antigenic sites to be described in the context of the intact virions. For poliovirus, the studies with neutralization-resistant mutants have included representative strains of all three serotypes, and have revealed significant serotypic and strain dependence in the relative dominance of antigenic sites. For poliovirus, these monoclonal studies also have been supplemented with studies of the immune response to synthetic peptides (Emini *et al.,* 1983, 1984; Blondel *et al.,* 1986; Chow *et al.,* 1985; Ferguson *et al.,* 1985; Minor *et al.,* 1986; Diamond *et al.,* 1985).

In the remainder of this chapter we will focus on the antigenic structure of poliovirus, presenting a brief summary of the virus structure and describing in some detail the location and nature of the antigenic sites. Where it is relevant, the results with poliovirus will be compared with those of rhinovirus 14 and the influenza antigens to identify general properties that these antigenic sites have in common, and which may be properties of other viral antigens as well. Finally, the three-dimensional distribution of antigenic sites will be discussed, insofar as it is relevant to understanding the mechanisms of viral escape from neutralization.

II. Poliovirus

Poliovirus is a member of the picornavirus family, which also includes the coxsackieviruses, the rhinoviruses, the cardioviruses (such as EMC, Mengo, and Theiler's virus), the aphthoviruses (foot-and-mouth disease virus), and hepatitis A virus. All known poliovirus isolates can be grouped into one of three serotypes by their behavior with reference panels of neutralizing antisera. The poliovirus particle is approximately 310 Å in diameter and has a molecular mass of 8.5 million daltons (Rueckert, 1985). The virion is composed of 60 copies of each of four capsid protein subunits: VP1 (M_r = 33,000), VP2 (M_r = 30,000), VP3 (M_r = 26,000), and VP4 (M_r = 7,400) arranged on a T = 1 icosahedral surface, and a single-stranded, messenger-sense RNA genome of approximately 7,500 nucleotides. The RNA contains a single large open-reading frame from which a 220-kilodalton polyprotein is synthesized. All known viral proteins are derived from this polyprotein by post-translational cleavages catalyzed by virally encoded proteases (Nicklin *et al.*, 1986). One of the early cleavages liberates a large protein (called P1) from the amino terminus of the polyprotein. P1 contains all four capsid proteins in the order VP4–VP2–VP3–VP1. Cleavage of P1 to yield VP1, VP3, and a precursor protein VP0 (in which VP4 and VP2 remain covalently linked) is associated with the formation of a stable pentameric assembly intermediate that can be isolated from infected cells. The final cleavage of VP0 to VP4 and VP2 occurs very late in assembly, may be linked to the encapsidation of the viral RNA, and makes the assembly process irreversible.

III. Poliovirus Structure

We have now determined the structures of two different strains of poliovirus, the Mahoney (neurovirulent) strain of type 1 and the Sabin (attenuated vaccine) strain of type 3 poliovirus. Although the structures of the two strains differ in detail [and particularly in the antigenic sites (Filman *et al.*, 1988)], overall the two structures are very similar.

The molecular structures of the three large capsid proteins (VP1, VP2, and VP3) are generally similar to one another. Each is comprised of a conserved core: an eight-stranded antiparallel β-barrel with flanking helices (Fig. 1a). At one end of each of the β-barrels the

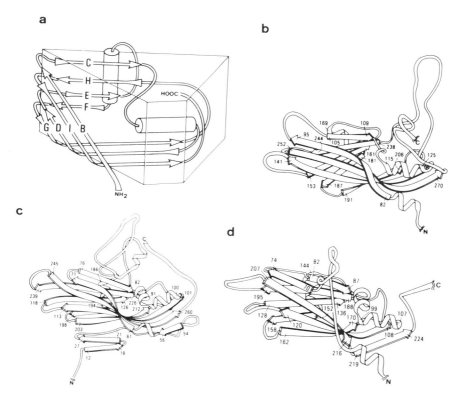

Fig. 1. Schematic representation of the capsid proteins VP1, VP2, and VP3. (a) Model of the conserved core common to all three major capsid proteins. Strands of the eight-stranded antiparallel β-barrel are shown as arrows and are labeled B-I in a manner consistent with the strand designations in the structurally similar cores of rhinovirus and several plant viruses. Flanking helices are indicated as cylinders. The triangular wedge emphasizes the overall shape of the cores. (b, c, and d) Ribbon diagrams of VP1, VP2, and VP3, respectively. Residue numbers have been included as landmarks. Extensions at the amino and carboxyl termini of VP1 and VP3 have been truncated for clarity.

β-strands are connected by short loops, giving the barrel the overall shape of a triangular wedge. In contrast to the great structural similarity exhibited by the core regions, each of the three major subunits has a different set of loops connecting the regular secondary structural elements of the cores, and different amino- and carboxyl-terminal extensions (Fig. 1b–d).

The description of the capsid proteins in terms of conserved cores and dissimilar connecting loops and terminal extensions is relevant to their structural roles in the virion. The conserved cores form the closed continuous shell of the virion. The amino-terminal extensions form a network on the inner surface of the protein shell that we believe serves to direct the assembly of the particle. The carboxyl-terminal extensions and many of the connecting loops decorate the outer surface of the virion. As we will show, these elaborations on the outer surface contain most of the antigenic sites of the virus, and may have evolved to furnish the virus with structurally inessential components that can be modified readily under immune selection without affecting the viability of the virus.

In the virus particle, five copies of VP1 pack around the 5-fold axes with the narrow ends of their wedge-shaped cores pointing toward the axes. Similarly, VP2 and VP3 alternate around the 3-fold axes with the narrow ends of their cores pointing toward the axes. The tilts of the cores up along the 3-fold and 5-fold symmetry axes result in prominent radial protrusions at the particle 5-fold and 3-fold axes. These protrusions are separated by a deep circular moat around each of the 5-fold peaks. A saddle-shaped depression across the particle 2-fold axes connects these circular moats. In its overall shape, the particle resembles the geometric figure shown in Fig. 2.

The protrusions at the 5-fold axes are accentuated by loops connecting the top three pairs of strands in the VP1 β-barrels. Likewise the smaller protrusions at the particle 3-fold axes are accentuated by exposed portions of the loops connecting the top two pairs of strands at the narrow end of the β-barrels of VP2 and VP3 and by small finger-like projection formed by residues 50–70 of VP3. A third major surface feature located near the particle 2-fold axes is formed by the large double-loop connection between the E and F strands of the beta barrel of VP2 (residues 126–186), by the carboxyl terminus of VP2, and by the large elongated loop connecting the G and H strands of the β-barrel of VP1 (residues 207–237). These three large features dominate the exposed outer surface of the virus. Each feature is approximately the same size as the antigen-binding portion of a Fab fragment, and each is separated from the others by deep depressions that exclude

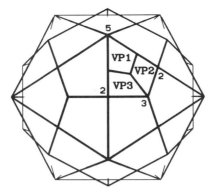

FIG. 2. A geometric figure representing the overall shape of the poliovirus particle. The figure was generated by superimposing an icosahedron and a dodecahedron. The symmetry axes of the particle and the positions of VP1, VP2, and VP3 within a single icosahedral asymmetric unit are indicated.

access to large probes such as antibody molecules. The overall appearance of the poliovirus particle is shown in Fig. 3.

IV. Antigenic Sites

The neutralizing antigenic sites of poliovirus have been characterized by sequencing mutants selected for their resistance to neutralization by monoclonal antibodies. Such studies have now been carried out for all three serotypes of poliovirus, although types 1 and 3 have been studied more extensively than type 2. The mutations that confer resistance to monoclonal antibodies map to a number of discrete regions in the capsid protein sequences, including residues 91–102 (in the B strand and the loop connecting β-strands B and C), 168 (in the loop connecting strands E and F), 221–226 (in the large elongated loop connecting strands G and H), 254 (in strand I), and 285–289 (in a loop near the carboxyl terminus) of VP1 (to date seen only in type 3 poliovirus); residues 72 (in the loop connecting strands B and C), 166–170 (in one of the two loops connecting strands E and F), and 270 (near the carboxyl terminus) of VP2; and residues 58–60 (in the finger-like protrusion preceding the B strand), 71, 73, and 76–79 (from the loop connecting strands B and C) of VP3 (see Table I). We have located each of the mutations in the three-dimensional structure of the virus. Based on the knowledge that the antigen binding site of a Fab fragment of an antibody is approximately 30 Å in diameter, and on the

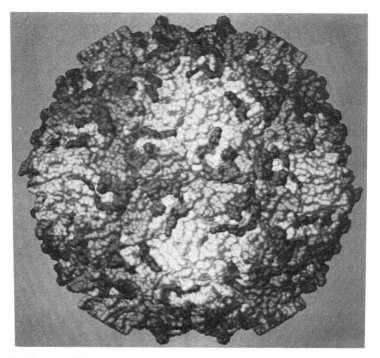

FIG. 3.   A space-filling model of the poliovirus particle. At the center of the particle
VP1 is white, VP2 is light grey, and VP3 is dark grey. All of the proteins are darker
toward the edge of the particle as a result of depth cueing and shadowing, which have
been included to provide an illusion of depth.

assumption that a Fab fragment is unlikely to span a deep depression
on the virus surface, we have found that the individual mutation sites
can be grouped into three general sites.

Site 1 is located at the top of the large protrusion near the 5-fold
axes of the particle. This site includes mutations from each of three
distinct peptide segments in VP1: residues 89–102 (in strand B and the
exposed loop connecting strands B and C), 252 (in strand D), and
residue 168 in the loop connecting strands E and F (Fig. 4a). Site 2 is
located at the top of the large protrusion near the particle twofold axes
(Fig. 4b). This site includes mutations from two separate polypeptide
segments of VP2: residues 166–170 (in the larger of the twin loops
connecting strands E and F), and residue 270 (near the carboxyl
terminus); and one polypeptide segment of VP1 (residues 221–226, in
the large elongated loop connecting strands G and H). Site 3 is located

in and around the smaller protrusion at the particle 3-fold axes (Fig. 4c). This site includes mutations in the finger-like protrusion of VP3 (residues 58–60) from the B strand of VP3 (residues 71 and 73) and from the loop connecting the B and C strands of VP3 (residues 76, 77, and 79). Because the remaining mutations in the polypeptide segment near the carboxyl terminus of VP1 (residues 285–289) are located halfway between sites 2 and 3, it has been impossible to assign them to either site based on distance measurements alone. Closer inspection of the structure and the location of the mutations, however, showed that this loop was somewhat separated from the remainder of site 2 by the ridge of the 164–170 loop of VP2, providing a weak structural argument for the inclusion of this peptide segment as a portion of site 3.

The neutralization-resistant mutants also have been grouped independently by immunological methods, testing each mutant for its ability to be neutralized by large panels of individual monoclonal antibodies (Minor *et al.*, 1985, 1986; Page *et al.*, 1988). The groupings obtained by these "cross-neutralization" studies are, in general, completely consistent with the groupings based on structural considerations alone. The cross-neutralization data have confirmed the inclusion of the residues 91–102, 168, and 254 segments of VP1 as portions of a single site (that is, that there are monoclonal antibodies that no longer neutralize a variant with mutations in the 91–102 segment of VP1 and that also fail to neutralize variants with mutations in residue 168 or residue 254 of VP1). Similarly, the cross-neutralization experiments support the inclusion of 164–170 and 270 from VP2 and 221–226 of VP1 as part of a second site. The behavior of the variants that map to site 3 is somewhat more complex. The cross-neutralization studies have confirmed the inclusion of residues 285–289 of VP1 (at least in type 3 poliovirus) along with residues 58–60, 71, and 73 as part of a third site. These studies also have provided evidence for a link between the portion of site 3 contributed by the B-C loop of VP3 (76–79) and the B-C loop of VP2 (residue 72). Curiously, however, the cross-neutralization studies have failed (at least as of this writing) to demonstrate a link between the portions of site 3 contributed by the finger-like insertion and B strand of VP3 with the portion contributed by the B-C loops of VP3 (residues 76–79 and VP2 (residue 72). The failure to demonstrate a linkage between these two portions of site 3 might be due to a failure to date to select the appropriate antibody and mutants, or, alternatively, it may indicate that these two subsites function as totally independent antigenic sites. For now we have decided to call the two subsites site 3A (VP1 285–289, VP3 58–60, 71, 73) and site 3B (VP3, 76–79, VP2 72).

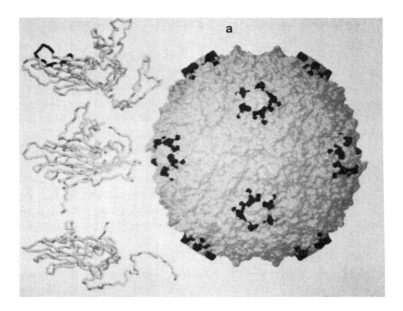

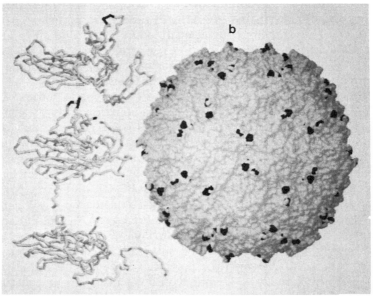

FIG. 4. The antigenic sites of poliovirus. Each panel shows a copy of VP1, VP2, and VP3 (left) and an intact particle (right). The sites of mutations that confer resistance to neutralizing monoclonal antibodies are highlighted in black. The mutations have been grouped by spatial considerations and by cross-neutralization studies into three sites as described in the text. (a) Site 1, (b) Site 2, (c) Site 3, and (d) all sites. In d it is clear that the antigenic sites taken together occupy the outermost features of the particle and are not present in the depressions on the virus surface.

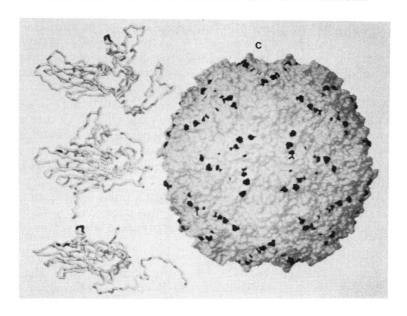

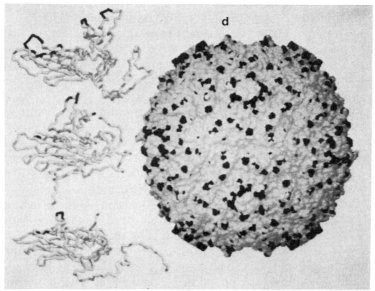

FIG. 4. (Continued)

Up to this point the description of the structure of the antigenic sites of poliovirus has ignored strain and serotypic differences. While this simplification is useful in delineating the diversity of the antigenic structure of the virus, it is, in fact, a serious oversimplification. Comparison of monoclonal escape experiments carried out on each of the three serotypes of poliovirus have indicated that there is a great deal of serotype specific variability in the extent to which any one of the sites is represented in the immune response to a given strain of poliovirus. An additional complication is that the vast majority of the monoclonal experiments have been performed with a single independent lineage within each serotype [the Mahoney lineage of type 1 (including the Mahoney strain and its attenuated derivative Sabin strain), the Sabin strain of type 2, and the Leon lineage of type 3 (including the Leon strain and its attenuated derivative Sabin strain)].

Early observations with the Leon strain of type 3 poliovirus and with its attenuated derivative Sabin 3 strain indicated that the vast majority of monoclonal antibodies to the (Leon derived lineage of) type 3 poliovirus were specific for site 1 (Minor et al., 1983, 1985). Indeed, because the systematic studies of type 3 poliovirus predated the studies of type 1, this site became widely known as the immunodominant site of poliovirus. In contrast, subsequent experiments performed with the (Mahoney lineage of) type 1 poliovirus have found that the vast majority of the murine neutralizing antibody response is directed against sites 2 and 3 (Diamond et al., 1985; Minor et al., 1986; Blondel et al., 1986; Page et al., 1988).

The greater importance of site 1 in the immune response to type 3 poliovirus (relative to type 1) can be explained in part by structural differences. In comparing the structures of the Sabin 3 and the Mahoney 1 strains, we have found that by far the largest structural difference occurs in the B-C loop of VP1 which comprises a major portion of site 1 (Filman et al., 1988). Within this 10-residue loop (95–104) differences between equivalent α-carbon positions as large as 8 Å have been found. The immunodominance of this loop in type 3 is likely to be related to our observation that this loop in the Sabin 3 structure is considerably more exposed than it is in the Mahoney 1 structure. In general, the largest structural differences between the two strains of poliovirus appear to be associated with substitutions involving proline in regions of local sequence divergence. In the 95–104 loop of VP1, there are two such proline substitutions between Sabin 3 and Mahoney 1 [pro (PM1) to glu (PS3) at position 95 and ser (PM1) to pro (PS3) at position 97], as well as several other sequence differences. In the Lansing and Sabin strains of type 2 poliovirus, the limited monoclonal studies that are available indicate that the immune response is dominated by site 1 (Minor *et al.*, 1986), while sequence comparisons show that both strains exhibit the Sabin 3 type pattern of prolines in this loop. On this basis, therefore, we would predict that these type 2 strains will likely be found to adopt a structure that is more similar to that observed in Sabin 3.

While the structural differences may provide a partial explanation for the observed serotypic differences in the degree of immunodominance of site 1, studies in which this site is selectively destroyed by proteolysis have indicated that other factors must be important as well (Icenogle *et al.*, 1986). A number of strains of poliovirus contain a specific trypsin site in the 95–104 loop of VP1 (Fricks *et al.*, 1985). Cleavage at this site has no effect on the infectivity of the virus *in vitro,* but eliminates the ability of monoclonal antibodies that recognize site 1 to bind or neutralize the virus. Measurement of the relative binding or neutralization titer of polyclonal sera against native or cleaved virus thus provides a convenient estimate of the percentage of the response that is directed against site 1. In agreement with the results of the monoclonal escape mutation experiments, these studies have shown that site 1 dominates the immune response of several inbred strains of mice to the (Leon-derived strains of) type 3 poliovirus, but not the (Mahoney-derived strains of) type 1 poliovirus. These studies also have shown that the degree of dominance varies reproducibly with the strain of mouse immunized, ranging from 75% in the SJL/J strain to 95% in the C57BL/6 strain. Studies with congenic strains of mice, however, failed to reveal any clear-cut relationship between the degree of dominance of site 1 in the anti-type 3 response and the MHC type of the mouse immunized. Similar studies with outbred species, including horse, rabbits, and monkey have shown that the degree of dominance of site 1 in the anti-type 3 response varied with the species immunized (30% in the horse and 10% in monkeys) and perhaps with the route of administration.

It may be especially significant that site 1 appears to play little role in the anti-type 3 response in oral (trivalent Sabin) vaccinees (Icenogle *et al.*, 1986). Indeed, several lines of evidence including studies that follow the mutations accumulated during the course of virus replication in oral vaccinees, studies of the relative titers against cleaved and uncleaved virus, and direct studies of the susceptibility of excreted virus to site 1-specific monoclonal antibodies suggest that the virus produced in the intestinal tract is itself proteolytically processed (Minor *et al.*, 1987; Roivainen and Hovi, 1987).

Although the interpretation of the monoclonal release mutation studies might at first seem straightforward, there are several potential difficulties in the interpretation of the results of these experiments. For example the discussion above indicates the potential difficulties posed by studies that are based primarily on the response of a single inbred species of animal (the mouse). In addition this type of experiment is very likely to yield an incomplete list of antigenic sites. The ability to observe a particular site or portion of a site depends both on the inclusion of an appropriate antibody in the panel used to select variants, and on the requirement that a mutation in the site not render the virus nonviable by interfering with other essential functions of the capsid proteins including folding, assembly, cell attachment, and cell entry.

The results described above represent the synthesis of studies in several laboratories. Particularly in the case of type 1 and type 3 poliovirus, these studies have included a large number of variants selected by and screened against a large number of monoclonal antibodies. The overall consistency between the results of these studies provides some confidence that the number of sites and their general location have been described adequately, at least for the murine response to poliovirus. However, in light of the limitations inherent in the method, it seems likely that the working definitions of the residues in each site, and possibly the connections between sites will continue to evolve as additional studies are done.

Finally, there is some question as to the precise relationship between the site of mutation and the site on the virus that is bound physically. While the simplest model for the mechanism by which a variant escapes neutralization is that the mutation alters a residue within the physical binding site in such a way so as to interfere with antibody binding, there has been some discussion of the possibility that a mutation outside of the actual binding site might permit an escape from neutralization either by altering the structure of the binding site, or by preventing structural transitions required for neutralization (Diamond *et al.*, 1985; Blondel *et al.*, 1986). An examination of the mutation sites in monoclonal selected mutants of poliovirus shows that most of the mutated residues are located in exposed regions of the structure. These regions appear to be highly accessible to direct interactions with antibody molecules, and, similarly, the majority of the side-chains that undergo mutation are themselves accessible to antibody-sized probes. One very striking example of this property is the VP1 91–102 component of site 1 in type 3 poliovirus. Within this region mutations are observed at residues 91, 93, 95, and 97–102. The observation of mutations only in odd-numbered residues at the amino-terminal portion of this site is a consequence of the location of residues 91–95 in the B strand of the β-barrel of VP1. In a β-sheet the side-chains occur on strictly alternating sides of the sheet. In the B strand of VP1, the odd-numbered side-chains are located on the exposed surface of the sheet, while the even-numbered side-chains are buried inside the β-barrel. In consequence, residues 91, 93, 95, and 97 are accessible to antibodies, whereas residues 92, 94, and 96 are not. In this instance, however, the observed distribution of mutations may not be a simple consequence of the exposure of the odd-numbered residues, since the even-numbered residues interact in a fairly specific way with other side-chains in the hydrophobic core of the β-barrel. Mutations in the even ordered residues would, therefore, be less likely to yield viable virus.

In an effort to put the question of exposure of the monoclonal release mutations on a more objective basis, we have evaluated the degree of exposure of all residues on the outer surface of the type 1 Mahoney structure using a novel algorithm developed by Drs. John Tainer and Elizabeth Getzoff at Scripps Clinic. This algorithm determines the radius of the largest spherical probe that can contact any given point on the virus surface without touching any neighboring points. This analysis has produced several interesting results (Page *et al.*, 1988). First, the majority of the residues that have been observed as monoclonal release mutations in type 1 poliovirus are exposed to spherical probes that are comparable in size to the antigen-binding portion of a Fab fragment. Second, all of the mutation sites that are exposed to a lesser degree are located close to fully exposed sites, and many of these participate in interactions that stabilize local loop structures within the antigenic sites in an obvious way. In no case have we observed a mutation that would require long-range propagation of a structural alteration to effect escape from neutralization. Third, the calculation has identified several groups of residues that lie close to the known antigenic sites, and that are highly accessible to antibody-sized probes, but that have not yet been observed as sites of monoclonal release mutations. These include the loops connecting the H and I strands of VP2 and VP3, the carboxyl terminus of VP1 (in or near site 3), and the loop connecting the D and E strands of VP1 (in or near site 1). The failure to select for mutations in any of these residues might be interesting if it is a consequence of a limitation in the ability of the residue to function as an antigenic or immunogenic site, or if mutations in the site reduce the viability of the virus. Alternatively, the failure to observe these mutations may simply reflect incomplete sampling due to the large but finite number of monoclonal antibodies and mutants in the screens. Eventually, these alternatives may be resolved experimentally by producing point mutations in these regions by site-directed mutagenesis of the infectious cDNA clones of the virus (G. Page and M. Chow, MIT, personal communication).

V. Use of Synthetic Peptides to Characterize Antigenic Sites

A number of investigators have used antibodies to synthetic peptides that correspond to capsid protein sequences for probing the antigenic sites of poliovirus. Many of the antigenic sites identified by these studies correspond to the sites defined by the monoclonal antibody studies. Specifically, synthetic peptides corresponding to the B-C loop (Emini *et al.*, 1983; Chow *et al.*, 1985; Ferguson *et al.*, 1985) and H-I loops at the narrow end of the β-barrel of VP1 and the E-F loop of VP1 (site 1) (Chow *et al.*, 1985), the G-H loop of VP1 (Chow *et al.*, 1985), and the E-F loop of VP2 (site 2) (Emini *et al.*, 1983), and the carboxyl-terminal loop of VP1 (site 3a) (Chow *et al.*, 1985) have been shown to induce a neutralizing response to poliovirus or to prime for a subsequent neutralizing response upon subsequent inoculation with a subimmunizing dose of virus. The general similarity between many of the sites identified by synthetic peptide antibodies and those identified by monoclonal release mutations has interesting implications for the classical distinction between sequential (linear) and conformational (three-dimensional) epitopes. Historically, synthetic peptide antibodies have been used to define sequential epitopes. In contrast the antigenic sites of poliovirus as defined by the collected monoclonal studies are clearly conformational. The simplest interpretation of these results is that the antipeptide antibodies are recognizing sequentially contiguous portions of conformational antigenic sites. Thus, at least in the case of poliovirus, the distinction between sequential and conformational sites may be largely semantic.

It is significant, however, that several of the peptides that have been shown either to elicit or to prime for a neutralizing response against poliovirus do not correspond directly to the sites identified by monoclonal antibodies. This is not entirely surprising because the synthetic peptide method is not subject to some of the constraints that limit the monocolonal experiments (e.g., genetic determinants of immunodominance and the requirement that mutants be viable). In particular, a peptide corresponding to the third loop (D-E loop) at the narrow end of the barrel of VP1 has been shown to prime for a neutralizing response

(Jameson *et al.*, 1985). This loop is highly exposed in the virion and its location is entirely consistent with this loop being a part of site 1. The failure to observe monoclonal escape mutations in this loop might simply reflect the limited (albeit large) sampling of mutations or restrictions on the viability of mutations within this loop. Indeed, this loop has been identified as a site of monoclonal escape mutations in rhinovirus 14 (see below).

For some of the antipeptide antibodies, however, the neutralizing response is not explained so readily because the peptides correspond to portions of the capsid protein that are located in the interior of the native virus. These include antibodies directed against several peptides corresponding to sequences in the amino-terminal extension of VP1 (Emini *et al.*, 1983; Chow *et al.*, 1985) and to a peptide corresponding to the F-G loop of the β-barrel of VP1 (Chow *et al.*, 1985). We suspect that the ability of these antipeptide antibodies to neutralize poliovirus is related to conformational alterations in the capsid structure that are either induced or more probably trapped by the antibodies.

When poliovirus attaches to susceptible cells, it is known to undergo a conformational rearrangement resulting in the release of the internal protein VP4, a decrease in sedimentation coefficient from 160S to 135S, changes in antigenicity, and a loss of infectivity due to the loss of the ability to attach to cells. A similar if not identical form of the virus is the predominant species found inside cells soon after infection, and the conformational change is widely believed to represent an early step in the uncoating of the virus. We have shown that this conformational rearrangement results in the extrusion of the amino terminus of VP1 and that neutralizing antibodies raised against synthetic peptides corresponding to the amino terminal extension of VP1 (residues 24–40, and 61–80) and to the F-G loop of VP1 (residues 182–201) have appreciably higher titers to altered virus than they do to native virus in immunoprecipitation assays (Fricks and Hogle, 1988). It may also be relevant that human oral vaccinees have appreciable titers against the amino terminus of VP1 (C.E. Fricks, M. Kubitz, and J. M. Hogle, unpublished observations). In contrast, hyperimmune mice and rabbits (both nonpermissive hosts for poliovirus) that have been immunized by intraperitoneal injection lack appreciable titers to the amino terminus of VP1. Although we have yet to determine whether or not the portion of the response in human vaccinees that is specific for the amino terminus of VP1 is neutralizing, this observation raises the interesting possibility that the antigenic sites recognized by a permissive host may be exposed during the binding of the virus to host-specific receptors, and thus may not be identical to the sites recognized by a nonpermissive host.

VI. Comparison of Antigenic Structures of Polio and Rhinovirus

Rhinovirus 14 and poliovirus share approximately 60% sequence identity at the amino acid level in the capsid region. Not surprisingly, the strong sequence homology is reflected in similarities in the three-dimensional structures of the virions and their component capsid proteins. Indeed, the major structural differences between viruses are confined almost entirely to the external loops (where there are several significant deletions and insertions in one structure with respect to the other) and, to a lesser extent, to the terminal extensions of the capsid proteins.

The structural distribution of antigenic sites in the two viruses is also strikingly similar. Like poliovirus, the antigenic sites of rhinovirus as mapped by monoclonal release mutations (Sherry *et al.,* 1986) are located in three general regions on the virus surface (Rossman *et al.,* 1985): one near the fivefold axis that includes the B strand and B-C loop of VP1, a second near the twofold axes that includes the E-F loops of VP2 and the G-H loop of VP1, and a third close to the particle threefold axis that includes the B-C loop of VP3. A detailed comparison of the antigenic sites of the two viruses, including the operational definition of subsites provided by cross-neutralization studies with panels of monoclonal antibodies is shown in Table I. Note that despite the striking similarity in the overall antigenic organization, there are significant differences in both the identities of the loops that participate in forming the sites and in their separation into subsites as defined operationally by cross-neutralization studies. Undoubtedly, some of these differences will turn out to be artifacts of the limited sampling provided by currently available mutation studies. For example, a complete analysis of escape mutants is now available for only one of the more than 100 serotypes of rhinovirus, whereas the mapping of antigenic sites of poliovirus represents a compilation of data from all three serotypes of that virus.

In at least one case, however, there is an obvious structural explanation for the difference in the fine structure of an antigenic site. Antigenic site 2 of poliovirus is dominated by the second of the two loops in the E-F loop of VP2 and by the elongated G-H loop of VP1. In contrast the analogous site in rhinovirus 14 includes residues from both portions of the E-F loop of VP2, while the G-H loop of VP1 appears to play a less significant role. These observations can be explained by

TABLE I

COMPARISON OF ANTIGENIC SITES IN POLIOVIRUS AND RHINOVIRUS[a]

Poliovirus[b]		Rhinovirus 14[c]	
Site 1	VP1 B strand B-C loop (91,93,95,97–102) E strand loop 168 H-I loop 254	Site 1 A B	B-C loop (91,95) B strand B-C loop (83,85) D strand D-E loop (138–139)
Site 2	VP1 G-H loop (221,223,224,226) VP2 E-F loop (164–170) VP2 C term (270)	Site 2	VP1 G-H loop (210) VP2 E-F loop (136) E-F loop (158–159, 161)
Site 3A	VP1 C term (285–288) VP3 pre-B (58–60)	Site 3	VP1 C term (287) VP3 B-C loop (72,75,76) VP3 H-I loop (203)
Site 3B	VP2 B-C loop (72) VP3 B-C loop (76,77,79)		

[a] Residue numbers (in parentheses) are specific for each virus. Loop designations are consistent with those shown in Hogle et al., 1985 for poliovirus and Rossmann et al., 1985 for rhinovirus 14.

[b] Data compiled from Minor et al., 1983, 1985, 1986; Diamond et al., 1985; Blundel et al., 1986; Page et al., 1988.

[c] Data compiled from Sherry et al., 1986; Rossmann et al., 1985.

structural differences between the viruses. In poliovirus the second E-F loop of VP2 is much larger than the first, which limits the exposure of the smaller of the two loops, while the G-H loop of VP1 is large and somewhat exposed. In rhinovirus, however, the two E-F loops of VP2 are nearly equal in size and in exposure, while the G-H loop of VP1 is some four residues shorter than the corresponding loop in poliovirus.

Although the antigenic sites of a number of picornaviruses are currently being studied, the only other such virus for which there is a relatively complete description of antigenic sites is foot-and-mouth disease virus. In FMDV the antigenic response appears to be directed predominantly against a single site that corresponds to residues 140–160 of VP1. The sequences of a number of picornaviruses have been aligned by a combination of computational sequence alignment and subjective assessments of likely structural similarities by Palmenberg and Rossman (A.C. Palmenberg, personal communication). These alignments indicate that residues 140–160 of VP1 in FMDV corresponds to the G-H loops of VP1 in poliovirus and rhinovirus. Detailed modeling of the structure of the FMDV surface based on existing picornavirus structures would be a highly speculative exercise, considering the apparent deletion of most of the E-F loop of VP2 in FMDV. The structural interpretation of the antigenic sites and possible explanations for the more limited distribution of antigenic sites in FMDV must therefore await the completion of crystallographic studies of FMDV which currently are in progress (D. Stuart, Oxford, and F. Brown and D. Rowlands, Wellcome Biotechnologies, personal communication).

VII. Relationship between Antigenic Sites and Possible Receptor Binding Sites

When the sites of neutralization resistant mutants are considered together, it is apparent that collectively, they occupy the protrusions that constitute the outermost surface features of both poliovirus (Fig. 4d) and rhinovirus. These protrusions are separated by depressions in which escape mutation sites have not been observed, and which exhibit a relatively greater degree of sequence conservation within each type of virus. This sequence conservation makes these depressions likely candidates for the site on the virus surface which is responsible for receptor recognition and binding. In a similar analysis of sequence changes due to antigenic drift and selection for neutralization escape *in vitro*, a depression on the surface of the influenza virus hemagglutinin was identified as the likely receptor binding site for influenza virus (Wiley *et al.*, 1981). In the case of influenza virus the receptor apparently consists predominantly of sialic acid linked to glycoproteins and/or glycolipids on the cell surface. Subsequent studies of sequence changes in virus strains with altered stereospecificity for the linkage of sialic acid and direct studies of crystalline complexes of the hemagglutinin with acid-containing trisaccharides has confirmed that this depression is indeed the receptor binding site (Weis *et al.*, 1988).

Using an extension of this argument Rossmann and his colleagues have focused on the largest of the surface depressions, namely the "canyon" surrounding the protrusion at the 5-fold axes as the most probable receptor site in poliovirus and rhinovirus (Rossmann *et al.*, 1985). They argue that this depression is unique in that it is sufficiently deep to exclude contact between antibodies and the residues at the base and lower walls of the depression, thus protecting the residues in the receptor site from immune selection. They emphasize that the protection from antibody binding, and hence from immune selection, makes this site a particularly attractive candidate for a receptor site. We believe, however, that the focus on this particular region may be premature.

Like all RNA viruses the picornaviruses are constantly producing errors during replication resulting in a sampling of mutations in all regions of the genome. Mutations in the receptor binding site are, in fact, being made constantly, but are for the most part lethal. These mutations, thus, can neither be selected for nor against by immune pressure. In addition, it is not necessary that the receptor site be entirely inaccessible to antibodies. The receptor site in the influenza hemagglutinin, for example, is too shallow to protect completely the residues involved in sialic acid binding. Instead it appears that the receptor site is protected by being surrounded by loops that can accommodate mutation (Weis *et al.*, 1988). The distribution of antigenic sites in both poliovirus and rhinovirus 14 is suggestive that a similar mechanism of protection may occur in the picornaviruses.

VIII. Future Prospects

In this chapter, we have described the structure of poliovirus, defining the nature of its antigenic sites and the structural basis for serotypic differences among polioviruses. We also have attempted to correlate this information with that obtained from the combined structural and immunlogical characterizations of other viral antigens, including rhinovirus and the hemagglutinin and neuraminidase surface glycoproteins from influenza virus, to derive more general principles governing the distribution of antigenic sites in viruses. These comparisons have shown that in all cases the antigenic sites are located on the exterior surface, in loops that are simultaneously the most immunogenic and the most mutable regions of the virus or virus structural protein. The comparisons suggest that the decoration of the surfaces of animal viruses with flexible loops may serve to force the host's immune system to respond to areas that can accommodate mutations, and may thus provide a common mechanism by which animal viruses evade immune surveillance.

In addition to these contributions to our understanding of the viral antigens and their interactions with the immune system at a very basic level, knowledge of the three-dimensional structure of poliovirus (and other viral antigens) presents considerable future prospects for very practical applications in the field of vaccine development. Indeed, some of these future prospects have already begun to be realized. These include the use of the three-dimensional structure to assist in the search for candidate peptide vaccines, the use of structural studies in the attempt to produce more physically stable vaccine strains, and the use of structure in the design of antigenic chimeras in which the genetically stable Sabin strain of type 1 poliovirus is used to present antigenic determinants of types 2 and 3 poliovirus or related viruses such as hepatitis A virus.

Much of the published work investigating the potential use of synthetic peptides as poliovirus vaccines predated the determination of the three-dimensional structure of the virus. Although these studies succeeded in identifying several peptides that were capable of eliciting a neutralizing response, the neutralizing titers obtained generally were disappointing. Knowledge of the structure provides several avenues for improving the immunogenicity of the synthetic peptides by providing: (1) a rational basis for the selection of candidate peptides, (2) a basis for the construction of peptides that are constrained to adopt a conformation more like that in the intact virus, and (3) a basis for the selection of combinations of synthetic peptides that represent individual polypeptide segments within the complex antigenic sites. Furthermore, a number of laboratories currently are mapping the sites responsible for stimulation of a T-cell (predominantly T-helper) response against poliovirus. As these results become available, the structure could prove invaluable in designing combinations of peptides that simultaneously express both B-cell and T-cell epitopes.

One of the major problems with the current attenuated poliovirus vaccines is that they are unstable at elevated temperature and thus require strict maintenance of a cold chain to deliver effective vaccine. All three Sabin vaccine strains are temperature sensitive, growing well at 37°C but not at 39° or 40°C. The temperature sensitivity of the Sabin strain of type 3 poliovirus has been particularly well characterized, and studies within our own laboratory have shown that the temperature sensitivity of Sabin 3 may be correlated with thermolability of the virus particle. Genetic studies of the Sabin 3 strain and its neurovirulent parent Leon 3 have shown that the temperature sensitivity of Sabin 3 maps to a single mutation, which results in the substitution of a phenylalanine (Sabin 3) for serine (Leon 3) at position 91 of the capsid protein VP3 (Minor et al., 1988). The side-chain of phenylalanine 91 of VP3 occupies an unusual location in the three-dimensional structure of Sabin 3 in that it is fully exposed to solvent on the external surface of the virion (Filman et al., 1988). Indeed, we have been able to see direct evidence of ordered solvent (presumably water) molecules around the phenyl side-chain in the election density maps of Sabin 3.

The solvation of a large hydrophobic side chain such as that of phenylalanine is energetically unfavorable, and we have hypothesized that the exposed phenylalanine destabilizes the virion by promoting any conformational change that allows this side-chain to be buried.

Recently a number of naturally occurring and laboratory-selected non-temperature-sensitive variants of Sabin 3 have been sequenced (Minor et al., 1988). A number of these variants were found to have second-site suppressor mutations which restore the non-temperature-sensitive phenotype. In collaboration with Philip Minor (NIBSC) and Jeffrey Almond (Reading), we have undertaken a combination of crystallographic and computational modeling studies of these second-site revertants to characterize more fully the structural factors that control thermal stability in poliovirus. Such studies eventually may provide information that will allow the construction of more thermo-stable attenuated vaccine strains.

Although the attenuated poliovirus vaccines are among the most safe, effective, and economical vaccines currently in use, a handful of cases of poliomyelitis continue to occur in countries with established vaccine programs. Virtually all of these cases are associated with an increased neurovirulence of the Sabin vaccine strains of type 2 and type 3 poliovirus upon replication in the intestine of vaccinees (WHO Collaborative Study, 1981). In contrast there has never been a well-documented case of poliomyelitis associated with the Sabin strain of type 1 poliovirus. Consistent with this observation genetic studies of the Sabin 3 strain and its neurovirulent parent Leon 3 have shown that only two mutations in Sabin 3 contribute significantly to its attenuation (Westrop et al., 1986), whereas the Sabin 1 strain has accumulated a number of attenuating mutations with respect to its neurovirulent parent Mahoney 1 (Omata et al., 1986). There has therefore been a suggestion that more stable vaccine strains for type 2 and type 3 poliovirus could be constructed by grafting the antigenic sites from type 2 or type 3 vaccine strains into the genetically more stable Sabin 1 strain.

Three separate groups have succeeded in constructing such antigenic hybrids (or chimeras) of poliovirus (Burke et al., 1988; Murray et al., 1988; Martin et al., 1988). In each case the infectious DNA clone of a type 1 strain was modified to replace the sequence of the B-C loop of VP1 (antigenic site 1) with the analogous antigenic site from a strain of type 2 or type 3 poliovirus. The resulting chimeric viruses displayed the expected reactivities when tested versus panels of type-specific antisera and monoclonal antibodies, and elicited neutralizing responses to both parental serotypes in small animals and in monkeys.

In each case, knowledge of the three-dimensional structure of the virus was an important consideration in the design of the chimera, and, in the type 1–type 2 chimera, the structure was useful in identifying an unfavorable sequence in the initial construct (Martin *et al.*, 1988). Elimination of the unfavorable sequence converted the chimera from a poorly growing virus to one that grows nearly as well as the parent strains. A number of laboratories now are attempting to use similar approaches to produce chimeras with hybrid sequences in antigenic sites 2 and 3.

The type 1–type 2 chimera was produced by replacing the sequences of antigenic site 1 of the Mahoney strain of type 1 poliovirus with the corresponding sequences from the Lansing strain of type 2 poliovirus. Whereas most strains of poliovirus, including the Mahoney strain, are specific for primates, the Lansing strain has been adapted to mice, where it causes a paralytic disease which is very similar to poliomyelitis in humans. Several years ago Vincent Racaniello and his colleagues at Columbia University showed that the ability to cause paralysis in mice mapped to the capsid region of the Lansing genome (La Monica *et al.*, 1986) and that mutations in the B–C loop (antigenic site 1) were capable of attenuating the neurovirulence of the Lansing strain in mice (La Monica *et al.*, 1987). Marc Girard and his colleagues at the Pasteur Institute have shown that the substitution of the Lansing sequences from antigenic site 1 into the Mahoney strain is in itself sufficient to confer mouse adaptation on the type 1–type 2 chimera (Martin *et al.*, 1988). These studies raise the exciting possibility that the three-dimensional structure of the virus capsid may provide a useful tool for designing viruses that have been attenuated via site-directed mutagenesis of the capsid proteins.

As a practical matter, it is important to note that the safety and efficicacy of the existing poliovirus vaccines will make testing and licensing of any new polio vaccine very difficult. Nonetheless, any significant improvement in the economy, deliverability, or safety of the vaccine could substantially reduce the estimated 250,000–2,000,000 cases of paralytic poliomyelitis that occur annually in unvaccinated or under-vaccinated populations in the Third World, and reduce the suffering and costs of litigation caused by the low level (5–10 cases per year in the United States) of vaccine-associated poliomyelitis in countries with extensive vaccine programs. Furthermore, poliovirus has traditionally served as a model system for other viruses, and we might therefore anticipate that advances made in vaccine development with poliovirus will prove useful in the development of vaccines against viruses for which no suitable vaccines currently exist. In particular, studies with poliovirus will be especially relevant to the related hepatitis A virus, which is sufficiently difficult to grow to make development and production of either killed or attenuated vaccines extremely difficult and nearly prohibitively expensive. Sequence alignments between members of the Picornavirus family are now sufficiently accurate to at least roughly correlate the sequence of hepatitis A virus with the known structures of poliovirus, rhinovirus 14, and mengovirus (Ann Palmenberg, University of Wisconsin, personal communication). Several groups are actively using these correlations to design candidate synthetic peptide vaccines against hepatitis A or to construct chimeric viruses in which the predicted antigenic determinants of hepatitis A are carried by attenuated polioviruses.

ACKNOWLEDGMENTS

J.M.H. acknowledges support from National Institutes of Health grant AI-20566. The authors would also like to thank the many investigators in the field who have contributed to the understanding of poliovirus and its antigenic properties, and especially Marie Chow (Massachusetts Institute of Technology) and Philip Minor [National Institutes of Biological Standards and Control (London)] who have been our collaborators in the structural studies of poliovirus. This is publication no. 5263MB from the Research Institute of Scripps Clinic.

REFERENCES

Amit, A. G., Mariuzza, R. A., Phillips, S. E. V., and Poljak, R. J. (1986). *Science* **233**, 747–753.

Babbit, B., Allen, G., Matsueda, E., Haber, E., and Unanue, E. (1985). *Nature (London)* **317**, 359–361.

Bjorkman, P. J., Saper, M. A., Samaouri, B., Bennett, W. S., Strominger, J., and Wiley, D. C. (1987a). *Nature (London)* **329**, 506–512.

Bjorkman, P. J., Saper, M. A., Samaouri, B., Bennett, W. S., Strominger, J., and Wiley, D. C. (1987b). *Nature (London)* **329**, 512–518.

Blondel, B., Crainic, R., Fichot, O., Dufraisse, G., Cardea, A., Girard, M., and Horaud, F. (1986). *J. Virol.* **57**, 81–90.

Burke, K. L., Dunn, G., Ferguson, M., Minor, P. D., and Almond, J. W. (1988). *Nature (London)* **332**, 81–82.

Buus, S., Colon, S., Smith C., Freed, J. H., Miles, C., and Grey, H. M. (1986). *Proc. Natl. Acad. Sci. U.S.A.* **83**, 3968–3971.

Chow, M., Yabrov, R., Bittle, J., Hogle, J. M., and Baltimore, D. (1985). *Proc. Natl. Acad. Sci. U.S.A.* **82**, 910–914.

Colman, P. M., Varghese, J. N., and Laver, W. G. (1983). *Nature (London)* **303**, 41–44.

Colman, P. M., Laver, W. G., Varghese, J. N., Baker, A. T., Tulloch, P. A., Air, G. M., and Webster, R. G. (1987). *Nature (London)* **326**, 358–363.

Diamond, D. C., Jameson, B. A., Bonin, J., Kohara, M., Abe, S., Itoh, H., Komatsu, T., Arita, M., Kuge, S., Nomoto, A., Osterhaus, A. D. M. E., Crainic, R., and Wimmer, E. (1985). *Science* **229**, 1090–1093.

Emini, E. A., Jameson, B. A., and Wimmer, E. (1983). *Nature (London)* **304**, 699–703.

Emini, E. A., Jameson, B. A., and Wimmer, E. (1984). *J. Virol.* **52**, 719–721.

Ferguson, M., Evans, D. M. A., Magrath, D. I., Minor, P. D., Almond, J. W., and Schild, G. C. (1985). *Virology* **143**, 505–515.

Filman D. J., Syed, R., Chow, M., Macadam, A., Minor, P. D., and Hogle, J. M. (1988). *Science*. Submitted.

Fricks, C. E., and Hogle, J. M. (1988). In preparation.

Fricks, C. E., Icenogle, J. P. Hogle, J. M. (1985). *J. Virol.* **54**, 856–859.

Hogle, J. M., Chow, M., and Filman, D. J. (1985). *Science* **229**, 1358–1365.

Hurwitz, J. L., Heber-Katz, E., Hackett, C. J., and Gerhard, W. (1984). *J. Immunol.* **133**, 3371–3377.

Icenogle, J. P., Minor, P. D., Ferguson, M., and Hogle, J. M. (1986). *J. Virol.* **60**, 297–301.

Jameson, B. A., Bonin, J., Murray, M. G., Wimmer, E., and Kew, O. (1985). *In* "Vaccines' 85" (R. A. Lerner, R. M. Chanock, and F. Brown, eds.), pp. 191–198. Cold Spring Harbor Lab., Cold Spring Harbor, New York).

Katz, J. M., Laver, W. G., White, D. O., and Anders, E. M. (1985). *J. Immunol.* **134**, 616–622.

La Monica, N., Meriam, C., and Racaniello, V. R. (1986). *J. Virol.* **57**, 515–525.

La Monica, N., Kupsky, W. J., and Racaniello, V. R. (1987). *Virology* **161**, 429–437.

Luo, M., Vriend, G., Kamer, G., Minor, I., Arnold, E., Rossman, M. G., Boege, U., Scraba, D. G., Duke, G. M., and Palmenberg, A. C. (1987). *Science* **235**, 182–191.

Martin, A., Wychowski, C., Couderc, T., Crainic, R., Hogle, J. M., and Girard, M. (1988). EMBO J. **7**, 2839–2847.

Minor, P. D., Schild, G. C., Bootman, J., Evans, D. M. A., Ferguson, M., Reeve, P., Spitz, M., Stanway, G., Cann, A. J., Hauptman, R., Clarke, L. D., Mountford, R. C., and Almond, J. W. (1983). *Nature (London)* **301**, 674–679.

Minor, P. D., Evans, D. M. A., Ferguson, M., Schild, G. C., Westrop, G., and Almond, J. W. (1985). *J. Gen. Virol.* **65**, 1159–1165.

Minor, P. D., Ferguson, M., Evans, D. M. A., and Icenogle, J. P. (1986). *J. Virol.* **67**, 1283–1291.

Minor, P. D., Ferguson, M., Phillips, A., McGrath, D. J., Huovilainen, A., and Hovi, T. (1987). *J. Gen. Virol.* **68**, 1857–1865.

Minor, P. D., Dunn, G., Evans, D. M. A., Magrath, D. I., John, A., Howlett, J., Phillips, A., Westrop, G., Wareham, K., Almond, J. W., and Hogle, J. M. (1988). EMBO J. Submitted.

Murray, M. G., Kuhn, R. J., Arita, M., Kawamura, N., Nomoto, A., and Wimmer E. (1988). *Proc. Natl. Acad. Sci. U.S.A.* **85**, 3203–3207.

Nicklin, M. J. H., Toyoda, H., Murray, M. G., and Wimmer, E. (1986). *Bio Technology* **4**, 33–42.

Omata, T., Kohara, M., Kuge, S., Komatsu, T., Abe, S., Semler, B. L., Kameda, A., Itoh, H., Arita, M., Wimmer, E., and Nomoto, A., (1986). *J. Virol.* **58**, 348–358.

Page, G. S., Mosser, A. G., Hogle, J. M., Filman, D. J., Rueckert, R. R., and Chow, M. (1988). *J. Virol.* **62**, 1781–1794.

Roivainen, M., and Hovi, T. (1987). *J. Virol.* **61**, 3749–3753.

Rossmann, M. G., Arnold, E., Erickson, J. W., Frankenberger, E. A., Griffith, J. P., Hecht, H.-J., Johnson, J. E., Kamer, G., Luo, M., Mosser, A. G., Rueckert, R. R., Sherry, B., and Vriend, G. (1985). *Nature (London)* **317**, 145–153.

Reuckert, R. R. (1985). *In* "Virology" (B. Fields, D. M. Knipe, R. M. Chanock, J. L. Melnick, B. Roizman, and R. E. Shope, eds.), pp. 705–738. Raven Press, New York.

Sheriff, S., Silverton, E. W., Padlan, E. A., Cohen, G. H., Smith-Gill, S. J., Finzel, B. C., and Davies, D. R. (1987). *Proc. Natl. Acad. Sci. U.S.A.* **84**, 9075–8079.

Sherry, B., Mosser, A. G., Colonno, R. J., and Rueckert, R. R. (1986). *J. Virol.* **57,** 246–257.

Varghese, J. N. Laver, W. G., and Colman, P. M. (1983). *Nature (London)* **303,** 35–40.

Weis, W., Brown, J. H., Cusack, S., Paulson, J. C., Skehel, J. J., and Wiley, D. C. (1988). *Nature (London)* **333,** 426–431.

Westrop, G. D., Evans, D. M. A., Minor, P. D., Magrath, D., Schild, G. C., and Almond, J. W. (1986). In "The Molecular Biology of Positive Strand Viruses." (D. J. Rowlands, B. W. J. Mahy, and M. Mayo, eds.), pp. 53–60. Academic Press, London.

Wiley, D. C., Wilson, I. A., and Skehel, J. J. (1981). *Nature (London)* **289,** 373–378.

Wilson, I. A., Skehel, J. J., and Wiley, D. C. (1981). *Nature (London)* **289,** 366–373.

WHO collaborative study. (1981). *J. Biol. Stand.* **9,** 163–184.

Yewdell, J. W., Bennink, J. R., Smith, G. L., and Moss, B. (1985). *Proc. Natl. Acad. Sci. U.S.A.* **82,** 1785–1789.

ADVANCES IN VETERINARY SCIENCE AND COMPARATIVE MEDICINE, VOL. 33

Immune Response to Vaccination

B.I. OSBURN AND J. L. STOTT

School of Veterinary Medicine, University of California, Davis, California

I. Introduction

The objective of any vaccination program is to provide the best possible protection for an animal against infectious disease. To accomplish this objective, consideration of the status of the vaccine, i.e., killed or modified live, the inclusion of adjuvants, and the frequency and routes of administration all must be taken into account. The status of the animals to be immunized must also be evaluated carefully. The age, genetics, health and nutritional status, environmental and management factors all play important roles in the eventual outcome of immunization programs. Any one, or a combination of any or all of the above, can influence the response of the immune system and subsequent success of vaccination programs.

In this review, the emphasis will be directed at reviewing the current concepts of the immune response that are important to successful immunization.

93

II. Lymphoid System

The lymphoid system consists of central and peripheral organs (Trnka and Morris, 1985). The central lymphoid organs consist of the bone marrow, thymus, and, in avian species, the bursa of Fabricius. These are the organs from which the lymphoid cells arise and undergo maturation. Immune responses do not normally occur in these organs. The peripheral lymphoid system consists of lymph nodes, spleen, and mucosal-associated lymphoid organs including the gut-associated tissues. In some species there are additional lymphoid organs such as the hemal lymph nodes of cattle. Peripheral lymphoid organs are the site of primary immune responses in most animals.

The lymphoid system can be categorized further as systemic and local immune systems. Lymphoid organs involved in systemic immunity include peripheral lymph nodes which drain the interstitial tissues of the limbs, trunk, and nonmucosal-associated viscera of the body. Another important organ involved in systemic immunity is the spleen, whose principal function is to filter blood (Trnka and Morris, 1985; Lascelles and McDowell, 1974).

Lymphoid organs associated with the mucosal immune system include the nasopharyngeal lymphoid tissue, Peyer's patches, mesenteric lymph nodes, and bronchial lymph nodes. Certain secretory organs such as salivary glands, gall bladder, and the mammary gland participate in local or mucosal immunity (Trnka and Morris, 1985; Lascelles and McDowell, 1974; Befus and Beinenstock, 1982; George and Griffin, 1983; Morag *et al.*, 1974; Duhamel *et al.*, 1986; Nagi and Babiuk, 1987).

Function

1. Central Lymphoid System

Bone marrow is the source of stem cells in postnatal life. During fetal life stem cells reside in the liver and in early embryonic life they reside in the yolk sac. The precursor lymphocytes arising from stem cells are destined to be either a T lymphocyte or B lymphocyte or a null-cell subset (Osburn, 1981; Osburn *et al.*, 1982). Although there are few differentiation antigens on these cells as they leave the bone marrow, the pre-T and -B lymphocytes are destined to enter other organs for further maturation.

Approximately 3–5% of the bone marrow-derived pre-T-lymphocytes enter the thymus gland through vessels in the outer cortex (Weissman,

1986; De Waal Malefijt *et al.*, 1986). While in the outer cortex these cells undergo division and subsequently come in contact with epithelial-derived thymic nurse cells (TNC) (De Waal Malefijt *et al.*, 1986). Lymphocytes are engulfed by the TNC and enter a vacuole where they may either be destroyed or acquire additional phenotypic markers. Surviving lymphocytes leave the outer cortex and enter the inner cortex where they are educated to recognize "self" through the presence of dendritic cells that express major histocompatibility complex (MHC) antigens. It is also in this location where 10–15% of the cells acquire lymph node homing determinants on the cell membrane and another 3–5% acquire Peyer's patch homing determinants. Thymus epithelial cells in the cortex and medulla secrete thymopoietins which facilitate maturation and differentiation of these lymphocytes (Weissman, 1986; De Waal Malefijt *et al.*, 1986). Approximately 1% of the lymphocytes that enter the thymus eventually will leave through the medullary lymphatics. These lymphocytes, upon contact with specific antigens, will enter the peripheral lymphoid organs where the final stages of differentiation occur.

B-cell differentiation and maturation are reasonably complete when B-lymphocytes leave the bone marrow in most domestic species (Kincaide and Phillips, 1985). The exception appears to be the avian species where pre-B-lymphocytes migrate to the bursa of Fabricius where differentiation occurs. The epithelial cells in this organ participate in the final stage of non-antigen-related lymphocyte maturation; the mature B cells subsequently enter the circulation and peripheral lymphoid tissues.

The lymph nodes in the peripheral lymphoid system are the site of most antigen-driven immune responses. Lymph nodes are encapsulated organs that filter the interstitial fluids bathing the tissues. Lymphatics channel the interstitial fluids to the lymph node where it enters the capsule through efferent lymphatics. Lymph then filters through the cortical, paracortical and medullary areas of the node. The cortical region contains many dendritic cells and lymphoid follicles containing predominately B-lymphocytes with some T-lymphocytes; paracortical regions are rich in T-lymphocytes. The post-capillary venules traversing these areas contain high endothelial cells through which the receptors on T lymphocytes attach and subsequently emigrate between the endothelial cells and the basement membrane to enter the lymph node. These cells remain in the lymph node for up to 24 hr, unless they are recruited to participate in an antigen-driven immune response.

Antigen-driven immune responses occur primarily in lymphoid

follicles. In these structures the dendritic macrophages or antigen-presenting cells (APC) will engulf, process, and present antigen on the cell membrane in context with Class II determinants of the MHC. T-helper (T_h) lymphocytes are activated upon antigen-specific engagement of the T-cell receptor with the antigen–MHC Class II protein complex (Hopkins *et al.*, 1985). Such activated T cells subsequently will interact with B lymphocytes that express Class II MHC determinants and specific IgM antigen recognition molecules on their cell membranes.

The cooperative interaction between these cells in response to antigen initiates a series of events resulting in a rapid proliferating and expansion of lymphocytes, most of which will respond only to the inciting antigen upon re-exposure. This proliferation activity leads to morphologic changes in the lymphoid follicle. The follicle expands, the center becomes pale as some lymphocytes die during the proliferation, and those that live will migrate to, and temporarily accumulate in, a dense cellular mantle surrounding the follicle. The progeny of both T and B lymphocytes originating in the follicle migrate from the cortex through the lymphatic channels to the medulla. Many of the B-lymphocytes further differentiate into plasma cells as they locate within the medullary cords. It is from this location that antigen-specific immunoglobulin is secreted into the afferent lymph. The T lymphocytes and some B-memory lymphocytes pass through the lymphatic channels and leave the lymph node by way of the afferent lymphatics. These lymphocytes then enter the blood vascular system by way of the thoracic duct. T lymphocytes constitute 65–70% of the peripheral blood lymphocyte pool. They are on a continuing, recirculating traffic pattern through peripheral lymph nodes, the spleen, and blood.

The mucosal immune system has a different lymphocyte traffic pattern and the introduction of antigen is by different routes than those in the peripheral system (Hall, 1980). The best-studied mucosal system is that involving the Peyer's patches and the associated gastrointestinal–mesenteric lymphoid system. Peyer's patches are specialized mucosal lymphoid tissues located in the ileum of mammalian species. These ovoid structures are located on the antimesenteric side of the ileum. On the mucosal surface they appear as depressed dimpled structures. This appearance is due to the low or blunted villous processes which are intermingled with long villous processes of the adjacent intestinal lamina propria. The somewhat blunted villous process of the Peyer's patch consists of modified epithelial cells known as M cells under which lymphoid cells extend to the submucosa. M cells contain microvilli on their epithelial surface. M cells are capable of sampling antigens from the intestinal lumen and transporting these antigens across the cell to the underlying lymphoid tissues. The lymphoid tissue in the Peyer's patches contains B and T lymphocytes as well as APCs. It is in these locations that the initial mucosal immune response occurs. Upon antigen-induced proliferation, both B and T lymphocytes leave the areas of lymphatics and enter the regional mesenteric lymph nodes.

Mesenteric lymph nodes are the site of additional maturation of antigen-stimulated B and T lymphocytes (Hall, 1980). APCs from Peyer's patches, or antigen from the intestine trapped by lymph node APCs, provide additional opportunities for expansion of lymphocyte clones in the cortical lymphoid follicles. The antigen-specific B- and T-lymphocyte populations leave the mesenteric lymph nodes through afferent lymphatics traveling to the thoracic duct and then into the blood vascular system. These cells have determinants on their surface that are specific for lymphocyte homing receptors on high endothelial cells in the intestinal mucosa. Both the T and B lymphocytes with these determinants leave the blood vascular system and emigrate into the lamina propria of the intestine and secretory organs such as salivary and mammary glands. Many of the B lymphocytes will differentiate into IgA-producing plasma cells. Some IgG- and IgM-bearing plasma cells are also found in these locations.

2. Cellular Interactions in Germinal Center

Within the lymphoid follicle there are a number of important cellular interactions that occur following primary exposure to antigen; these events hopefully will culminate in expansion of clones of memory cells that will provide the basis for a rapid secondary immune response and protective immunity following a second exposure. The development of an immune response occurs through cellular interactions that primarily occur through the release of soluble mediators, many of which are termed interleukins (IL). Antigen presentation to T_h lymphocytes occurs via T-cell receptor recognition of processed antigen complexed with the pleiomorphic regions of the class 2 major MHC proteins on the surface of the APC (Celvens et al., 1988; Janeway et al., 1988). Macrophages represent the major APC, however, B lymphocytes may also bind antigen via surface immunoglobulin, internalize, and process antigen as well (Jones, 1987). Although it has been demonstrated that such B cells can present antigen in a class 2 restricted fashion to T cells, it is uncertain if such interactions result in induction of T memory. The physical T_h–APC interaction is realized via the specific binding of the α-β heterodimer, which is associated with the CD3 complex (human), of the T-cell receptor to the antigen–class 2 protein complex. Initiation of this interaction is genetically dependent upon the ability of an animal's class 2 proteins to bind a given processes antigen and the presence of a T-cell receptor that can recognize the antigen–class 2 protein complex. Additional binding capabilities, though not antigen-specific, are realized through the binding of CD4 (human) T-cell differentiation antigen to a constant region of the class 2 protein on the APC. A third interaction occurs between the CD2 (human) T-cell differentiation antigen (erythrocyte receptor) and the APC lymphocyte function antigen (LFA-3). These three interactions, in association with the T-cell receptor for IL-1 becoming occupied via elaboration of this monokine by the APC (macrophage) (Le and Vilcik, 1987), initiates the T-cell activation process (Vitetta $et\ al.$, 1987). Upon initial activation signal(s), IL-2 is produced by the T cell and acts in an autocrine fashion inducing surface expression of high-affinity IL-2 receptors. This series of events culminates in activation and clonal expansion of antigen-specific T_h cells. In addition to IL-2, the activated T cells produce an array of lymphokines including IL-3, IL-4, IL-5, and IL-6 as well as interferon-gamma (IFN-γ), all of which may be rather permissive relative to the cells they can act upon in initiating a balanced immune response (Coffman $et\ al.$, 1988; Issekutz $et\ al.$, 1988; Janeway $et\ al.$, 1988; Kishimoto and Hirano, 1988; Vitetta $et\ al.$, 1987). IL-2, in addition to expanding the T_h population, also facilitates activation and/or expansion of the T cytotoxic (T_c) subset, B cells, macrophages, natural killer (NK) cells, and lymphokine-activated killer (LAK) cells (Smith, 1980, 1984). IL-3, often referred to as colony-stimulating factor (CSF), represents a growth factor for a variety of bone marrow cells (especially myeloid precursors) and B cells. IL-4, previously termed B-cell stimulatory factor (BSF-I), enhances differentiation of B cells into IgE- and IgG_1-producing plasma cells; this effect may be at the level of directing Ig class switching. Similarly, IL-5 (T-cell replacing factor, TRF) tends to support induction of an IgA response, as well as potentiating growth of eosinophils. Many of the $in\ vitro$ responses induced by IL-4 or IL-5 are enchanced when used in concert. IL-6 (IFN-β_2) has been reported to facilitate multiple activities, in addition to its antiviral effects, due to the presence of receptors on multiple cells types. Among these actions are promotion of B-cell, T_c-cell, myeloid, and thymocyte differentiation/proliferation, either alone or in concert with other lymphokines. IFN-γ is also produced by activated T cells and has a wide array of effect, many of which are dependent upon the concentration used in *in vitro* assays. This mediator is capable of activating macrophages (Smith, 1980), with concomitant enhanced expression of class 2 genes; this activity was previously described as macrophage activating factor (MAF). IFN-γ also enhances NK cell activity, is involved in inducing DTH responses by acting as a lymphocyte attractant, inducing macrophage expression of IgG Fc receptors and promoting production of IgG_{2a}; the latter two features facilitate ADCC. At high concentrations, IFN-γ may oppose the effects of IL-4 and suppress production of IgE and IgG_1.

The molecular cloning and expression, of the above-mentioned lymphokines have facilitated our understanding of their source, induction, and effects using *in vitro* techniques. The effects of these lymphokines are quite diverse, and may depend upon concentration used and the presence of additional mediators. Studies in murine systems suggest there are two populations of T_h cells, each preferentially elaborating a given set of lymphokines. As more knowledge is gained relative to cell–cell interactions and the role of associated lymphokines involved in directing a specific type of response, advances in selecting or enhancing desired immune responses for the purpose of immunoprophylaxis and/or disease treatment may become a reality.

3. Immunoglobulins

Immunoglobulin classes secreted by B cells are IgM, IgG, IgA, and IgE (Butler, 1983). IgM is the first immunoglobulin produced in response to antigenic stimulation. IgM is a large immunoglobulin found in the blood vascular system and in small quantities in secretions including colostrum. It is not found in interstitial tissues unless there has been damage to the vascular wall. IgM consists of five immunoglobulin molecules held together by joining (J) chains such that each IgM molecule has 10 antigen combining sites. IgM levels in serum ranges from 70 to 500 mg/100 ml in domestic animals.

IgG is the most common immunoglobulin in serum, interstitial fluids, and colostrum; the latter is particularly important in ruminant species. Serum levels range from 300 to 2,900 mg/100 ml. IgG is a single molecule with two antigen receptor sites. Some subclasses of IgG fix complement whereas other subclasses are cytophilic for neutrophils, macrophages, some lymphocyte subpopulations, and for transient periods on mast cells and basophils. IgG is important for neutralization of viruses and toxins, complement fixation, and opsonization. IgG_1 is the predominant immunoglobulin in bovine and ovine colostrum.

IgA is the third most common immunoglobulin in serum. In serum, the molecules are monomeric with a molecular weight of 160,000–180,000. Serum levels range from 10 to 50 mg/100 ml. IgA is the predominant immunoglobulin in secretions. Secretory IgA is a dimer with a molecular weight of 380,000. The two molecules are held together by a J-chain and the dimer picks up secretory (5) piece as it passes through the lining epithelial cells. This immunoglobulin class is very important in mucosal immunity.

IgE is present in very small (2.3 mg/100 ml) quantities in serum. The immunoglobulin is cytophilic for mast cells and basophils. Its principal role is to trigger antigen-related release of vasoactive substances from mast cells and basophils. This facilitates the leakage of other immunoglobulins and inflammatory cells into the area. Excessive release of vasoactive substances from these cells will lead to either local or systemic anaphylaxis.

III. Infection and Immunity

Much of what is known relative to protective immune responses to bacterial, viral, and parasitic infections has been accumulated through various developmental vaccine studies. Strategies employed have included attenuation of pathogen virulence, microbial recombination, subunit protein preparations, synthetic peptides, and expression of pathogen proteins from cDNA *in vitro* or *in vivo* using live virus vectors. Such approaches have greatly facilitated our understanding of the protective immune response(s), and their protein specificities, capable of inducing protective immunity. Using combinations of antibody-mediated epitope mapping, construction of hydrophobicity plots from cDNA sequencing, and synthesis of sequential overlapping peptides, the epitopes capable of inducing antibody responses are being elucidated (Hopp and Woods, 1981; Novotny *et al.*, 1987; Steward and Howard, 1987). Similar to advances in defining antibody responses and specificities, antigenic T-cell epitopes are being elucidated (Townsend *et al.*, 1986). Using cDNA sequences derived from the cloning of pathogen genes, it has been possible to predict T-cell epitopes based upon identification of those sequences that have the potential to code for peptides that can form amphipathic α-helixes (Margalit *et al.*, 1987). With identification of invariant epitopes, advances in development of vaccines capable of inducing immunity that would not be complicated by serotype, strain, or antigenic variants may become a reality. Advances in our understanding of T- and B-cell specificities, at the molecular level, associated with the availability of cDNA clones representing various lymphokines, will continue to provide major insights to immune responses. Synthesis or cDNA expression of immunogenic peptides representing both B- and T-cell epitopes, in association with exogenously derived lymphokines, may facilitate mononuclear leukocyte subpopulation targeting for elicitation of desired immune responses. Because the subject of vaccine technologies is dealt with in subsequent chapters, only a basic overview of bacterial, viral, and parasitic immunity will be presented.

A. BACTERIAL IMMUNITY

An array of immune responses has been defined for protective immunity against bacterial infections (Moon *et al.*, 1980). Bacteria may have a wide array of structural and nonstructural products capable of causing disease. Toxins produced by bacteria are capable of causing profound pathogenic effects unless the toxin is rendered incapable of interacting with the target cell receptor. Humoral immunity, with a specific antibody directed to the active attachment sites of the toxin molecule, prevents the toxin from attaching to the cell receptor. Examples of effective anti-toxin antibodies would include those directed to tetanus, botulism, choleratoxin, and the heat-labile and heat-stable toxins of enterotoxigenic *Escherichia coli* (Darner, 1980; Dobrescu and Huygelen, 1976; Furer *et al.*, 1982; Klepstein *et al.*, 1982; Gyles and Maas, 1987).

Pili which are present on some bacteria are associated with virulence. The adhesion sites on pili are important for bacterial attachment to cells (Gaastra and de Graff, 1982; Kemm, 1985). Once this occurs, bacteria toxins are released in close proximity to cell receptors with subsequent expression of disease. Similarly, capsular polysaccharides are associated with colonization of intestinal epithelium. Antibodies, directed to the adhesins present on the capsular polysaccharide, block bacterial attachment to intestinal epithelial cells, thereby preventing other virulence factors from exercising their pathogenic properties on the host (Gyles and Maas, 1987; Brenton *et al.*, 1983; Bylsma *et al.*, 1987).

Endotoxins are lipopolysaccharides (LPS) associated with the cell membranes of Gram-negative bacteria. The LPS of Gram-negative bacteria act as a toxin, activating a number of systems including the clotting, kinin, lipo-oxygenase, arachidonic acid, and complement systems. The consequences are far reaching and include shock, disseminated intravascular coagulopathy, and fever. Antibodies directed to core antigens on the LPS molecule have definite protective properties (Ziegler *et al.*, 1975; Davis *et al.*, 1978; Fenwick *et al.*, 1986).

Bacterial cell membranes contain a variety of antigens. Antibodies generated to these antigens include agglutinating, opsonic, cytotoxic, and complement-fixing antibodies (Allen and Porter, 1983; Kohler, 1978). Agglutinating antibodies will cause clumping of bacteria into large complexes. These may then be sequestered in organs containing macrophages or in foci within tissues. The aggregated masses have less mobility and are more easily phagocytosed by macrophages and neutrophils. Opsonic antibodies attach to antigens on bacterial cell walls by the Fab receptors. The Fc portion of the antibody molecule attaches to complementary receptors on neutrophils and macrophages, facilitating their ability to phagocytose the bacteria. Antibodies of the immunoglobulin class IgM, or subclasses of IgGs with complement-fixing (CF) properties, provide additional ways of controlling bacteria. Complement-fixing antibodies also facilitate opsonization through C_{3b}-activated receptors. This immune adherence protein binds the bacteria to the C_{3b} receptors on neutrophils and macrophages, thus facilitating phagocytosis. Activation of the complement cascade by complement fixing (CF) antibody can lead to lysis of bacteria via the membrane attack complex (MAC). The MAC leads to perforations in the cell membrane with subsequent loss of osmoregulation, cellular swelling, and lysis.

Cytotoxic antibodies directed to bacteria provide another means of controlling bacterial infections. Lymphocyte subclasses, particularly the killer or K lymphocyte, express receptors for the Fc portion of the immunoglobulin molecule of certain IgG subclasses. These antibody-armed lymphocytes will attach to bacterial cell membranes. Upon attachment, the K cell releases "perforins" which function very similar to the MAC of complement, resulting in cell membrane perforation. Again, the cell lyses due to loss of osmoregulation.

Some genera of bacteria possess cell membrane properties that favor cell-mediated immune responses. The role of mycolic acids, associated with the cell membranes of *Mycobacteria* spp. in cell-mediated immunity have been studied in greater detail than the cell membranes of other bacterial genera (Orme and Collins, 1984; Hussein *et al.*, 1987). The mycolic acids function in concert with specific antigens to stimulate a vigorous cell-mediated response. This response is dependent on T lymphocytes, macrophages, and interleukins. To initiate the response, antigen-specific T_h lymphocytes must interact with antigen. This interaction will lead to the release of lymphokines such as IL-2 and IFN from T_h lymphocytes. These lymphokines facilitate the immune response by activating macrophages and NK cells as well as by recruiting and stimulating the proliferation of lymphocyte subpopulations. The mycolic acids also tend to stimulate granuloma formation, which will localize and wall off the infectious agent.

B. Viral Immunity

Traditionally viral immunity has been assessed by measuring evidence of humoral responses. Neutralizing antibody has been equated with resistance to infection. Within the last few years there has been increasing evidence that cell-mediated immunity plays an important role in viral immunity (Ghalib et al., 1985; Wiktor, 1978).

Antigens localized on the outer coat of virus particles are important for attachment to cells. These viral antigens, and their cellular receptor sites, are different for various viruses. The immune response of the host generates antibodies to antigens on the surface of viral particles. Antibodies directed specifically to these antigens on the virus necessary for attachment to cell receptors will serve to block the virus attachment (Mims and White, 1984). These virus-neutralizing antibodies (VNA) present in body fluids or on mucosal surfaces provide the first line of immunological defense by preventing viral attachment to cells. This is accomplished through steric hindrance or by preventing or altering the uncoating of viral nucleic acids once the virus is in the cell (Mims and White, 1984). The latter may lead to more rapid destruction by lysosomal enzymes. There is also evidence that these antibodies may interfere with transcription of mRNA from viral nucleic acids within the cell (Mims and White, 1984). Other protective humoral immune responses may include antibodies to fusion proteins which hinder the spread of paramyxovirus from cell to cell, and through slowing the release of infectious virus from cells as occurs with antibodies directed to the neuraminidase-associated with influenza virus (Mims and White, 1984).

The Fc portion of the antibody molecule plays a very important role in controlling viral infections. Some subclasses of IgG utilize the Fc portions of the molecule to enhance uptake of virus through opsonization by macrophages and neutrophils (Grewal et al., 1977; Grewal and Rouse, 1979; Rouse and Babiuk, 1974, 1978). The phenomenon of antibody-dependent cell cytotoxicity can also target virus infected cells for destruction (Rouse et al., 1976; Jeggo and Brownlie, 1984; Belden and Peng, 1987; Mims and White, 1984).

The complement system participates in many ways in preventing or minimizing viral infections. Complement-fixing antibodies directed to surface epitopes can participate in the formation of complexes, facilitating phagocytosis by the macrophage system. The activation of complement component 3 will lead to the formation of C_{3b} which binds to the surface of macrophages and neutrophils, again enhancing opsonization. Activation of the entire or alternate complement pathways, directed either to the virus or to viral-associated antigens on cell membranes, will lead to lysis and destruction of the virus or cells.

Sensitized animals may have T_c, which recognize and destroy virus-infected cells (Jeggo and Brownlie, 1984; Stott *et al.*, 1985; Brown, 1987; Blancon *et al.*, 1979; Mandel, 1979; Miller-Edge and Splitter, 1986). Most T_c express the CD8 (human) differentiation antigen and this structure probably plays a role in binding to a constant region of the class 1 MHC protein expressed on the target cell membrane. Antigen specificity is dictated at the level of the T_c receptor (variable regions of the α- and β-chain heterodimer) and this structure recognizes and binds processed viral antigen expressed on the target cell membrane in association with class 1 proteins. Using a variety of model systems, T_c specificities have been found to be directed at not only those classic viral glycoproteins (envelope, hemagglutinin, etc.) associated with the cell membrane, but also against core and nonstructural viral proteins (Bennink *et al.*, 1987). Attempts currently are being made to identify invariant T-cell epitopes on viral proteins for use as candidate immunogens for inducing cross-strain and cross-serotype immunity. The mechanism(s) whereby T_c kill their targets, while themselves being protected, is not fully understood. Pore-forming protein, commonly termed perforin, may be released by the T_c in the form of cytoplasmic granules. This release is directed to the region of T_c–target cell contact, and in the presence of Ca^{2+} intercalates into the target membrane, polymerizes, and pores are formed resulting in cell lysis. Additional cytotoxic mechanisms also appear to exist and may include a T_c-derived signal that is received by the target cell with subsequent DNA fragmentation of a suicidal nature.

Another cell which plays an important role in cytotoxic response is the NK cell. NK cells are activated by IFN-γ and IL-2. NK cells seek out tumor or virus-infected cells that have altered cell membranes. The NK cells identify such cells and release cytoxic factors, similar in nature to those released by T_c, which lead to lysis of affected cells.

C. Parasitic Immunity

Protective immunity in parasitic infection requires both humoral and cellular components. The most effective responses lead to destruction of the infectious or primary infecting stage of the parasites life cycle. For instance, the most effective responses to the helminth *Schistosoma* are directed at the infective larvae schistosomule. Similar effective responses in plasmodium infections are to the sporozoite and merozoites.

Humoral immune responses may act in a variety of ways to interfere with parasitic infections. Antibodies, primarily IgG or IgM, directed to antigens associated with the oral or excretory orifices of parasites may effectively prevent nourishment and eventual death of the parasite. Antibodies directed to receptor sites on infectious sporozoites or initial bodies may prevent the protozoan parasites from attaching to host cells. These parasites may then be eliminated by macrophages through opsonization. Recent studies on schistosoma immunity suggests that the IgE isotype represents an important protective immune response (Caprou *et al.*, 1987). The mechanism for effecting this immunity is through the cytotoxic antibody associated with antibody-dependent cell cytotoxicity. The principal effector cells are monocytes/ macrophages and eosinophils that have been primed by lymphokines such as IFN-γ and tumor necrosis factor. The IgE antibody is most effective when it is directed to a carbohydrate-rich antigen present on the schistosomula. The attachment of these cells to the schistosomula by IgE leads to the release of lysosomal products and oxygen metabolites which cause death of the parasite and eventual lysis.

T_c responses have been identified to occur in some parasitic diseases; however, their role in protective immunity is only now being defined (Lillehoj, 1986). Extensive murine and human studies have been directed at defining immune responses, and epitope specificities, directed at the circumsporozoite (CS) protein of *Plasmodium* species (Good *et al.*, 1988). A central repetitive segment of the CS protein has been identified as an immunodominant B-cell epitope that is relatively conserved within species, and antibodies directed at this epitope can block entry of the sporozoite into target cells. However, the protective capacity of this response is variable, and increasing evidence would suggest an important role for cell-mediated immunity. Protective T-cell responses in malarial immunity may be represented by a combination of lymphokine (IFN-γ and IL-2)-producing T_h cells and T_c cells. Mice lacking B cells and/or Ig can be successfully immunized and T-cell transfers, specifically T_c (CD8), can protect animals against live parasite challenge.

IV. Summary

Effective immune responses requires a synchronization of a number of different physiological and immunological events. Effective vaccines simulate natural invasion of the body by microbes or parasites. The route of administration of vaccines contributes to the effectiveness of preventing or controlling local or systemic infections. Immune responses to microbial agents usually involve more than one mechanism. For instance, toxins may be neutralized by a single antibody, while cellular interactions are required for destruction of more complex microorganisms. These systems have been illustrated in this review.

REFERENCES

Allen, W. D., and Porter, P. P. (1983). *Dev. Biol. Stand.* **53,** 147–153.
Befus, A. D., and Beinenstock, J. (1982). *J. Am. Vet. Med. Assoc.* **181,** 1066–1073.
Belden, E. L., and Peng, H. M. (1987). *Vet. Immunol. Immunopathol.* **16,** 157–171.
Bennink, J. R., Yewdell, J. W., Smith G. L., and Moss, B. (1987). *J. Virol.* **61,** 1098–1102.
Blancon, J., Andral, L., Lagrange, P. H., and Tsiang, H. (1979). *Infect. Immun.* **24,** 600–605.
Brenton, C. C., Fusco, P., Wood, S. W., Jayappa, H. G., Goodnow, R. A., and Strayer, J. G. (1983). *Vet. Med. (Kansas City, Mo.)* **78,** 962–966.
Brown, F. (1987). *Prog. Vet. Microbiol. Immunol.* **3,** 59–72.
Butler, J. E. (1983). *In* "Bovine Immunoglobulins: An Augmented Review" (F. Kristensen and D. F. Antczak, eds.), pp. 43–152. Elsevier, Amsterdam.
Bylsma, I. G. W., van Haaten, M., Frik, J. F., and Ruitenberg, E. J. (1987). *Vet. Immunol. Immunopathol.* **16,** 235–250.
Caprou, A., Dessaint, J. P., Capron, M., Ouma, J. H., and Butterworth, A. E. (1987). *Science* **238,** 1065–1072.
Clevens, H., Alarcon B., Wileman, T., and Terhost, C. (1988). *Annu. Rev. Immunol* **6,** 629–662.
Coffman, R. L., Seymour, B. W. P., Lebman, D. A., Hiraka, D. D., Christiansen, J. A., Shrader, B., Cherwinski, H. M., Finkelman, F. D., Bond, M. W., and Mossman, T. R. (1988). *Immunol. Rev.* **102,** 5–28.
Darner, F. (1980). *Vet. Med. (Prague)* **27,** 207–221.
Davis, C. E., Ziegler, E. J., and Arnold, K. (1978). *J. Exp. Med.* **147,** 1007–1017.
De Waal Malefijt, R., Leere, W., Roholl, P. J. M., Wormmeestar, J., and Hoeben, K. A. (1986). *Lab. Invest.* **55,** 25–34.
Dobrescu, L., and Huygelen, C. (1976). *Zentralbl. Veterinaer med.* **23,** 79–88.
Duhamel, G. E., Bernoco, D., Davis, W. C., and Osburn, B. I. (1986). *Vet. Immunol. Immunopathol* **14,** 1021–1022.
Fenwick, B. W., Cullor, J. S., Osburn, B. I., and Olander, H. J. (1986). *Infect. Immun.* **53,** 298–304.
Furer, E., Cryz, S. J., Donner, F., Nicolet, J., Wanner, M., and Germainer, R. (1982). *Infect. Immun.* **35,** 887–894.
Gaastra, W., and de Graff, F. K. (1982). *Microbiol. Rev.* **46,** 129–161.
George, R. J., and Griffin, F. T. (1983). *Ir. Vet. J.* **37,** 39–42.
Ghalib, H. W., Schore, C. E., and Osburn, B. I. (1985). *Vet. Immunol. Immunopathol.* **10,** 177–183.
Good, M. F., Berzofsky, J. A., and Miller, L. H. (1988). *Annu. Rev. Immunol.* **6,** 663–688.
Grewal, A. S., and Rouse, B. T. (1979). *Int. Arch. Allergy Apl. Immunol.* **60,** 169–177.
Grewal, A. S., Rouse, B. I., and Babiuk, L. A. (1977). *Infect. Immun.* **15,** 698–703.
Gyles, C. L., and Mass. W. K. (1987). *Vet. Microbiol. Immunol.* **3,** 139–158.
Hall, J. G. (1980). *Monogr. Allergy* **16,** 100–111.

Hopkins, J., McConnell, I., Bujdase, R., and Munro, A. J. (1985). *In* "Immunology of the Sheep" (B. Morris and M. Miyasaka, eds.), pp. 441–459. Editiones Roche, Basel.

Hopp, T. P., and Woods, K. R. (1981). *Proc. Natl. Acad. Sci. U.S.A.* **78**, 3824–3828.

Hussein, S., Curtis, J., Akuffo, H., and Turk, J. L. (1987). *Infect. Immun.* **55**, 564–567.

Issekutz, T. B., Stoltz, J. M., and Meide, P. V. D. (1988). *Immunol. Today* **9**, 140–144.

Janeway, C. A., Carding, S., Jones, B., Murray, J., Portoles, P., Rasmussen, R., Rojo, J., Saizawa, K., West J., and Bottomly, K. (1988). *Immunol. Rev.* **101**, 39–80.

Jeggo, M. H., and Brownlie, J. (1984). *Immunology* **52**, 403–410.

Jones, B. (1987). *Immunol. Rev.* **99**, 5–18.

Kemm, P. (1985). *Rev. Infect. Dis.* **7**, 321–340.

Kieng, M. P., Desmettne, P., Soulebot, J.-P., and Lathe, R. (1987). *Prog. Vet. Microbiol. Immunol.* **3**, 73–111.

Kincaide, P. W., and Phillips, R. A. (1985). *Fed. Am. Soc. Exp. Biol. Fed. Proc.,* **44**, 2874–2889.

Kishimoto, T., and Hirano, T. (1988). *Annu. Rev. Immunol.* **6**, 485–512.

Klepstein, F. A., Engert, R. F., and Clements, J. D. (1982). *Infect. Immun.* **37**, 550–557.

Kohler, E. M. (1978). *Vet. Med. (Kansas City, Mo.)* **73**, 352–356.

Lascelles, A. K., and McDowell, G. H. (1974). *Transplant. Rev.* **19**, 170–208.

Le, J., and Vilcik, J. (1987). *Lab. Invest.* **56**, 234–248.

Lillehoj, H. S. (1986). *Vet. Immunol. Immunopathol.* **13**, 321–330.

Mandel, B. (1979). **15**, 37–49.

Margalit, H., Spouge, J. L., Cornett, J. L., Cease, L., DeLisi, K. B., and Berzofsky, J. A. (1987). *J. Immunol.* **138**, 2213–2229.

Miller-Edge, M., and Splitter, G. (1986). *Vet. Immunol. Immunopathol.* **13**, 301–319.

Mims, C. A., and White, D. O. (1984). *In* "Viral Pathogenesis and Immunology," pp. 87–131. Blackwell, Oxford.

Moon, H. W., Kohler, E. M., Schneider, R. A., and Whipp, S. C. (1980). *Infect. Immun.* **27**, 222–230.

Morag, A., Beutner, K. R., Morag, B., and Ogra, P. L. (1974). *J. Immunol.* **113**, 1703–1709.

Nagi, A. M., and Babiuk, L. A. (1987). *J. Immunol.* **105**, 23–37.

Novotny, J., Handschumacher, M., and Bruccoleri, R. E. (1987). *Immunol. Today* **8**, 26–31.

Orme, I. M., and Collins, F. M. (1984). *Cell. Immunol.* **84**, 113–120.

Osburn, B. I. (1981). *Adv. Exp. Med. Biol.* **137**, 91–103.

Osburn, B. I., MacLachlan, J. J., and Terrell, T. C. (1982). *J. Am. Vet. Med. Assoc.* **181**, 1049–1056.

Rouse, B. T., and Babiuk, L. A. (1974). *Infect Immun.* **10**, 681–687.

Rouse, B. T., and Babiuk, L. A. (1978). *Can. J. Comp. Med.* **42**, 414–427.

Rouse, B. T., Wardley, R. C., and Babiuk, L. A. (1976). *Infect. Immun.* **13**, 1433–1441.

Smith, K. A. (1980). *J. Exp. Med.* **151**, 1551–1558.

Smith, K. A. (1984). *Annu. Rev. Immunol.* **2**, 319–334.

Steward, M. W., and Howard, C. R. (1987). *Immunol. Today* **8**, 51–58.

Stott, J. L., Barber, T. L., and Osburn, B. I. (1985). *Am. J. Vet. Res.* **46**, 1043–1049.

Townsend, A. R. M., Rothbard, J., Gotch, F. M., Bahadur, G., Wraith, D., and McMichael, A. J. (1986). *Cell (Cambridge, Mass.)* **44**, 959–968.

Trnka, Z., and Morris, B. (1985). *In* "Immunology of the Sheep" (B. Morris and M. Miyasaka, eds.), pp. 1–18. Editiones Roche, Basel.

Vitetta, E. S., Bossie, A., Fernandez-Botran, R., Myers, C. D., Oliver, K. G., Sanders, V. M., and Stevents, T. L. (1987). *Immunol. Rev.* **99**, 193–239.

Weissman, I. (1986). *Lab. Invest.* **55,** 1–4.

Wiktor, T. J. (1978). *Deve. Biol. Stand.* **40,** 255–264.

Wiley, D. C., Wilson, I. A., and Skehel, J. J. (1981). *Nature (London)* **289,** 373–375.

Ziegler, E. J., McCutchan, J. A., Douglas, H., and Braude, A. I. (1975). *Trans. Assoc. Am. Physicians* **88,** 101–108.

The Development of Biosynthetic Vaccines

MARC S. COLLETT

Molecular Genetics, Inc., Minnetonka, Minnesota

I. Introduction

Expectations for biotechnology have been and continue to be great. Much of the excitement for the application of biotechnology to the development of new and improved vaccines arose from the coalescence of two disparate areas of research. By the 1970s, it had become apparent that isolated structural components (particularly proteins) of infectious pathogens were generally immunogenic. Such noninfectious "subunit vaccines" often evoked protective immune responses with fewer undesirable side effects generally associated with inactivated whole-agent vaccines. However, at the time, their production for practical purposes was prohibitively expensive. During this same period, advances in molecular biology and recombinant DNA technologies, particularly with respect to the development of generalized microbial expression systems, provided the potential for inexpensive, high-level production of virtually any gene product of interest, pro-

109

karyotic or eukaryotic. A perfect match! Thus was heralded the new era of "recombinant DNA subunit vaccines," complete with venture capital, new "biotech" start-up enterprises, and a multitude of implied promises. However, many of these promises were excessive and unfounded from the start; promises of rapid solutions to complex disease problems were placed in unrealistic timeframes. Since that initial period (*ca.* 1978–1983), tremendous advances have been made in our basic understanding of a great many infectious agents. Through the variety of methods of genomic analysis and molecular cloning, genes for antigens can be readily identified and isolated. Genes can then be engineered into a variety of expression systems to yield relatively abundant quantities of the antigens or portions thereof. Resulting polypeptides have numerous valuable uses as research tools for probing and unraveling features of disease pathogenesis and host defense mechanisms, as well as for further development into diagnostic reagents and vaccines. The technologies currently in the hands of the modern vaccinologist allow the investigation of pathogens from new perspectives and provide a variety of fundamentally new approaches for the development of effective vaccines. In this chapter, the use of biological systems will be considered for the production of immunogens, specifically proteins, for application toward new vaccine development.

It is necessary first to establish the meaning of "biosynthetic vaccine" as it will be used here. A biosynthetic vaccine is a formulation containing a noninfectious, protective subunit immunogen that is produced in or by a biologic system. Additionally, "immunogen" is limited here to mean "immunogenic polypeptide." This definition excludes vaccines consisting of modified (attenuated, recombinant, or genetically altered) live agents, inactivated (killed) whole agents, and chemically synthesized or nonproteinaceous immunogens. Antiidiotype immunogens, which fit the above definition, are considered elsewhere in this volume (see chapter by Altman and Dixon). The scope of this chapter is further narrowed to only consider biosynthetic vaccine development related to viral and bacterial pathogens. Parasitic agents are addressed separately (see chapter by Barbet).

The concept of a subunit vaccine, containing only those immunogenic components necessary to elicit a protective response and excluding others unnecessary for immunity, has several attractive features. First and foremost is the element of safety. Subunit vaccines lack infectious material. No infection, either acute, persistent, or latent, can be established in the vaccinee/vaccinate, substantially reducing complications arising from vaccination of immunocompromised or pregnant individuals. Adventitious agents can be eliminated. Extraneous antigens are lacking, reducing, or eliminating pyrogenic, allergenic, immunosuppressive, and other undesirable reactogenicity. Subunit vaccines also exhibit considerable stability, potentially allowing for wide distribution and prolonged storage. Another advantage of the subunit approach is that it allows a ready identification of vaccinees/vaccinates. Simple serologic tests can readily distinguish vaccination from infection. Such a vaccine is therefore compatible with, and essential for, disease control and eradication programs.

The employment of biologic systems to produce these subunit components is appreciated due to the often complex nature of the immunogens. Biologic systems not only can efficiently produce these complex macromolecules on a large scale, but in the best cases, can also carry out the often required and complicated modifications and structural configuring of polypeptides important for immunogenic potency.

The use of gene cloning technologies to bioproduce immunogens provides two additional advantages for vaccine development. The first is the added measure of safety in genes encoding appropriate immunogenic proteins of dangerous or highly pathogenic agents transferred to harmless microbes for safe mass production. Second, subunit vaccines can now be (and are being) considered for "exotic" and "unculturable" pathogens, thus expanding the scope of diseases that may be controlled by vaccination.

However, the new biosynthetic subunit vaccine candidates are not without their shortcomings. Expense is still a major consideration; this is not necessarily the cost of the product itself, but of the research and development costs incurred toward obtaining the same. Also important is the question of efficacy. Noninfectious, nonreplicating immunogens are inherently less immunogenic than replicating intact agents. Whereas "live" vaccines often only require a single inoculation, subunits frequently require multiple administrations before protective immunity is established. Although much of the reduced immunogenicity of subunit vaccines may relate to immunogen choice, structure, and presentation, subunit vaccines generally must incorporate immunostimulants, such as adjuvants, to make their efficacy acceptable.

The following is an overview of systems available for the biological production of subunit immunogens and their application to vaccine development for select bacterial and viral pathogens. This is followed by a discussion of considerations important in the design of biosynthetic subunit vaccines. This review has considered literature published through May 1987.

II. Biosynthesis of Subunit Immunogens

A. NATURAL PATHOGEN

The subunit approach to vaccines is based largely on experimental data demonstrating protection of vaccinates/vaccinees with some extracted or fractionated component produced by the etiologic agent itself. If the pathogen can be propagated readily and stably *in vitro* under defined culture conditions, this "authentic" bioproduction system can serve as the source of subunit vaccine components. In fact, many current and effective products, such as bacterial toxin (Dorner and McDonel, 1985) and pilus (Tramont and Boslego, 1985) vaccines, are so produced. This approach is certainly not as glamorous as the "high-tech" recombinant DNA strategies discussed below. Yet, in certain cases, this "conventional" means of bioproduction can provide new, useful, and effective subunit vaccines in the very near term. Additionally, evaluation of the components of authentic pathogens can serve as the basis for identifying immunogenic proteins potentially useful in alternative modes (second generation) of vaccine development. Equally important, such analyses can aid in defining critical features of antigen structure and presentation necessary for potent subunit immunogenicity (Neurath and Rubin, 1971).

There may be several reasons for the low profile of this approach to biosynthetic subunit vaccines. One, it has been overshadowed by the fascination with, and perceived potential of, the new "modern high-technology" approaches. Second, it has been considered too expensive for commercialization, particularly with many viral subunit vaccines. The purification of viral components from infected cells or cell culture fluids has been judged uneconomical for the mass production of subunit vaccines. However, given the clear advantages in many situations of an effective subunit vaccine, and in view of certain other considerations (described below), the propagation of authentic pathogens as practical production systems for biosynthetic subunit vaccines must be weighed.

Advances in the large-scale propagation of mammalian cells and their viruses have been made employing various bioreactor systems (see Hu and Dodge, 1985). Downstream processing procedures, including concentration, extraction, and purification of the relevant subunit components from large cultures, have become more efficient. Use of high performance and affinity chromatography procedures provide fast and powerful purifications of components to levels of purity not previously readily attainable. This increased level of component purity now allows the use of potent adjuvants with little risk of eliciting complicating allergic reactions. All of these advances could be expected to decrease the unit cost of a mass-produced subunit vaccine. Moreover, this approach is associated with only modest research investment and rapid commercial development. In contrast, high-technology recombinant DNA strategies toward vaccine development have often required greater than anticipated investments of both money and time. Finally, given the current controversial environment surrounding attempts to introduce products generated via recombinant DNA approaches, subunit vaccines produced by "midlevel" technologies are spared from such "obstructionism" (Fox, 1987a).

B. EXPRESSION SYSTEMS EMPLOYING RECOMBINANT DNA TECHNOLOGIES

Clearly, the preceding discussion is not applicable to many pathogens for which affordable, safe, efficacious vaccines are needed. Examples, include diseases in which the infectious agent is either unable to be cultured, can be propagated only poorly, or yields only low levels of the desired immunogen. Also inappropriate are the circumstances of exotic or highly hazardous pathogens, whose large-scale culture would create numerous safety concerns. Recombinant DNA approaches to biosynthetic subunit immunogen production provide a necessary alternative in these situations.

Using recombinant DNA methodologies, a wide variety of biological expression systems have been developed for potential use in the production of a cloned gene product. These systems are constantly evolving, and continually being tailored and modified for specific applications. These expression systems generally have the following common denominators. The gene encoding the desired polypeptide, or portion thereof, is inserted into an "expression vector" by standard recombinant DNA techniques. The expression vector, generally a plasmid, represents the variable, individualized component of most expression systems. The resultant recombinant expression plasmid is then introduced into the system's host cell using any of a variety of DNA-mediated transfer procedures. Cells expressing the desired polypeptides are identified, selected, and propagated in pure culture. Generally, the goal in each system is to express high levels of the desired gene product. Consequently, a tremendous research effort has gone into the study and understanding of regulation and control parameters for gene expression and product stability in a variety of cell systems. The purpose here is not to review gene isolation and recombinant DNA methodologies, nor the work in the optimization of gene expression (Maniatis *et al.*, 1982; Reznikoff and Gold, 1986). Rather, an attempt is made to overview the salient features of the expression vectors most often employed in their respective cell systems.

1. Prokaryotes

Engineered gene expression began, not surprisingly, in the molecular biologist's workhorse, *Escherichia coli*. Early studies of the molecular genetics of *E. coli* and its bacteriophages provided the fundamental insights to understanding gene expression: initially the basic elements and factors involved and, subsequently, the parameters for optimized overproduction of almost any desired gene product. The general considerations that follow for expression vector design and maximized protein production in *E. coli* are applicable and relevant to all other systems of high-level gene expression, both prokaryotic and eukaryotic.

Most *E. coli* expression systems employ plasmid vectors, although there are also useful bacteriophage expression vectors for special applications (e.g., generation of gene expression libraries; Young and Davis, 1983; Young *et al.*, 1985a). The *E. coli* plasmid vectors generally consist of three basic segments: a replicon, a selectable marker, and an expression unit for heterologous genes. A generalized expression unit is composed of a strong promoter for transcriptional initiation, a ribosome-binding site (RBS) and an initiation codon for protein synthesis if not supplied by the inserted gene, followed by useful restriction endonuclease sites for insertion of desired genes. The expression unit is completed with translational and transcriptional termination signals. The variety within these basic elements and the combinations thereof are numerous. Most of the components and many vectors are available commercially.

Most plasmid expression vectors are derived from ColE1 plasmids such as pBR322 or pAT153 (Polisky, 1986). These plasmids are easy to manipulate and are stable. The ColE1 replicon maintains plasmid levels at greater than 50 copies per cell, and as such provides the immediate advantage of high gene dosage. Heterologous proteins expressed at high levels in *E. coli* are most often made from genes transcribed from one of three promoters: lambda (λ) P_L, *E. coli* tryptophan (trp), or *E. coli* mutant lactose (lac UV5). Why these three? Simply, at the time many expression vectors were being designed and constructed, these promoters were already well defined, well studied, and cloned (available). Since that time, numerous other promoters, both natural and synthetic, have been defined and successfully employed in *E. coli* expression vectors (Reznikoff and McClure, 1986). Comparative studies of promoter strength have been carried out (Deuschle *et al.*, 1986). Such studies show that the three above-mentioned promoters are not the strongest, and, in fact, are relatively weak when compared to the ribosomal operon and coliphage T5 and T7 promoters. However, an important feature shared by the λ P_L, trp, and lac promoters is that they are all regulatable. Cells harboring expression vectors employing these promoters may be grown to high densities in the absence of gene expression, and then be induced to produce the desired product. This attribute is important since constitutive expression, particularly overexpression, of many prokaryotic and eukaryotic proteins in *E. coli* is deleterious, or even lethal, to the bacteria. In this light, a derivative promoter, ptac, is important. Ptac is a hybrid between the trp and lac UV5 promoters and is considerably stronger than either and still regulatable (deBoer *et al.*, 1983; Amann *et al.*, 1983). Most certainly other hybrid promoter systems are in the making.

Strong regulatable promoters on multicopy plasmids may allow for high levels of transcription initiation. However, the level of resultant mRNA is dependent on its stability, which can significantly affect protein production (Buell and Panayotatos, 1986). The factors involved in determining mRNA stability (and decay) are not well understood, but are thought to involve features of RNA secondary structure. High-level protein expression is also influenced by the efficiency of translational signals. Factors involved here are the actual sequence of the bacterial RBS (Shine–Dalgarno sequence; Steitz, 1979), the spacing and sequence between the RBS and initiation (ATG) codon (Guarente *et al.*, 1980), codon usage, especially at the beginning of the protein, and again, the secondary structure of the mRNA (Stormo, 1986). Finally, the presence of a transcription termination signal has been shown to affect positively the ultimate level of protein production, presumably by preventing disruption of normal plasmid replication functions by readthrough transcription (Gentz *et al.*, 1981; Remaut *et al.*, 1981).

The best combination of the above regulatory sequences for maximum expression of any given gene is not predictable. This is most probably due to the influences of mRNA secondary structure and stability, and biased codon usage (deBoer and Kastelein, 1986) imparted by the actual sequence of the cloned gene involved.

High-level expression of recombinant genes imposes a heavy energy drain on the bacteria, generally resulting in reduced cell growth rates.

If a mutant arises that has in some way ceased to express the recombinant gene, not only will product yield decrease, but the variant will have a faster growth rate and can quickly overgrow the culture. Several approaches have been developed to maintain expression plasmid stability, including the use of multicopy or regulatable replicons (Uhlin *et al.*, 1979), partitioning functions (Skogman *et al.*, 1983), regulated promoters, and finally, selectable markers. Expression plasmid loss can be largely obviated by incorporating a function on the plasmid that is required by the employed host strain for viability. Such selection markers include functions that complement antibiotic susceptibilities or essential biosynthetic deficiencies of the host, the latter markers being more suitable for commerical production purposes (Nilsson and Skogman, 1986).

The ultimate level of protein production also depends on the stability of the synthesized product. The features that contribute to polypeptide stability and turnover are poorly understood. Often "abnormal" polypeptides are targeted for rapid proteolysis (Goff and Goldberg, 1985; Goldberg and Goff, 1986). Several methods have been used in attempts to overcome heterologous protein degradation in *E. coli*. One has been to optimize all other parameters of regulated gene expression to an extent that an induced rapid burst of expression, extending over no more than two cell generations, will overwhelm cellular proteases. In many instances, the rapid and high-level expression of proteins (both "normal" and "abnormal") leads to their precipitation within the cell and the formation of large amorphous aggregates resistant to the action of cellular proteases (Buell and Panayotatos, 1986). Alternatively, bacterial strains may be selected as production hosts that are deficient in certain protease activities (Buell *et al.*, 1985). Finally, expression of unstable proteins in *E. coli* may be stabilized by producing them as fusion polypeptides. In this situation, the desired gene in the expression vector is inserted in phase with prokaryotic gene sequences positioned either amino terminally, carboxyl terminally, or both. These gene fusions may consist of only a few additional amino acids (5–12 residues), small portions of prokaryotic genes (e.g., *cro, c*II, *trpE,* MS2 polymerase), or large polypeptides such as β-galactosidase (Maniatis *et al.*, 1982).

All of these parameters considered, engineered protein yields in *E. coli* vary from undetectable levels up to 50% of the total cullular protein. These highest levels are indeed phenomenal, but they are not the rule. On the other hand, heterologous protein sequences that appear to be unexpressible or only very poorly expressed in *E. coli*, for whatever reasons, do in fact exist: not all desired gene sequences can be produced in *E. coli*. Expression levels of between 2% and 10% of the total cell protein are obtained most frequently. Many overproduced proteins in *E. coli* are found in insoluble intracellular aggregates composed largely of the denatured expression product. Upon disruption of cells, these inclusions can be separated readily from soluble *E. coli* material. However, their dissolution requires the use of strong denaturants (e.g., guanidine hydrochloride, sodium dodecyl sulfate) and thus complicates further purification. Some proteins, most often those with molecular weights less than 25,000, if stably produced, have been obtained in more native configurations.

The biologic activity of many, but certainly not all, *E. coli*-produced recombinant proteins has been disappointing. Of particular concern are observations that these proteins are often significantly less immunogenic than their authentic counterparts. Many reasons have been put forth to explain these results, such as denatured nonnative conformation, inability to form proper disulfide linkages, lack of secondary protein modifications, and so on, many of which might be remedied by protein production in alternative expression systems.

The use of *Bacillus subtilis* as a host for the expression of heterologous genes would have several advantages over use of *E. coli: B. subtilis* is nonpathogenic to humans, does not produce endotoxins, has been used historically for the production of industrial and food products normally synthesized by the microbe, and has the ability to secrete proteins into the growth medium. This latter feature would simplify product recovery and purification, reduce or eliminate intracellular accumulation of proteins potentially toxic to the bacteria, and could allow products to assume more "native" conformations due to the ability to form correct disulfide bonds outside the reducing environment of the cytoplasm.

Numerous plasmid vectors have been characterized and are useful for cloning in *Bacillus*. Shuttle vectors, which are combination vectors having both *Bacillus* and *E. coli* plasmid replicons and selectable markers, allow manipulation of recombinant molecules in *E. coli*. Once the final plasmid construct is assembled and produced in *E. coli,* it is then tranformed into the *Bacillus* host.

A number of prokaryotic and eukaryotic genes have been introduced successfully into expression vectors containing *Bacillus* promoters, ribosome-binding sites, and secretion signal sequences. The reported levels of secreted protein production were quite variable, from less than 1 mg/liter and up to 50 mg/liter (Hardy *et al.*, 1981; Palva *et al.*, 1983; Honjo *et al.*, 1985; Shiroza *et al.*, 1985; Ulmanen *et al.*, 1985; Thompson and Vasantha, 1986). Low yield and poor quality of secreted heterologous proteins have been attributed mostly to the production by *Bacillus* of at least three extracellular proteases during the sporulation or stationary phases of bacterial growth. Several approaches to overcome this problem have been taken (Wong *et al.*, 1986), including use of a strong vegetative promoter in the secretion vector, introduction of the vector into protease-deficient mutant strains (Kawamura and Doi, 1984), and use of rich medium to maintain the cells in a nonsporulating growth stage. Use of asporogenous host strains can also reduce intracellular protein turnover (Ruppen *et al.*, 1986).

Among other bacterial systems for heterologous protein expression worthy of mention are the broad host range, high-copy-number cloning vectors that can be stably maintained in a wide range of Gram-negative bacteria (Bagdasarian *et al.*, 1981). When the *E. coli* tac promoter was incorporated into these vectors, it was found to function with similar efficiency and control in *Pseudomonas* as in *E. coli* (Bagdasarian *et al.*, 1983). The availability of alternaive Gram-negative host species in which protein expression may be directed by well-characterized *E. coli* promoters may overcome certain shortcomings associated with production in *E. coli*.

2. Fungi

Baker's yeast, *Saccharomyces cerevisiae*, has become an extremely important system for the bioproduction of heterologous proteins. Its attractiveness, like that of *Bacillus*, stems from its proven history as an industrial microorganism for efficient large-scale fermentation and its lack of toxic metabolites (Spencer and Spencer, 1983). In addition, yeast and other fungi are able to carry out many of the post-translational modifications that many eukaryotic proteins seem to require for full function.

Yeast expression systems have advanced rapidly, and several recent reviews are available (Kingsman *et al.*, 1985; Smith *et al.*, 1985; Knowlton, 1986; Das and Shultz, 1987). Expression systems have been developed to produce heterologous proteins that appear either intracellularly or are secreted into the culture medium. Expression vectors based on autonomously replicating plasmids typically have the ColE1 replicon and a selectable marker for manipulation in *E. coli*, the yeast two-micron sequences for high copy replication in the fungi, and one or more auxotrophic selectable markers. An alternative to these multicopy vectors are the integrating vectors which lack the yeast replicon.

Numerous yeast promoters, both constitutive and regulatable, have been isolated. The properties of these promoters are very different from those of prokaryotic promoters, and more closely resemble the promoter elements found in higher eukaryotic cells (Struhl, 1986, 1987). Promoters from highly expressed yeast genes (e.g., PGK, ADH1 and 2, PHO5, GAL1, GPD, and MFα1) are generally the strongest for heterologous gene expression. However, the levels of foreign protein production are most often considerably lower than predicted on the basis of promoter strength. For example, the PGK gene on a multicopy plasmid can produce PGK at levels of up to 50% of the total yeast protein, however use of this strong promoter to direct heterologous gene expression results in yields of only 1–5% (Tuite et al., 1982; Mellor et al., 1983). Many factors may be involved to explain these observations, including the effects of 5'- and 3'-flanking sequences, mRNA stability, and protein product stability (Mellor et al., 1985; Kniskern et al., 1986).

Unlike intracellular protein expression, promoter strength is not directly related to secreted protein production levels. In fact, secreted protein levels can be improved severalfold by replacing a strong promoter (e.g., MFα1) with a moderate strength or weak promoter (e.g., CYC1, ACT) on a multicopy vector (Ernst, 1986). Integration of the transcriptional unit has also been shown to increase the efficiency of secretion (Smith et al., 1985). Finally, it must be pointed out that not all proteins expressed from these yeast secretion vectors are in fact secreted (Das and Shultz, 1987).

Yeast strains other than Saccharomyces are also being tailored for heterologous protein production. The methylotrophic Pichia pastoris represents a notable example. The methanol-regulated AOX1 promoter from P. pastoris has been engineered to produce, on an industrial scale, the hepatitis B surface antigen at a level of 2–3% (400 mg/liter) of the total cell soluble protein in this strain (Cregg et al., 1987). Expression systems in filamentous fungi (e.g., Aspergillus niger and A. nidulans) are also being developed and may be capable of producing gram/liter levels of secreted proteins (Van Brunt, 1986).

3. Insect Cells

A virus-based expression system has been developed for the production of heterologous proteins in cultured insect cells (Miller, 1981; Smith et al., 1983b; D. W. Miller et al., 1986). The baculovirus Autographa californica nuclear polyhedrosis virus (AcNPV), possessing a covalently closed circular DNA genome of about 130 kilobase pairs, replicates in the nucleus of infected cells. Large polyhedral occlusion bodies accumulate and consist of enveloped virus particles embedded in a crystalline protein matrix. This matrix is composed almost exclusively of a 29-kD polyhedrin protein (Kelly, 1982; Miller *et al.*, 1983). Polyhedrin synthesis begins about 18 hr post-infection and continues until cell death, at which time polyhedrin may constitute 25–50% of the total protein of the infected cell. Therein lies one attraction of this system: the power of the polyhedrin promoter to drive high-level expression of heterologous genes. Key to the exploitation of this system was the demonstration that polyhedrin was nonessential for replication of the virus in cell culture (Smith *et al.*, 1983a). Thus, it became feasible to delete the polyhedrin gene and introduce foreign genes into the viral genome downstream of the strong polyhedrin promoter. The resultant recombinant virus should then be able to replicate in insect cells and produce high levels of the inserted heterologous gene product in the place of polyhedrin.

Because the genome of AcNPV is so large, its direct manipulation by recombinant DNA procedures *in vitro* is not practical. Therefore, introduction of foreign genes into the viral genome is accomplished by allelic replacement, which involves intracellular recombination of cotransfected wild-type viral DNA and a plasmid transfer vector containing the gene of interest. Various transfer vectors have been constructed; they are basically derivatives of *E. coli* plasmids into which the polyhedrin promoter and flanking AcNPV DNA sequences have been inserted. Unique cloning sites for gene insertion have been introduced either downstream of the promoter transcription initiation site of polyhedrin mRNA, or downstream of a translation initiation codon (Smith *et al.*, 1983b; D. W. Miller *et al.*, 1986; Matsuura *et al.*, 1987). The flanking viral sequences in these plasmids are required for subsequent recombination with the homologous sequences in the wild-type viral DNA upon co-transfection of cells. Frequencies of recombinant virus in the progeny following co-transfection are generally in the range of 0.1–1.0% (D. W. Miller *et al.*, 1986), although higher frequencies have been reported (Smith *et al.*, 1983a). Cells infected with recombinant viruses are distinguished readily in that plaques lack the highly refractile polyhedra characteristic of wild-type virus plaques. Other detection methods are also available (D. W. Miller *et al.*, 1986). The recombinant viruses generally replicate as well as wild-type virus and appear stable.

The level of heterologous protein production in recombinant baculovirus-infected cells is unpredictable. In wild-type virus-infected cells, polyhedrin levels reach into the hundreds of milligrams per liter range. Most heterologous gene expression levels do not approach polyhedrin levels, although there are exceptions (Overton *et al.*, 1987; Matsuura *et al.*, 1987), and are usually in the 1–10 mg/liter range (D. W. Miller *et al.*, 1986).

In addition to the potential for high-level expression of heterologous genes, this system is attractive for mammalian virus immunogen production due to the similarities in macromolecular processing pathways between insect and mammalian cells. Although no spliced mRNA transcripts have been noted for AcNPV (Lubbert and Doerfler, 1984; Friesen and Miller, 1985), this expression system can process and express intron-containing genes (Jeang et al., 1987). The proteolytic processing and secretory machinery of insect cells and mammalian cells are similar (G. E. Smith et al., 1983a,b; R. A. Smith et al., 1985; D. W. Miller et al., 1986); however, protein glycosylation is different. Insect cells lack sialic acid and contain negligible levels of galactosyl and sialyl transferase activities (Butters et al., 1981). Furthermore, N-linked glycosylation is only of the high mannose type (Kornfeld and Kornfeld, 1985).

The utility of this expression system for the large-scale commercial production of immunogen subunits remains unexplored. Insect cell culture requirements are similar to those of mammalian cells, although there is little need for CO_2 and the growth temperature is reduced. Due to the lytic nature of this expression system, production could be compared to, and should be cost competitive with, authentic virus subunit vaccine production methods. It may also be interesting to explore the possibility of capturing the strength of the polyhedrin promoter in a stable, chromosomally integrated form, so as to create continuous cell culture production capability in insect cells (analogous to mammalian cell expression systems discussed below). The advantages of subunit preparation in the absence of mammalian cell infectious or adventitious agents may be relevant. Also possible with this system is the use of insect larvae for protein production (Overton et al., 1987). "You could dream of tanks of worms, beetles, and caterpillars making your vaccines of the future" (Anonymous, 1987)!

4. Mammalian Cells

Generalized mammalian cell expression systems evolved from early investigations attempting to devise models for the study of eukaryotic gene expression. Simple mammalian DNA viruses offered the initial inroad toward this end. The papovavirus (SV40, polyoma) genomes were most thoroughly studied, readily manipulable (similar to bacterial plasmids), and completely sequenced. Although SV40 dominated the early work (Elder et al., 1981), other mammalian virus cloning vectors were soon developed (see Gluzman, 1982).

Many of the early systems involved the construction of a recombinant viral genome in which a viral gene downstream of a promoter was deleted and replaced with the cloned gene of interest. The resultant defective chimeric viral genome was transfected into cells in the presence of a helper virus. This helper virus was capable of complementing the defect, thus allowing the recombinant viral DNA to replicate, express protein, and be packaged into infectious virus particles. Due to amplification (some 10^5-fold) during the vegetative growth phase, these and later virus-based vectors can produce substantial quantities of protein (Berkner et al., 1987; Davidson and Hassell, 1987). In the case of SV40 viral vector systems, insert DNA is restricted to about 2.5 kb (Elder et al., 1981); retrovirus vectors and adenovirus derivatives can accommodate 6-kb and 10- to 20-kb segments of foreign DNA, respectively (Shimotohno and Temin, 1981; Wei et al., 1981; Thummel et al., 1981; Cepko et al., 1984). Study of these virus vectors has contributed greatly to our understanding of mammalian cell mRNA biogenesis and the signals involved, as well as translational control parameters (Elder et al., 1981; Gluzman, 1982). However, use of many of these viruses is limited to cells permissive for virus replication. Futhermore, cell death is often the result of infection.

Many current mammalian cell expression strategies are based on the desire to establish stable, continuous cell lines capable of producing the desired product. Systems generally employ plasmid shuttle vectors containing the ColE1 replicon and a selectable marker for manipulation in E. coli, and mammalian cell transcription units for expression of some mammalian cell selectable marker and the gene-of-interest. The two individual mammalian gene expression units (gene-of-interest and selectable marker) are most often linked on the same plasmid, but may also be co-introduced into cells on separate plasmids (Wigler et al., 1979). Alternatively, both the gene-of-interest and the selectable marker gene may be transcribed as a single polycistronic mRNA (Kaufman et al., 1987).

Mammalian cell expression units generally consist of a viral or cellular enhancer-promoter, insertion cloning sites, and RNA splicing and polyadenylation signals. Translational initiation and termination signals may also be present. The elements of mammalian promoter regions, including enhancers, upstream elements, TATA boxes, and cap sites, have been recently reviewed (Wasylyk, 1986). Many current vectors employ enhancer-promoter units derived from viruses: SV40 (Mulligan and Berg, 1980), adenoviruses (Thummel et al., 1981; Kaufman, 1985), cytomegalovirus (CMV) (Boshart et al., 1985), and retroviruses (see Gluzman, 1982). Others have incorporated cellular elements that have been characterized, such as the metallothionein (Hamer and Walling, 1982; Karin et al., 1983) and heat shock promoters (Dreano et al., 1986, and references cited therein). Several of these enhancer-promoters are regulatable (metallothionein and heat shock, mouse mammary tumor virus long terminal repeat; Huang *et al.*, 1981; Lee *et al.*, 1981), while the others are constitutive. Attempts have been made to compare the strength of different enhancer-promoters (see, for example, Riedel *et al.*, 1984; Foecking and Hofstetter, 1986). Complicating such comparisons are not only specific influences of the cloned gene sequences involved, but also the long-distance effects (several thousand basepairs) of enhancer elements, particularly when there may exist more than one such element on a given expression units are exchangeable (e.g., heterologous enhancer and cell-specific manner (Spandidos and Wilkie, 1983; Khoury and Gruss, 1983; Yaniv, 1984). Most of the components of mammalian gene expression units are exchangeable (e.g., heterologous enhancer and promoter elements may be combined), making useful combinations almost limitless.

Selectable markers for mammalian cells are not only critical for identification and isolation of cells having received the expression plasmids, but are often important for maintenance of the introduced genes in the resultant cell lines. In many cases, selection of animal cell transfectants has relied on complementation by the selection genes of mutations in the recipient cell. For example, incorporation of the herpes simplex virus thymidine kinase (HSV-*tk*) gene into the vector system allows for selection of the tk$^+$ phenotype from transfected tk$^-$ human or mouse cells (Bacchetti and Graham, 1977; Wigler *et al.*, 1977). Similarly, the dihydrofolate reductase (*dhfr*) gene may be engineered for use to isolate dhfr$^+$ cells from transfected Chinese hamster ovary (CHO) cells deficient in *dhfr* (Subramani *et al.*, 1981; Kaufman and Sharp, 1982). Use of such markers is limited, however, by the availability of mutant mammalian cell types to serve as gene recipients. A solution is offered by dominant-acting genetic marker systems. Very efficient expression of the *dhfr* gene (M. J. Murray *et al.*, 1983) or use of an altered *dhfr* gene (Simonsen and Levinson, 1983) have been employed for dominant selection of wild-type hamster and mouse cells in the presence of methotrexate (MTX). Expression of bacterial xanthine-guanine phosphoribosyl transferase (gpt) (Mulligan and Berg, 1981), kanamycin-neomycin phosphotransferase (neo) (Colbere-Garapin *et al.*, 1981; Southern and Berg, 1982), and the gene that confers resistance to hygromycin B (Bernard *et al.*, 1985) provide efficient dominant selection systems in a variety of mammalian cells. More recently, systems based on expression of adenosine deaminase (ADA) (Kaufman *et al.*, 1986) and asparagine synthetase (AS) (Cartier *et al.*, 1987) have been described.

An additional feature of several of these selectable marker systems

relevant to protein production in mammalian cells is their ability to
amplify the marker gene, and consequently any associated genes.
Upon passage of transfected cells in increasing concentrations their
respective selection agents, the *dhfr* (Schimke, 1984; Stark and Wahl,
1984), ADA (Kaufman *et al.*, 1986), and AS (Cartier *et al.*, 1987)
systems can be used to amplify gene copy number and protein
expression levels. Gene amplification may also be accomplished
through the use of mammalian virus replicons. Recombinant plasmids
carrying a viral origin of replication should be amplified in mammalian cells provided the necessary cofactors are supplied in the host cell.
The development of the COS monkey cell line (Gluzman, 1981), which
constitutively produces SV40 T antigen, allows for the episomal
replication of recombinant plasmids bearing the SV40 origin of replication. Efficient extrachromosomal replication of these plasmids,
however, required that certain "poison sequences" of the bacterial
plasmid be deleted (Lusky and Botchan, 1981). Similar bacterial
sequence inhibitory effects have been observed with eukaryotic cloning vectors incorporating the replicon and transforming region of
bovine papilloma virus (BPV) (Sarver *et al.*, 1981, 1982; Allshire and
Bostock, 1986). An extension of the use of viral replicons to amplify
transfected genes, thereby increasing their expression, is represented
by mammalian host-vector systems in which replication is regulatable.
Cell lines have been constructed that constitutively express temperature-sensitive T antigens. Such cells allow for the thermal regulation of gene copy number and expression of recombinant plasmids
containing papovavirus replicons (Portela *et al.*, 1985; Rio *et al.*, 1985;
Kern and Basilico, 1986).

With expression systems that incorporate strong enhancer-promoter
elements and gene amplification mechanisms, engineered mammalian
cell lines have been established that produce significant quantities of
desired immunogens. These systems are clearly targeted toward the
production of subunit components of mammalian pathogens. Depending on the pathogen (virus) and the specific subunit of interest,
reported expression levels generally have been comparable to or lower
than those of authentic virus infections (see discussion of specific viral
diseases below). However, several attractive features of these systems
present themselves. Immunogen production in cells homologous to
those of the natural infection, in the absence of the pathogen, estab-
lishes safety, and generally assures proper modifications and the
generation of "native" antigenic structures. Often the desired gene
product can be engineered to be secreted into the culture fluid,
allowing for a continuous (as opposed to batch) type production system,

with accompanying ease of product recovery. Currently, many viral vaccines are produced by production-scale cell culture, and scale-up technology for cultivation of anchorage-dependent and suspension mammalian cell cultures continues to progress (Hu and Dodge, 1985; Hu *et al.*, 1985; Pullen *et al.*, 1985; Tharakan and Chau, 1986). However, considerable advances are still required to promote engineered mammalian gene expression systems from laboratory scale to efficient production scale (Sterling, 1987).

Gene expression in the mammalian cell systems described above requires nuclear transcription, processing, and transport to the cytoplasm of the desired gene product mRNA. This means that considerations of specific transcript stability and of RNA splicing and processing signals are required for construction of optimized expression units. However, there are many viral pathogens that replicate exclusively in the cytoplasm of infected cells, and whose RNA transcripts are normally not exposed to the mRNA biogenesis machinery of the nucleus. The fate of transcripts from such viruses in the nuclear environment is not known *a priori*. It may be possible, for example, that a normally cytoplasmic virus transcript fortuitously contains a splice acceptor or donor site. Functional recognition of such a sequence may severely compromise efforts to employ the above mammalian cell expression approaches for production of useful quantities of that gene product. An alternative mammalian cell expression system of specific usefulness in these situations may be provided by the vaccinia virus expression vectors (Panicali and Paoletti, 1982; Mackett *et al.*, 1982; Mackett and Smith, 1986). Vaccinia viruses replicate to high titers exclusively in the cytoplasm of a wide variety of cell types. Quantitation of engineered protein production levels by vaccinia virus recombinants has rarely been reported, but appears to be comparable to that of other recombinant mammalian cell expression systems. Although generally considered from the point of view of useful live virus vaccines (see chapter by Esposito and Murphy), this expression system may offer certain distinct advantages for the mammalian cell production of select components for subunit vaccines.

III. Progress toward the Generation of Useful Vaccines

From the above overview, it should be clear that a wide variety of expression systems are available to the genetic engineer for potential bioproduction of subunit vaccine immunogens. Although not discussed, it should be noted that expression systems in plants are under active development. Their future application toward vaccine production should not be dismissed! Which expression system is best for biosynthetic vaccine production? There is no simple answer. Each application is unique (and complicated), and must be considered on an individual basis. Below, a limited number of pathogens has been chosen to illustrate progress in the use of the various expression systems for biosynthetic vaccine development. Throughout this discussion, one is encouraged to keep in mind the distinction between "expression success" of the systems for a given antigen and "immunization success" of the resultant immunogens.

A. Bacterial Diseases

Traditionally, vaccines for diseases of bacterial etiology have consisted of either inactivated whole cells, cell wall extracts or preparations, or crude culture broth filtrates. In all cases, these vaccines contain complex arrays of components, many of which are irrelevant and potentially toxigenic, contaminating the essential "protective immunogens." These essential immunogens are often undefined, but are generally considered to be those components involved in bacterial attachment and colonization (fimbriae, adhesins, outer membrane proteins) and those responsible for pathogenicity (toxins, virulence factors). Reviews of bacterial vaccines are available (Germanier, 1984; Tramont and Boslego, 1985; Dorner and McDonel, 1985). Application of molecular cloning and expression methodologies to the study of bacterial pathogens allows for the identification and isolation of many critical immunogens and virulence factors (Macrina, 1984). This in turn affords one the ability to establish the role of these determinants in pathogenesis and immunity, providing a rational approach to subunit vaccine development.

1. Enterotoxigenic E. coli and Cholera

Diarrheal diseases caused by enterotoxigenic *E. coli* (ETEC) are important afflictions of human and domestic livestock throughout the world. A great deal is known about the pathogenic mechanisms of ETEC (Levine *et al.*, 1983; Levine, 1984). The required bacterial colonization is mediated by mucosal adhesins which may be fimbrial or nonfimbrial. Anti-adhesin vaccines, composed of purified pili, have been quite successful in preventing scours in newborn piglets and calves. Similar studies with humans have met with less spectacular results (Levine, 1984; Tramont and Boslego, 1985). Here, the pathogens themselves represented the immunogen bioproduction system.

Microbial engineering, however, may provide production advantages. First, as protection is afforded only against homologous strains, simultaneous expression of multiple adhesins may offer considerable production cost savings. Second, increasing strain stability and/or product yields would be valuable. Often pilus expression in the natural pathogenic hosts can be strongly affected by growth conditions, differentially regulated, or unstable (metastable) (de Graaf *et al.*, 1980; van Verseveld *et al.*, 1985; Orndorff *et al.*, 1985).

However, simply elevating the level of fimbriae expression requires some understanding of the genetic organization of the operon in question. For example, the K88 operon, when placed into plasmid pBR322 under the control of the P1 promoter, increased K88 pilus expression several fold over that of the natural promoter, up to 2% of the total cell protein. But replacement of the P1 promoter with the stronger trp promoter was lethal to the bacteria (Kehoe *et al.*, 1983). Expression of K88 surface fimbriae is dependent on the presence of at least five cistrons encoded within the K88 operon. When just the K88 subunit gene was placed under control of the trp promoter, with the other cistrons under P1 control, levels of K88 antigen of up to 30% of the total cell protein could be produced stably under normal culture conditions (Winther *et al.*, 1985). Claims for the "first" vaccines to be produced through recombinant DNA technology stem from construction of *E. coli* strains overproducing the K88 and K99 antigens (Shuuring, 1982).

Another consideration important in protection against bacterial-induced diarrheal diseases involves neutralization of enterotoxins. The majority of ETEC produce heat-labile (LT) and heat-stable toxin (ST), either singly or together. These toxins from heterologous ETEC serotypes appear to be highly related to one another. Immunization with either of these components can confer protection against ETEC strains producing the respective toxin (Klipstein *et al.*, 1981; Klipstein and Engert, 1981; Kauffman, 1981). A chemically synthesized peptide consisting of the 18 amino acids of ST and a 26-amino-acid epitope of the LT-B subunit is being evaluated as a candidate vaccine in humans (Klipstein *et al.*, 1986; see chapter by Esposito and Murphy). Engineered bacteria may also provide ETEC toxin immunogens. *E. coli* strains have been constructed which express only the immunodominant, nontoxigenic LT-B subunit to high levels (Winther and Dougan, 1984; Miller *et al.*, 1985). By placing the LT-B coding sequences under the control of the lac promoter and introducing this plasmid construction into a phage λ lysogenic strain of *E. coli,* Miller *et al.* (1985) were able to produce LT-B in the culture supernatant at a level of up to 8.5% of the total soluble protein. In view of the work of Klipstein, Houghten, and co-workers (Houghten *et al.*, 1985; Klipstein *et al.*, 1986), fusion of the sequence for the 18 amino acids of ST to such a plasmid might lead to bioproduction of an even more potent vaccine component.

E. *coli* strains overproducing the ETEC LT-B subunit might also be useful for production of cholera and combination cholera-*coli* vaccines. Cholera toxin (CT) is structurally, functionally, and immunologically similar to ETEC LT (Dallas and Falkow, 1980; Holmgren, 1981; Yamamoto *et al.*, 1984; Jacob *et al.*, 1984), and immunization of rats with purified LT-B provided equally strong protection against LT-producing E. *coli* and *Vibrio Cholerae* (Klipstein *et al.*, 1984). Components other than CT that may be useful immunogens for cholera include adhesion antigens and outer membrane proteins (Levine, 1984; Manning, 1987). The gene encoding a soluble hemagglutinin has been cloned from *V. cholerae* and expressed in E. *coli* (Franzon and Manning, 1986; Van Dongen and de Graaf, 1986). The role of this antigen in immunity is imminently testable. Similarly, the recent cosmid cloning and expression in E. *coli* of the protective O antigen of *V. cholerae* (Manning *et al.*, 1986) adds yet another potentially valuable component for an effective E. *coli*-produced broad spectrum vaccine against bacterial diarrhea.

2. Pertussis

In most parts of the world, the current pertussis (whooping cough) vaccine consists of killed whole cells of *Bordetella pertussis*. Such vaccines are known for their side-effects, and development of an acellular vaccine is clearly warranted (for reviews, see Robinson *et al.*, 1985; Fox, 1987b). Work has centered on understanding the roles of individual bacterial components in the pathogenesis of pertussis, with focus on surface proteins that mediate adhesion to the respiratory mucosa [e.g., agglutinogens and filamentous hemagglutinin (FHA)] and various toxins [pertussis toxin (PT), demonecrotic toxin]. Immunization with either PT or FHA appears to be protective, and when combined, is synergistic (Munoz *et al.*, 1981; Sato *et al.*, 1981; Oda *et al.*, 1984; Arciniega *et al.*, 1987). These components, prepared from B. *pertussis* culture supernatants, have formed the basis for a Japanese subunit vaccine (Sato *et al.*, 1984). However, further development of a component vaccine for pertussis has been hampered by the fastidious growth requirements of the organism and its ability to modulate expression and degradation of virulence factors important for immunity. Therefore, attempts are being made to clone, characterize, and express the PT and FHA genes in more suitable hosts.

PT is a hexameric protein made up of five dissimilar subunits (S1 through S5). Recently, two laboratories reported cloning and sequencing the entire PT gene (Locht *et al.,* 1986; Locht and Keith, 1986; Nicosia *et al.,* 1986). The cistrons for all five toxin subunits are coded by closely linked cistrons in a 3.1-kb chromosomal DNA region. Identification of a promoter-like structure located 5' of the coding sequences suggests that the toxin is expressed through a polycistronic mRNA. Expression of the native PT genes in *E. coli* has been disappointing. As the original genomic clones failed to express PT, attempts were made to express the entire operon or parts of it employing an *E. coli* expression plasmid containing the P_L promoter (Nicosia *et al.,* 1987). Although *E. coli* efficiently transcribed the cloned PT genes, it was unable to produce significant amounts of the proteins. High-level expression of the individual subunits as fusion proteins was achieved when each of the toxin genes was joined to a fragment of DNA coding for the amino terminus of the MS2 DNA polymerase, under the control of the P_L promoter. This suggests that translation initiation and/or initial codon usage of the *B. pertussis* genes may be problematic in *E. coli.* Protein degradation may also be involved in the low yields of PT proteins in *E. coli.* Barbieri *et al.* (1987) found expression of the S1 subunit increased 10-fold (to about 1 mg/liter of culture) when their expression plasmid was introduced into a strain of *E. coli* deficient in protein degradation. Unfortunately, immunization with each of the five *E. coli*-produced PT subunit fusion proteins, or mixtures of them, failed to protect mice against an intracerebral challenge (Nicosia *et al.,* 1987).

The FHA gene, encoding a 210- to 220-kD protein in *B. pertussis,* has been cloned in *E. coli* from a cosmid gene bank (Brown and Parker, 1987). Low-level protein expression was noted, presumably due to the *E. coli* kanamycin gene promoter. Also screening a cosmid library, Shareck and Cameron (1984) reported the expression of two *B. pertussis* outer membrane proteins in *E. coli;* however, their nature and levels of synthesis were unclear. Further understanding of the control of *B. pertussis* gene expression and manipulation of these cloned sequences in *E. coli,* or other suitable host cells will be required before potentially valuable polypeptides will be available for immunologic evaluation.

3. Anthrax

Efforts are being made to develop a more potent and less reactogenic human anthrax vaccine using recombinant DNA procedures. Anthrax and anthrax vaccines have a long history (Hambleton *et al.,* 1984). The current human vaccines consist of alum-precipitated supernatant

fluids of *Bacillus anthracis* cultures. These preparations contain predominantly the so-called protective antigen (PA) (Ristroph and Ivins,
1983), which, together with lethal factor (LF) and edema factor (EF),
form the tripartite exotoxin. PA vaccines fail to induce optimal
immunity, as antibody responses to the other toxin components
enhance protection. Additional immunologic responses may be necessary to provide complete protection against all strains of *B. anthracis*
(Little and Knudson, 1986). The genes for all three toxin components
reside on a single plasmid (Robertson and Leppla, 1986). The PA and
LF genes have been cloned individually into *E. coli* (Vodkin and
Leppla, 1983; Robertson and Leppla, 1986). Their products, expressed
from their natural bacillus promoters, were produced in *E. coli* at very
low levels and, furthermore, were not secreted. However, introduction
of the PA gene into *B. subtilis* resulted in the appearance of PA in the
culture fluids at levels greater than those seen in *B. anthracis* (Ivins
and Welkos, 1986), making this an attractive source for at least one
component of a new vaccine.

4. Gonococcal Infections

Gonococcal infections remain an enormous worldwide public health
problem, and so the potential for immunoprophylaxis of gonorrhea is
being explored (Gotschlich, 1984). Because vaccines composed of whole
killed gonococci were not efficacious, vaccine development has explored the usefulness of isolated outer membrane constituents and
extracellular products as potential vaccine components. The major
candidates for a subunit gonococcal vaccine include pili, and outer
membrane proteins designated protein I and III, and IgA protease. Pili
are responsible for bacterial adhesion to epithelial cells, and protein I
(a porin) may be involved in endocytosis. The role of protein III and IgA
protease are unknown (Blake and Gotschlich, 1983).

Intact gonococcal pili from different strains, and even within single
strains, exhibit a high level of antigenic diversity. In human trials,
purified intact pili when administered parenterally were able to elicit
a protective response at mucosal surfaces against homologous, but not
heterologous challenge. Gonoccocal pili do appear to possess a common,
although immunorecessive antigenic determinant (Schoolnik *et al.*,
1983). Antibodies to this common, receptor-binding domain of the pilus
protein were able to bind both homologous and heterologous pili (Virji
and Heckels, 1985). Furthermore, this region, as an isolated CNBr
fragment or a synthetic peptide, was able to elicit cross-reactive
antibodies in experimental animals (Schoolnik *et al.*, 1983; Rothbard
and Schoolnik, 1985). The protective nature of these immunogens

remains to be demonstrated. The gene for a gonococcal pilus protein has been cloned into *E. coli* and was expressed apparently under the direction of the natural *N. gonorrhoeae* promoter (Meyer *et al.*, 1982). However, the pilin subunits were not assembled into pilus structures. Expression of this gene, and additional gonoccocal pilus genes, in a more appropriate host (e.g., *Pseudomonas aeruginosa,* see below) should provide a ready production system for promising immunogens.

Gonococcal protein I, being immunogenic and existing in a limited number of serotypes, is also an attractive vaccine candidate. However, it was recently shown that protein I, and another neisserial antigen, H.8, were not immunologically accessible on all gonococci from the same culture (Robinson *et al.*, 1987). Cloning of the protein I gene has not yet been reported. All gonococcal strains contain protein III, but its utility in vaccines remains unexplored.

Another consideration for gonococcal vaccines is an immunogenic portion of the secreted gonococcal IgA protease (Gotschlich, 1984). The structural gene for this protease has been cloned into *E. coli* from the chromosomal DNA of two strains of *N. gonorrhoeae* (Koomey *et al.*, 1982; Halter *et al.*, 1984). Differences in the restriction maps of the two genes indicate strain-specific variation. Recently, it has been reported that *N. gonorrhoeae* can produce two types of IgA protease (Mulks and Knapp, 1987). The cloned IgA protease was expressed, presumably from the *N. gonorrhoeae* promoter, and in one case, was secreted in a functional form from *E. coli* at a level approaching that of the natural host (Halter *et al.*, 1984). This latter gene has been sequenced (Pohlner *et al.*, 1987). Production of this protein, or fragments thereof, should allow immunological studies contributing to a better understanding of the role of IgA protease in pathogenesis and its potential usefulness in a vaccine.

5. Ovine Footrot

The pili of *Bacteriodes nodosus* have been established as the major protective immunogen for ovine footrot (Stewart *et al.*, 1982). However, *B. nodosus* is a fastidious anaerobic Gram-negative bacterium and exhibits inconsistent pilus production in bulk liquid cultures, making vaccine manufacture expensive. Thus, efforts have been made to produce pili in a more suitable host. The pilin structural gene exists at a single locus in the *B. nodosus* chromosome (Elleman *et al.*, 1986b) and has been cloned in *E. coli* and sequenced (Anderson *et al.*, 1984; Elleman *et al.*, 1984, 1986a,b). Analogous to what was observed for gonococcal pilin (Meyer *et al.*, 1982), expression of the *B. nodosus* pilin gene in *E. coli* resulted in the production of intracellular monomeric subunits that failed to assemble into morphological pilus structures. The immunogenicity of this material was quite low (Elleman *et al.*, 1986a). However, expression of the gene, under the control of the λ P_R promoter, in *Pseudomonas aeruginosa* resulted in high-level production of distinct morphological pili on the outer surface of the cell (Elleman *et al.*, 1986c; Mattick *et al.*, 1987). Furthermore, the *B. nodosus* pili expressed in *P. aeruginosa* were highly immunogenic and served as an effective vaccine.

The successful production of assembled, highly immunogenic pili of *B. nodosus* in *P. aeruginosa*, but not in *E. coli*, in all likelihood relates to the fact that the former two bacteria possess pili of the same category—type 4 (Ottow, 1975). Other species possessing type 4 pili include *Moxarella* and *Neisseria*, among others. Type 4 pilins exhibit considerable amino-terminal sequence homology despite the large evolutionary distances between the different species expressing them. In fact, this homology has been used to isolate a pilin gene from *M. bovis* using a DNA probe based on the sequence of a *N. gonorrhaeae* pilin gene (Marrs *et al.*, 1985). This conservation might indicate compatibility in subunit processing and pilus assembly mechanisms among bacterial species from different genera. Thus, *P. aeurgenosa* may also serve as an appropriate surrogate host for the ready production of immunogenic pili from *M. bovis* and *N. gonorrhoeae*. Compatibility of one pilus type within Enterobacteriaceae has been shown by expression of *Klebsiella pneumoniae* pili in *E. coli* and *Salmonella typhimurium* (Purcell and Clegg, 1983).

6. Syphilis

Due to the inability to cultivate the spirochete *Treponema pallidum in vitro*, there is currently no vaccine for syphilis. This shortcoming has also hindered progress in understanding the pathogen itself, the molecular components of *T. pallidum* involved in pathogenesis, and the immune response to infection (Lukehart, 1985). This status is changing with the application of recombinant DNA technologies to this system. Several research groups have established *T. pallidum* genomic DNA libraries in *E. coli* (Stamm *et al.*, 1982, 1983; Walfield *et al.*, 1982; Norgard and Miller, 1983; van Embden *et al.*, 1983). These recombinant *E. coli* clones have been screened for the expression of *T. pallidum*-specific antigens using various syphilitic immune sera from infected rabbits or humans, and more recently with monoclonal antibodies (Swancutt *et al.*, 1986; Norgard *et al.*, 1986). The employed methodologies required that the expression of *T. pallidum* antigens be dependent on the functionality of treponeme transcriptional and translational signals in *E. coli.* This notwithstanding, a handful of individual clones were found to be positive. Many of the cloned treponeme-specific antigens so far identified appear to be specific for pathogenic subspecies of *T. pallidum.* Several may be cell-surface antigens of the spirochete, although this localization for some has been questioned (Swancutt *et al.,* 1986).

Further characterization of the cloned antigen genes is ongoing (Hansen *et al.,* 1985; Dallas *et al.,* 1987). The gene encoding a 39-kD treponemal cell-surface antigen has been engineered into an *E. coli* expression vector employing the lpp and lac promoters. Although these manipulations increased the expression of this antigen, the levels still appeared to be quite low. Sufficient protein was purified, however, and used to generate antisera, which in turn identified the native treponemal protein counterpart (Dallas *et al.,* 1987). A protease-resistant recombinant *T. pallidum* antigen (4D), identified from a Charon 30 phage gene bank, was expressed in *E. coli* as a soluble 190-kD oligomer composed of 19-kD monomers (Fehniger *et al.,* 1984, 1986). Expression of this antigen in *E. coli* (presumably under treponeme control) was estimated to be 50-fold higher than in *T. pallidum* cells, with yields of purified 4D antigen in the range of 1–3 mg/liter (Fehniger *et al.,* 1984). Rabbit antisera to the recombinant 4D antigen immobilized *T. pallidum* cells *in vitro* (Fehniger *et al.,* 1984) and provided partial protection of rabbits against intradermal challenge (Fehniger *et al.,* 1985, as cited in Radolf *et al.,* 1987). Evidence of a role for another cloned *T. pallidum* antigen (47 kD) in disease pathogenesis is also compelling (Norgard *et al.,* 1986).

7. Mycobacterial Infections

Like *T. pallidum, Mycobacterium leprae* can be propagated only in experimental animals, in this case, armadillos. Vaccination with the bacillus Calmette-Guerin (BCG, an avirulent strain of *M. bovis*) is of questional efficacy not only for *M. leprae* (Stewart-Tull, 1984), but also for *M. tuberculosis* (Collins, 1984). *Mycobacterium leprae,* grown in armadillos, can be purified from armadillo tissue. In fact, it has been noted that 125,000 *M. leprae* (whole-cell) vaccine doses can be prepared from a single armadillo (Stewart-Tull, 1984). How many armadillos does it take to support a vaccine campaign to control leprosy? In addition to the high cost of an armadillo preparation, cross-reactivity between human serum and liver proteins with armadillo antigens makes alternative approaches for leprosy vaccine development mandatory.

Several technologies are being employed to identify and characterize important mycobacterial proteins involved in protective immunity and immunopathology. In addition to various animal and human immune sera, a large number of monoclonal antibodies have been generated and used to identify the major mycobacterial protein antigens (Enger *et al.*, 1985; Buchanan *et al.*, 1987). As protective immunity and resistance to mycobacterial infection is dependent on T cells and cell-mediated immunity (Lagrange, 1984), human T-cell clones have been established to test antigen reactivity (Mustafa *et al.*, 1986; Ottenhoff *et al.*, 1986; Emmrich and Kaufman, 1986; Oftung *et al.*, 1987). Finally, genomic DNA libraries have been constructed in *E. coli* for *M. leprae* (Young *et al.*, 1985b; Clark-Curtiss *et al.* 1985), *M. tuberculosis* (Young *et al.*, 1985a), and *M. bovis* (Thole *et al.*, 1985). Gene bank constructions that relied on mycobacterial transcription and translation signals resulted in the identification of relatively few antigen-expressing clones (Clark-Curtiss *et al.*, 1985; Thole *et al.*, 1985). Furthermore, those that were positive produced protein only at levels near the limits of detection. Presumably the *E. coli* machinery for gene expression does not recognize the mycobacterial signals efficiently, although this may not be the case for all mycobacterial genes (Shinnick, 1987). Expression of mycobacterial genes in *Streptomyces* might be considered. *S. lividans* efficiently utilizes a high proportion of mycobacterial promoters and translational signals (Kieser *et al.*, 1986). By placing an *E. coli* promoter in front of the mycobacterium DNA inserts, antigen expression levels could be increased (Clark-Curtiss *et al.*, 1985; Thole *et al.*, 1985). Use of the λgt11 expression system, in which foreign insert DNA expression is under the control of *E. coli* transcription and translation signals and the expressed antigens are stabilized by fusion to *E. coli* β-galactosidase, yielded greater numbers of antigen-producing clones when screened with a battery of monoclonal antibodies (Young *et al.*, 1985a,b). These libraries have also been screened for antigens recognized by human T-cell clones (Mustafa *et al.*, 1986; Emmrich *et al.*, 1986; Oftung *et al.*, 1987). Results from these approaches have identified several interesting proteins. One of these, a 65-kD protein, is a prominent component of both *M. leprae* and *M. tuberculosis* and appears to be a major B-cell and T-cell antigen and immunogen in humans (Emmrich *et al.*, 1986; Husson and Young, 1987). The gene for this protein has been cloned and sequenced from *M. leprae* (Young *et al.*, 1985b; Mehra *et al.*, 1986), *M. bovis* (Thole *et al.*, 1985, 1987), and *M. tuberculosis* (Shinnick, 1987; Husson and Young, 1987). The protein product of the *M. bovis* gene, reliably expressed in *E. coli* under P_L promoter control, has been purified (yield, 3 mg/gram of cells) and shown to elicit a positive skin reaction in sensitized guinea pigs (Thole *et al.*, 1987).

8. Streptococcal Infections

Many streptococci possess antigens that are cross-reactive with mammalian heart tissue. The presence of these determinants in a streptococcal vaccine would have the potential for inducing an autoimmune response. Therefore, development of safe streptococcal vaccines will require a detailed knowledge of the immunogenic properties of their components and may best be produced in an alternative host. The surface fibrillar M protein, a major virulence factor of many streptococci and a prime candidate protective immunogen, happens to be a major heart cross-reactive component (Dale and Beachey, 1982). Another problem with this antigen is the fact that there are over 70 different serotypes of M protein. Thus, attempts are being made to identify protective, non-cross-reactive, and hopely, common determinants on the M proteins. The screening of *E. coli* phage and cosmid libraries of *S. pyogenes* DNA has resulted in the identification of the M protein genes for several serotypes (Scott and Fishetti, 1983; Spanier *et al.*, 1984; Kehoe *et al.*, 1985). The M proteins expressed in *E. coli* (presumably from streptococcal transcriptional–translational signals) possessed both immunoprotective epitopes and heart cross-reactive determinants (Scott and Fischetti, 1983; Poirier *et al.*, 1985). Using antisera generated to synthetic peptides, several protective epitopes on the type 24 M protein have been identified that do not evoke antibodies cross-reactive with cardiac tissue (Beachey *et al.*, 1984). However, these antisera were also unreactive with heterologous serotypes of M protein. A putative carboxy-terminal anchor–cell wall attachment region revealed by analysis of the complete sequence of the type 6 M protein gene appears to be highly conserved (Hollingshead *et al.*, 1986; Scott *et al.*, 1986). Evaluation of the immunogenicity of these conserved determinants with respect to protection and heart cross-reactivity hopefully will define the M protein sequences to be incorporated into an efficient expression system.

Many strains of steptococci also produce toxins, to which an antitoxin immune response may be more broadly cross-reactive and cross-protective. Thus, it is relevant that the streptolysin O determinant of *S. pyogenes* (Kehoe and Timmis, 1984), and the pneumolysin gene of *S. preumoniae* (Paton *et al.*, 1986; Walker *et al.*, 1987) have been cloned and expressed in *E. coli*.

S. mutans and *S. sanguis*, as well as *Actinomyces viscosus*, have been implicated in dental caries and periodontal disease. There are several candidate protective antigens that are not heart cross-reactive, including adhesins and glucosyltransferase proteins. Several of the genes for these proteins from the above organisms have been cloned and expressed in *E. coli* (Holt *et al.*, 1982; Robeson *et al.*, 1983; Donkersloot *et al.*, 1985; Pucci and Macrina, 1985; Fives-Taylor *et al.*, 1987). In fact, one group claimed "we have been able to clone all of the major antigens that might be of value as components of an *S. mutans* subunit vaccine" (Morrissey *et al.*, 1985)!

9. Bovine Brucellosis

The current live *Brucella abortus* strain 19 vaccine is reasonably efficacious, but has several serious drawbacks including its ability to establish chronic infection in vaccinated cattle and its pathogenicity for humans. Development of an effective subunit vaccine, compatible with a differential diagnostic, is essential for the goal of eradication of bovine brucellosis from the United States. The fastidious *B. abortus* is a facultative intracellular parasite, and in that sense resembles mycobacterial pathogens. Both B-cell and T-cell components appear to be involved in immunity, but their specificities and relative roles in protection remain unclear (Cheers, 1983; Montaraz and Winter, 1986). *Brucella* lack fimbriae and there are no known virulence factors. Therefore, outer membrane components have been explored for protective determinants. Extracted outer membrane preparations of *B. abortus* were capable of eliciting both an antibody response and T-cell blastogenesis (Winter *et al.*, 1983) and were protective in mouse and lemming model systems (Dubray and Bezard, 1980; Tabatabai and Deyoe, 1984). Results were less impressive in cows (Tabatabai and Deyoe, 1984). The several prominent proteins in these preparations were tightly associated with lipopolysaccharides (LPS) (Verstreate *et al.*, 1982). And, it has recently been shown that monoclonal antibodies specific for the O polysaccharide of *B. abortus* can confer protection, albeit short-lived (Montaraz *et al.*, 1986). Thus, the role of the cell-surface protein components in immunity remains unclear. Several groups have constructed *B. abortus* genomic libraries in *E. coli* (Beef, 1985; J. Mayfield, personal communication, 1987). Several of the surface protein genes have been identified and some are apparently expressed quite well (5–10% total cell protein) in *E. coli* using either their natural *Brucella* promoters or engineered *E. coli* promoters (L. Tabatabai; J. Mayfield, personal communications). However, as yet, none of the cloned antigens have exhibited protective activity. The cloning of additional *B. abortus* proteins continues; however, the unsettling issue of whether there exists a protective protein immunogen remains. Perhaps cloned surface antigens conjugated to the protective determinant of *B. abortus* LPS might be worthy of exploration. Additionally, the approaches being taken in the cases of *M.*

tuberculosis and *M. Leprae* may be appropriate here to identify important determinants of B-cell (as per Montaraz *et al.*, 1986) and T-cell immunity in *B. abortus* infection.

B. Viral Diseases

Development of subunit vaccines for viral diseases might appear to be inherently simpler than those for bacterial diseases, merely due to the difference in the genetic complexity of the pathogens. Myriad bacterial genes and gene products, as well as the variety of surface components and virulence factors, often make the identification and definition of the important and critical immunogenic components of bacterial pathogens difficult. In contrast, the coding capacities of some viral pathogens yield only a handful of virus-encoded gene products. All viral genomes, if not already molecularly cloned and completely sequenced, are in the process of being cloned and sequenced; and if not, they could be, if so desired. Yet possession of the entire nucleotide sequence of a viral genome, or the ability ot obtain the same, does not predestine the successful, straightforward production of an efficacious subunit vaccine. Once a viral genome, viral RNA transcript, or any portions thereof have been cloned, the choices for engineered expression of polypeptide products are numerous. Both prokaryotic and eukaryotic expression systems have potential utility for production of mammalian viral antigens.

1. Hepatitis B

The greatest success story to date in the area of biosynthetically produced subunit vaccines is that of hepatitis B virus (HBV), so much so that a yeast-produced, genetically engineered subunit vaccine has recently received FDA approval, becoming the first human recombinant vaccine to be sold in the United States. A similar product is already being marketed in Singapore, Belgium, and Switzerland (Van Brunt, 1987). Numerous other recombinant HBV subunit products produced in yeast (*S. cerevisiae* and *P. pastoris*) or mammalian cells (CHO, mouse, and others) are in various stages of clinical trials. Such success is the result of not only a tremendous research effort, but also of certain unique features of the virus itself.

Clearly, HBV poses a major, world-wide public health problem, control of which will require an extensive vaccination campaign. However, such a campaign is compromised by the fact that HBV cannot be propagated in cell culture or in the usual laboratory animals. The complete 42-nm virion, the Dane particle, is composed of a 3,200-nucleotide DNA genome surrounded by a core antigen (HBcAg). This nucleocapsid (27 nm) is enclosed, in turn, by a lipo-protein envelope consisting of cellular lipid and the viral surface antigen (HBsAg). The HBsAg also occurs as subviral 22-nm particles. These particles, shed into the plasma of infected individuals, are immunogenic and have provided the basis for safe and effective "plasma-derived" vaccines (Francis, 1983; Stevens et al., 1984). However, these vaccines, being derived from sera of chronically infected humans, are in limited supply, must be stringently controlled for the presence of other human infectious agents, are consequently expensive, and finally, require a three-dose regimen to establish an acceptable level of immunity. In this context, the enormous efforts expended in recombinant DNA approaches toward a biosynthetic HBV subunit vaccine are warranted.

The HBV surface antigen (S) gene actually encodes three proteins; the major S protein, which lacks pre-S sequences, and two proteins, which are amino-terminal extensions of S possessing either pre-S2 sequences (middle protein) or pre-S1 plus pre-S2 sequences (large protein) (Tiollais et al., 1985). Expression of the HBsAg in E. coli was less successful than anticipated. With one exception (Fujisawa et al., 1985), the resultant product was produced at only low levels, and was either unstable, toxic, or both to the bacteria (Burrell et al., 1979; Edman et al., 1981; Mackay et al., 1981; Fujisawa et al., 1983; Pumpen et al., 1984). However, both yeast and mammalian cell expression systems have been employed successfully for the production of HBsAgs. HBsAg proteins expressed in yeast cells were unglycosylated and found to form intracellular particles similar to, but slightly more heterogeneous in size than, the 22-nm particles found in human carrier plasma. The HBsAg expressed from recombinant vectors in mammalian cells was also assembled into particles. However, these particles contained glycosylated protein, were more uniform in size and morphology, and were secreted.

The first-generation yeast expression systems included only the S gene (Valenzuela et al., 1982; Miyanohara et al., 1983; Murray et al., 1984; McAleer et al., 1984), indicating that assembly into 22-nm-like particles required no other viral gene products. These particles were found to be immunogenic, and are the basis of the first recombinant vaccines (Jilg et al., 1984). Similarly, initial constructs for mammalian cell expression of HBsAg consisted of only the S gene sequences (Dubois et al., 1980; Hirschman et al., 1980; Moriarty et al., 1981; Crowley et al., 1983; Laub et al., 1983; Siddiqui, 1983). However, the pre-S2 region (of the middle protein) was shown to possess a receptor for polymerized human serum albumin (pHSA), which is believed to be important in HBV hepatotropism (Machida *et al.*, 1983), and encompasses epitopes that enhance the immunogenicity of HBsAg (Milich *et al.*, 1985). Furthermore, antibodies to pre-S2 synthetic peptides were protective (Neurath *et al.*, 1986; Itoh *et al.*, 1986a). Thus, more recent constructs in yeast (Valenzuela *et al.*, 1985a; Itoh *et al.*, 1986b) and mammalian cells (Guifang *et al.*, 1984; Michel *et al.*, 1985) have included the pre-S2 region with the S gene, and should yield a product with added protective efficacy. The large protein represents only a minor component of 22-nm particles derived from human plasma, and appears to regulate intracellular compartmentization of HBsAgs and inhibit secretion of HBsAgs in mammalian cells (Persing *et al.*, 1986; McLaughlan *et al.*, 1987; Ou and Rutter, 1987). However, expression in yeast resulted in the formation of the characteristic particles that carry pre-S1, pre-S2, and S protein epitopes, as well as the pHSA receptor (Dehoux *et al.*, 1986). The role of the pre-S1 sequences in the pathogenesis and immunology of HBV is unknown.

The HBcAg may also have a role in a future HBV vaccine. HBcAg has been expressed in *E. coli* (Edman *et al.*, 1981; Stahl *et al.*, 1982) and found to be aggregated into 27-nm particles similar in appearance to authentic viral cores (Cohen and Richmond, 1982). Both bacterially derived and plasma-derived HBcAg have been shown to induce some level of protective immunity (Murray *et al.*, 1984; Iwarson *et al.*, 1985). Expression of HBcAg at extremely high levels (40% of the soluble protein) in yeast has been reported (Kniskern *et al.*, 1986). The product was found assembled in 28-nm particles morphologically indistinguishable from HBcAg particles in human plasma.

2. Foot-and-Mouth Disease and Hepatitis A

Foot-and-mouth disease (FMD) is one of the most economically important diseases of world livestock, and one of the first to be targeted for development of a recombinant DNA vaccine (Bachrach, 1985). Currently, in most parts of the world the disease is controlled by vaccination. Inactivated virus vaccines produced in baby hamster kidney (BHK) cell suspension cultures are effective and inexpensive. However, several disadvantages of these vaccines (refrigeration requirement, difficulty in the cell culture propagation of some strains, safety concerns in production and complete virus inactivation) gave rise to the desire to produce a recombinant vaccine. From the beginning, the viral capsid protein VP1 has been the candidate polypeptide for a subunit FMDV vaccine, stemming from the data of Laporte *et al.* (1973) and Bachrach *et al.* (1975). Enter the cloners, armed with reverse transcriptase and *E. coli* expression vectors, and "magic": "Last week Agriculture Secretary John Block announced that researchers . . . had produced a safe, effective vaccine against the disease" (*Science,* June 29, 1981, p. 5). Block continued: "This breakthrough can mean annual savings of billions of dollars and an increase in the supply of meat" (*Wall Street Journal,* June 19, 1981). Currently, however, there are no recombinant-derived FMDV vaccines on the market.

By 1981, three groups had reported the cDNA cloning of VP1 genes (Boothroyd *et al.,* 1982; Kleid *et al.,* 1981; Kupper *et al.,* 1981). Since then, the VP1 genes from all important virus serotypes have been cloned and expressed in various forms in bacterial systems. Curiously, there are no reports of VP1 expression in yeast or mammalian cells (see, however, chapter by Brown). Most of these bacterially produced polypeptides, but not all (e.g., type O), were reported to be immunogenic and protective (for reviews, see Della-Porta, 1983; Bachrach, 1985). However, the biological activity of these recombinant products was no greater than that of authentic VP1 isolated from virions, both of which were very much less effective than the current inactivated vaccines. For example, two inoculations of 250 μg of an *E. coli*-produced VP1 analogue or 140 μg of authentic VP1 showed protection in cattle (Kleid *et al.,* 1981), while a single inoculation of 1–5 μg of inactivated virus was protective (Brown, 1982). Clearly, features of antigen configuration and presentation are important for picornavirus immunogenicity (see chapter by Hogle and Filman). Quite interestingly, synthetic peptide immunogens of certain defined epitopes on the FMDV VP1 polypeptide were more immunogenic than the intact protein (Bittle *et al.,* 1982; DiMarchi *et al.,* 1982; see Chapter 5). Immunogenic activity was enhanced substantially when two epitopes, one from an internal region and the other from the carboxyl terminus of VP1, were combined. These epitopes, when biosynthetically linked to β-galactosidase and produced in *E. coli,* also showed high protective activity (F. Brown, personal communication, 1987). By constructing β-galactosidase expression vectors consisting of one of these FMDV determinants repeated 1, 2, 4, or 8 times, fusion protein immunogenicity was found to be dependent on the number of repeats (Broekhuijsen *et al.,* 1986). Analogous two-epitope tandem repeat constructs will be interesting to evaluate.

A major complication of FMDV vaccine development relates to the number of viral serotypes associated with the disease. Use of minimal or select epitopes as immunogens will require that individual serotype-specific components be produced and combined in the final product. In contrast to the serotypic complexity of FMDV, the human picornavirus hepatitis A virus (HAV), exhibits little antigenic variation. In fact, HAV possesses a single immunogenic neutralization site located on VP1 (Hughes *et al.*, 1984; Stapleton and Lemon, 1987). Further definition of this determinant, with help from the recently determined nucleotide sequence of HAV (Cohen *et al.*, 1987a,b) may allow the construction of a single, potent, microbially produced immunogen.

3. Herpesvirus Infections

There are numerous herpesvirus infections of both humans and livestock for which effective vaccines are needed. Concern over the oncogenic potential of the viral DNA, and the possibilities for attenuated virus vaccines to establish latent infections or to recombine with non-vaccine strains *in vivo* (Javier *et al.*, 1986), has made the subunit vaccine approach attractive. Vaccine development has centered on the viral glycoproteins, since host immune responses are largely directed toward these (Norrild, 1980; Spear, 1985; Hall and Katrak, 1986; Rager-Zisman *et al.*, 1987). For developing a subunit vaccine, it may be pertinent to understand the role of the individual glycoproteins in the induction of the protective immune response.

Types 1 and 2 HSV (HSV-1, HSV-2) encode five to seven glycoproteins. Three of these, gB, gC, and gD, are considered prime subunit vaccine candidates. Glycoprotein D is of particular interest. Antiserum or monoclonal antibodies prepared to this protein are type-common. They can neutralize both HSV-1 and HSV-2, and are protective against both viruses in mouse passive transfer–challenge experiments. Furthermore, gD purified from virus-infected cells induces protective immunity in mice immunized with this protein. Expression in *E. coli* of both gD1 and gD2 sequences has been reported (Watson *et al.*, 1982, 1984; Weis *et al.*, 1983). Production levels of tripartite (cro–gD1–β-galactosidase) fusion proteins were high (4–10% total cell protein). However, when the β-galactosidase sequences were removed, expression of the resultant cro–gD1 proteins fell dramatically. It was found that the carboxy-terminal transmembrane and anchor sequences of gD1 were deleterious to expression, as well as to *E. coli* growth. Removal of these sequences allowed for increased expression. Interestingly, analogous gD2 constructs possessing the gD2 transmembrane and anchor sequences did not exhibit these inhibitory effects (Steinberg *et al.*, 1986).

The HSV gC1 gene appears to also possess sequences that when expressed in *E. coli* inhibit growth (Amann *et al.*, 1984). However, these sequences were localized to the central region of this glycoprotein. Expression of gC1 sequences in *E. coli* was observed only with constructs employing the tac promoter directing transcription of a tripartite (cI–gC–β-galactosidase) fusion protein (Amann *et al.*, 1984).

Mammalian cell lines have been constructed to express individual HSV glycoproteins. Berman *et al.* (1983) constructed an expression vector in which the entire gD1 coding region was placed under the control of the SV40 early promoter. The plasmid also contained the SV40 dhfr transcription unit for dominant selection in dhfr-deficient CHO cells. Cell lines that resulted from transfection of this plasmid expressed the processed and glycosylated gD protein constitutively on their cell surface. By constructing an analogous expression vector in which the gD gene was truncated by removal of the carboxy-terminal 93 amino acids, these workers found that the resultant cell lines produced a gD protein that was glycosylated and transported to the extracellular medium (Lasky *et al.*, 1984). The carboxy-terminal deletion removed the transmembrane anchor domain. Earlier work with the vesicular stomatitis virus G protein (Rose and Bergman, 1982) and the influenza HA protein (Sveda *et al.*, 1982) demonstrated that removal of such membrane-binding domains resulted in the secretion of these proteins in transient expression systems. Using a similar mammalian cell expression plasmid as described above for gD1, CHO cell lines have been established which express the complete gB1 gene or a truncated version lacking 194 carboxy-terminal amino acids (Pachl *et al.*, 1987). Again, the complete gB1 protein was cell associated, and the truncated polypeptide was secreted. Similar data were reported for mammalian cell expression of gB2 (Stuve *et al.*, 1987). Use of *dhfr* selection in these expression systems allowed for gene copy amplification upon methotrexate selection. In one example, a methotrexate-selected cell line was isolated in which the truncated gB1 gene copy number was amplified 10-fold, and the expression level of gB1 protein had increased 60-fold (Pachl *et al.*, 1987). Comparison of the gB expression level in this cell line with Vero cells lytically infected with HSV-1 indicated that the engineered cell produced about four times more protein in a 48-hr period (the lytic cycle time for HSV-1).

The immunogenicity of these genetically engineered HSV glyco-proteins has been evaluated by several means. The *E. coli*-produced gD1 fusion proteins elicited antibodies in rabbits capable of neutraliz-ing both HSV-1 and HSV-2 infectivity *in vitro* (Weis *et al.*, 1983; Watson *et al.*, 1984), and conferred significant protection against heterologous (HSV-2) challenge in a model system (C. J. Heilman, personal communication, 1987). Similarly, the secreted form of gD1 produced in CHO cells induced neutralizing antibodies to HSV-1 and HSV-2 and was protective in mice against lethal challenge with either virus (Lasky *et al.*, 1984). CHO cell-produced and -secreted gB1 also induced neutralizing antibodies and protected mice against a lethal HSV-1 challenge (Pachl *et al.*, 1987). The CHO cell gD1 and gB1 proteins have been shown to activate, and be recognized by, human T cells (Zarling *et al.*, 1986a). A recent study compared the human immune T-cell and lymphokine responses in individuals with recurrent herpes labialis to inactivated whole virus, purified authentic gD1, gB1, and gC1, purified CHO cell-produced truncated gD1, and purified *E. coli*-produced form of gD1 (Torseth *et al.*, 1987). The results revealed several interesting points. First, both the CHO cell and *E. coli* recombinant proteins induced T-cell transformation to similar levels, suggesting that there was no absolute dependence on protein glycosylation for this response. In both cases, however, the immune responses were lower than those induced by authentic gD. Certain combinations of glycoprotein antigens elicited greater responses than the individual proteins alone. But, in only a few measurements were the responses comparable to those induced by the whole-virus immunogen. These results suggest that additional antigens in the whole-virus preparation contribute significantly to immune-specific T-lymphocyte responses (Torseth *et al.*, 1987).

This leads to the final system to mention for the bioproduction of HSV immunogens: authentic HSV-infected cells. As HSV replicates quite well in cultured cells, this system can serve as a source for any or all of the relevant glycoproteins and may be commercially applicable. Currently, an HSV-2 subunit vaccine consisting of gB, gC, gD, gE, and gG is being tested for immunogenicity and efficacy in humans (Mertz *et al.*, 1984; Ashley *et al.*, 1985, 1987). Preparation of this vaccine involved detergent solubilization of HSV-2-infected chick embryo fibroblasts, clarification, DNase treatment, and glycoprotein purification on lectin affinity columns (Mertz *et al.*, 1984).

Pseudorabies virus (PRV) of swine and bovine herpes virus 1 [BHV-1; infectious bovine rhinotracheitis virus (IBR)] are important pathogens of their respective species. They also replicate quite well in cell culture. Several of the glycoproteins genes of PRV have recently been identified. The genes for glycoproteins gI (Mettenleiter *et al.*, 1985) and gX (Rea *et al.*, 1985) were identified by mRNA hybrid selection–translation approaches. The gene for gp50 was identified through the use of a monoclonal antibody resistant (mar) variant virus and mapped by marker rescue (Wathen and Wathen, 1984). This gene has subsequently been sequenced and shown to be homologous to HSV gD (Petrovskis *et al.*, 1986a). Using "shotgun expression" cloning of the PRV genome into an *E. coli* expression plasmid, Robbins *et al.* (1984, 1986) identified and characterized the glycoprotein gIII gene, which appears to be analogous to HSV gC. The phage expression cloning vector λgt11 was used by Petrovskis *et al.* (1986b) to construct a PRV-phage expression library. They were able to identify the previously mapped gI and gX genes, as well as a new glycoprotein gene encoding gp63. Taking advantage of the homologous sequences between PRV and HSV-1 (Davison and Wilkie, 1983), Robbins *et al.* (1985) identified the PRV gII gene, which is homologous to HSV gB. All of these genes have been sequenced and most have been engineered to expression in *E. coli* systems. The resultant proteins have been used to generate antisera to confirm gene product identification. Certain of these proteins have also been used to evaluate their immunogenicity in swine. The authentic glycoproteins gII, gIII, and gp50, immunoaffinity-purified from PRV-infected swine cells, each were individually protective in swine challenged with virulent PRV. *E. coli*-produced analogs of gII and gIII protected either not at all or poorly; although their combination did confer a significant measure of protection (T. Zamb; D. Reed, personal communications, 1986). Glycoprotein gX has been expressed in *E. coli* as a trpE–gX–β-galactosidase fusion protein (Rea *et al.*, 1985) and in CHO cells (Bennett *et al.*, 1986). However, it appears that the gX protein may not be useful for vaccine purposes (as cited in Thomsen *et al.*, 1987). The gp50 gene has also been expressed in CHO cells (Petrovskis *et al.*, 1986a).

The BHV-1 glycoproteins have been characterized biochemically and immunologically (van Drunen Littel-van den Hurk *et al.*, 1984; van Drunen Littel-van den Hurk and Babiuk, 1985, 1986). Immunoaffinity-purified glycoproteins gI, gIII, and gIV (BHV-1 and PRV glycoprotein nomenclatures are independent; Hampl *et al.*, 1984; van Drunen Littel-van den Hurk and Babiuk, 1986) were used individually or in combinations to immunize calves. Animals immunized with gIV alone or in combination with gI or gII responded with the highest neutralization and antibody-dependent cell cytotoxicity titers. All animals vaccinated with gI, gIII, gIV, or any combination thereof were protected from lethal BHV-1/*P. haemolytica* challenge (van Drunen Littel-van den Hurk *et al.*, 1986; T. Zamb, personal communications, 1986). The BHV-1 genes encoding these glycoproteins have been identified, cloned, sequenced, and expressed in *E. coli* (T. Zamb, personal communication, 1986).

Given the current state of knowledge of the important glycoproteins of BHV-1 and PRV, ongoing and future engineering of their genes in mammalian expression systems will lead to stable cell lines potentially suitable for vaccine bioproduction of appropriate imunogens. However, as may be the case for HSV, useful immunogens may be purified readily from virus-infected cultures using powerful monoclonal antibody affinity columns in a cost-effective manner to yield efficacious "first-generation" vaccines immediately.

Other herpesviruses that replicate more poorly in culture are more urgent targets for the application of genetic engineering. Three such viruses are Epstein-Barr virus (EBV), varicella-zoster virus (VZV), and CMV. The genomes of EBV (Baer et al., 1984) and VZV (Davison and Scott, 1986) have been completely sequenced (172 and 125 kb, respectively). Much work is currently ongoing to define those open reading frames that encode immunologically important proteins. A key immunogen for EBV appears to be the surface glycoprotein gp350. Depending on the method of purification of authentic gp350, Epstein and co-workers found this immunogen to be either highly efficacious or unable to confer protection in a cottontop tamarin lymphomagenic model system (Epstein et al., 1985, 1986). The gene for gp350, and the related glycoprotein gp220 generated by internal slicing of the gp350 transcript, has been mapped and defined (Hummel et al., 1984; Biggin et al., 1984; Beisel et al., 1985). Portions of the gp350 gene have been expressed in E. coli, and the resultant polypeptides were used to generate antisera that possessed virus neutralizing activity (Beisel et al., 1985; Motz et al., 1986). Expression and secretion of gp350 from an unspliced message in yeast have been reported (Schultz et al., 1986). Mammalian cell expression of the gp350 gene also has been carried out. Using a eukaryotic expression plasmid in which the SV40 early promoter controlled gp350 gene transcription and the adenovirus major late promoter directed the dhfr gene, CHO cells were transfected and selected for the dhfr$^+$ phenotype (Motz et al., 1986). Although cells grew very slowly and many died, the stable cell clones that were finally established synthesized only low levels of both gp350 and gp220, localized to the cell membrane. Similar results were reported by Whang et al. (1987) for gp350 expression in a variety of cell types using expression vectors that incorporated either the CMV immediate early, murine leukemia virus long terminal repeat (MuLV LTR), murine mammary tumor virus (MMTV) LTR, metallothionein, or VZV gpI promoters to drive gp350 gene transcription. Apparently, high-level expression of the EBV gp350 protein was toxic to cells. Removal of the 3' membrane anchor sequence in these expression vectors allowed for the secretion of gp350/220 from transfected GH3 cells, but not from CHO or L cells (Whang et al., 1987). A continuous GH3 cell line has been established that produces 2.5–5 mg of gp350/220 per liter of culture fluid (time interval not specified) (Whang *et al.*, 1987). Another EBV glycoprotein gene, identified as being homologous to HSV-1 gB, has been placed into *E. coli* and mammalian cell expression systems. Antisera generated to the *E. coli* fusion protein failed to neutralize virus but did allow further characterization of this antigen (Gong *et al.*, 1987). Clearly there are additional important EBV glycoproteins that remain to be identified.

VZV encodes three major groups of glycoproteins capable of stimulating the development of virus-neutralizing antibodies, and many of the genes for these proteins have been identified (reviewed in Davison and Scott, 1986). The few CMV genes mapped to date are summarized in Jahn *et al.* (1987). However, as more sequencing and homology data accumulate, CMV glycoprotein genes should become available for expression engineering.

4. Acquired Immunodeficiency Syndrome

Efforts to develop safe and efficacious therapies for acquired immunodeficiency syndrome (AIDS) are certainly intense (Fauci, 1986). AIDS is the clinical result of infection by a human lentivirus termed human immunodeficiency virus (HIV; Coffin *et al.*, 1986). The RNA genome of this virus encodes at least six gene products. Most current strategies for the development of an AIDS vaccine are focusing on the viral envelope (*env*) gene and its glycoprotein products. This approach is based largely on analogy to oncovirus protective immunogens. However, serious consideration of the unique features of lentivirus infection and pathogenesis (Haase, 1986) must be taken into account in the development of AIDS vaccines. The primary gene product of *env* is a 160-kD glycoprotein precursor (gp160) that is proteolytically processed to the external glycoprotein gp120 and the transmembrane gp41 protein. It has been shown that purified authentic gp120 can induce virus-neutralizing antibody (Robey *et al.*, 1986), whereas antibodies to gp41 do not influence *in vitro* virus infectivity (Matthews *et al.*, 1986). However, the relevance of *in vitro* neutralizing antibody activity to protective immunity and clinical disease is highly suspect (Fauci, 1986). The HIV envelope glycoproteins (produced by recombinant vaccinia viruses, see chapter by Esposito and Murphy) also stimulate T-cell responses with both helper and cytotoxic activities (Zarling *et al.*, 1986b).

Portions of the HIV *env* gene have been expressed in *E. coli,* yeast, baculovirus–insect, and mammalian cell systems. A large segment of the *env* gene encompassing portions of both gp120 and gp41 was expressed in *E. coli* under the direction of the P_L promoter, yielding an antigenic 68-kD protein as well as several smaller polypeptides believed to be internal initiation products (Crowl *et al.*, 1985). Various portions of the gp120 and gp41 gene sequences were also expressed in *E. coli* by Putney and co-workers (1986), however, the precise nature of their expression system was not disclosed. These workers reported a production level by one construct containing 37% of the coding region of gp120 to be 3 grams of purified protein from 500 grams of *E. coli* cells (compared to 1 mg of purified authentic gp120 obtained from 500 grams of infected cells). These bacterially produced polypeptides elicited antibodies reactive with authentic gp120, however only the construct expressing the carboxy-terminal half of gp120 induced neutralizing antibody activity. The level of activity was similar to that induced by authentic purified gp120 or deglycosylated gp120, suggesting that protein glycosylation was not necessary for the induction of this response (Putney *et al.*, 1986). Portions of the gp120 and gp41 coding regions were expressed in yeast cells under transcriptional control of the GAPDH or PYK promoters, or a regulatable ADH-2/ GAPDH hybrid promoter (Barr *et al.*, 1987b). Expression of a major portion of gp41 was toxic to the cells. However, a small region of gp41 when fused with sequences of human superoxide dismutase (SOD) provided a stable fusion product. Although levels of expression were not mentioned, all of the yeast-produced *env* analog proteins were present in the insoluble fraction of cell lysates. When solubulized, they were antigenic and immunogenic. The HIV envelope gene has been used to construct a recombinant insect virus vector (S-L, Hu, personal communication, 1987). A glycosylated 150-kD protein was produced, as well as immunoreactive polypeptides of 130 kD and 41 kD. These proteins were identified as analogs of the mature gp120 and gp41, suggesting that in this insect cell system, proteolytic processing of the *env* gene product was occurring. Evaluation of the immunogenicity of these envelope glycoprotein analogs is in progress. Mammalian cell lines have been engineered to produce a secreted form of the HIV envelope glycoprotein (Lasky *et al.*, 1986). Using expression vectors similar to those employed for the production of HSV glycoproteins (SV40 early promoter; dhfr selection in CHO cells), these workers found that attempts to express the full-length *env* protein, and even carboxy-terminal truncated versions, resulted in "inefficient expression" (Lasky *et al.*, 1986). To improve expression, they replaced the hydrophobic amino-terminal domain of the HIV *env* gene with the HSV gD signal sequence. The resultant construct contained 25 amino acids of gD and lacked 30 residues of gp160. Expression of this chimera in CHO cells resulted in the synthesis of an unprocessed protein that was localized intracellularly and was not present on the cell surface. Removal of the entire transmembrane region (i.e., gp41) in a subsequent construction allowed for the intracellular production of a 100-kD *env* analog possessing simple glycosylation and the secretion of a 130-kD form with complex *N*-linked carbohydrate. It was estimated that this secreted gp130 was produced by transfected, methotrexate-amplified CHO cells at a level of 1 mg/liter, although no time interval was specified (Lasky *et al.*, 1986). Sera from guinea pigs immunized with gp130 showed virus-neutralizing activity.

The use of the HIV envelope glycoprotein for effective vaccine purposes may be complicated. There is considerable heterogeneity and antigenic variation in the *env* gene among the numerous HIV isolates. Antisera generated to either authentic gp120 or the recombinant gp130 *env* protein neutralized the virus isolate from which the immunogen was obtained, but failed to prevent infection by other HIV isolates (Matthews *et al.*, 1986; Weiss *et al.*, 1986). Certainly multiple gp120 immunogens could be combined to generate a broader-spectrum immune response. However, lentiviruses are known for their envelope gene polymorphism. The progressive antigenic drift of *env* glycoproteins within an infected individual, demonstrated with animal lentivirus infections, raises serious concerns about lentiviral glycoprotein-based vaccines (Stanley *et al.*, 1987). It is known that sera from HIV-infected humans are more cross-neutralizing than anti-glycoprotein antisera, however there appears to be a curious reluctance to consider antibodies to antigens other than the viral glycoprotein as responsible for this broader immune response (Weiss *et al.*, 1986; Matthews *et al.*, 1986). Certainly, sera from AIDS patients contain antibodies to other HIV-encoded polypeptides. Using "shotgun" expression cloning in *E. coli*, Chang *et al.* (1985a,b) showed that patients possessed antibodies not only to *env* sequences, but also to polypeptide sequences specified by the *gag* and *pol* regions. These regions are believed to be more conserved than those of the *env* gene. The *gag* gene encodes a 55-kD precursor which is processed into a 17-kD protein, the core protein p24, and the basic core ribonucleoprotein p15. The *gag* proteins have been generally considered useful for diagnostic purposes. However, quite relevant is the observation that antibodies to *gag* gene product p17 were as effective in their *in vitro* virus-neutralizing activity as sera from AIDS patients (Sarin *et al.*, 1986; Naylor *et al.*, 1987). The p24 region of the *gag* gene has been expressed in *E. coli* under the control of the trp promoter in the absence of any fused bacterial protein sequences to produce a diagnostic reagent (Dowbenko *et al.,* 1985). The entire *gag* region with portions of the 5' end of the *pol* gene have been found to express the *gag* precursor protein in both the baculovirus–insect cell (Madisen *et al.,* 1987) and yeast cell (Kramer *et al.,* 1986) systems. In both situations, the precursor subsequently was processed to yield polypeptides resembling intermediate and mature forms of the *gag* gene products, suggesting that the viral protease activity is encoded within the 5' end of the *pol* gene and is functional in both expression systems. Both this protease and the HIV reverse transcriptase (RT) are considered important targets for therapeutic strategies against AIDS. Most current strategies are chemotherapeutic in nature, however, and not immunoprophylactic. But, at least 80% of HIV-positive individuals possess antibodies to RT (Veronese *et al.,* 1986). The HIV RT has been expressed functionally in both *E. coli* (Tanese *et al.,* 1986; Farmerie *et al.,* 1987) and yeast (Barr *et al.,* 1987a). Correct proteolytic processing in *E. coli* required the *pol* protease sequences and resulted in a striking stabilization of the RT in expressing cells (Farmerie *et al.,* 1987).

IV. Considerations in the Design of Biosynthetic Subunit Vaccines

Molecular cloning and gene expression technologies are well established. Although in specific cases further refinements are needed, the basic systems are available for the identification, characterization, and production of useful vaccine components. Be this as it may, there are several points that deserve emphasis in the rational design of effective biosynthetic subunit vaccines. These considerations are not new, but still represent very important issues for the future of biosynthetic vaccines. Indeed, they have a bearing on the selection and character of immunogens to be expressed, and the choice of the bioproduction system in which to express them.

A. PROTECTIVE IMMUNITY AND NEUTRALIZING ANTIBODY

The essence of any vaccine must be that it is safe and capable of eliciting a protective response in the targeted host. Here, the emphasis is placed on "protection." Depending on the disease situation, this could mean protection from clinical disease or protection from infection by the pathogen, an important destinction in particular cases. And certainly, a criterion for protective efficacy must be established for each disease for which a vaccine is to be developed. The point is that "protection" does not mean, as is often stated or implied, that vaccine constituents are "immunogenic," "antigenic," "immunodominant," or finally, that they elicit "neutralizing antibodies." Protective immunity can be established only by challenge of the vaccinated host for which the vaccine is intended with the respective pathogen under conditions resembling those of the natural infection. The ability to conduct this test varies with each disease situation. Furthermore, host challenge–protection experiments are often carried out at a very late stage in vaccine development. Generally, we rely on laboratory animal disease models to evaluate candidate vaccines during their development. Undoubtedly, many highly efficacious vaccines have been developed for rodents! However, even here, some pathogens lack a model disease system (e.g., leprosy, HIV) in which case evaluation is further compromised. We are frequently aware of these shortcomings, but all too often loose sight of their consequences. Vaccine composition and potency cannot yet be fully predicted from experiments in nonhost animals or from *in vitro* assays.

Obviously, protection of the host from disease may be mediated by any combination of the multiple arms of the immune system. Any rational design of a subunit vaccine requires an appreciation of the relative roles of both antibody-dependent and antibody-independent immune mechanisms in the natural disease, as well as their elicitation by subunit immunogens. What type of immunity is critical to, or required for, protection in the targeted host? And from the vaccine development and testing point of view, what is the desired immunologic end point, and what determinants are required to attain that end point?

Often the value of candidate subunit immunogens is predicted on the basis of *in vitro* assays that measure serum antibody levels in response to vaccination. These include neutralization assays, RIAs, ELISAs, and others. The relevance of these *in vitro* assays with respect to immunity against the natural disease is often unknown. Of major concern here is that reliance on these assays during the course of vaccine development runs the risk of overlooking immunogens that may be very prominent or even critical factors in the elicitation of the protective immune response.

The one assay generally considered the most reliable predictor of an important or relevant immune response *in vivo* involves the measurement of "neutralizing antibody." Correlations between an *in vitro* serum neutralizing activity and animal protection do exist in some systems. These are given substantially more credence if "neutralizing" monoclonal antibodies are able to protect against disease upon passive transfer to animals. In such cases, important determinants for inclusion in a vaccine may be defined.

However, there are other situations in which neutralizing antibody activity and protection from disease bear no apparent relation. Lentivirus infections offer a timely example (Kennedy-Stoskopf and Narayan, 1986). In the case of AIDS, where the desired immunologic response remains unknown, there is no apparent distinction between infected asymptomatic individuals and those with clinical disease with respect to the presence and level of "neutralizing" antibodies (Fauci, 1986). Yet, evaluation of many candidate immunogens in this system is being based on their ability to elicit "neutralizing" antibodies. In more defined circumstances, certain purified proteins, although eliciting significant neutralizing antibody responses in animals, have failed to protect them upon experimental challenge. Examples include VP1 polypeptides of FMDV (Meloen and Barteling, 1986; DiMarchi *et al.*, 1986; D. Moore, personal communication, 1987), cell-associated HSV gB (Blacklaws *et al.*, 1987), EBV gp350 (Epstein *et al.*, 1986), the G1 glycoprotein of Rift Valley fever virus (RVFV; J. Smith and J. Dalrymple, personal communication, 1986). There are even examples of monoclonal antibodies that exhibit high-titer neutralizing activity *in vitro,* but fail to confer protection against challenge on passive transfer (e.g., yellow fever virus, Brandriss *et al.*, 1986; RVFV, J. Smith and J. Dalrymple, personal communication, 1986).

Conversely, protection may be provided in the absence of neutralizing activity. "Nonneutralizing" monoclonal antibodies have been shown to be protective in studies with Sindbis virus (Schmaljohn *et al.*, 1982), Venezuelan equine encephalitis virus (Mathews and Roehrig, 1982), HSV (Balachandran *et al.*, 1982), Semliki Forest virus (Boere *et al.*, 1985), and yellow fever virus (Schlesinger *et al.*, 1985; Brandriss *et al.*, 1986; Gould *et al.*, 1986). Active immunization with purified nonstructural protein NS1 of yellow fever virus (Schlesinger *et al.*, 1985, 1986), and of dengue virus (Schlesinger *et al.*, 1987), provided significant protection against challenge without eliciting any detectable neutralizing antibody. Additional examples exist, but suffice it to say that it is becoming difficult to accept *in vitro* neutralizing antibody data as a credible criterion for the selection of subunit components, or for establishing vaccine potency or predicting efficacy.

B. CELLULAR IMMUNE RESPONSE AND IMMUNOGEN CHOICE

For certain diseases, the importance of cellular immunity in the protective response has long been recognized. For others, it has only recently been appreciated, and for some, remains to be investigated. Quite simply, for any pathogen that exists in a cell-associated form, consideration and evaluation of cell-mediated immune responses are essential to any strategy of vaccine development. However, only recently have the antigen specificities of these responses been investigated. Enlightening prospects for subunit vaccine development have resulted from these studies.

The cytotoxic T lymphocyte (CTL) response to influenza A virus infection has been studied intensely. There appear to be two general populations of anti-influenza CTLs—strain-specific and cross-reactive. The cross-reactive CTLs have been shown to protect against lethal heterotypic challenge (Yap *et al.*, 1978; Lukacher *et al.*, 1984; Taylor and Askonas, 1986). Current influenza vaccines, whether purified hemagglutinin (HA)–neuraminidase (NA) or inactivated whole virus, stimulate primarily strain-specific antibody and helper T-cell responses (Ada *et al.*, 1981), but fail to induce cross-reactive CTLs in mice (Reiss and Schulman, 1980; Webster and Askonas, 1980). Clearly, induction of cross-reactive CTLs could have important implications in improved vaccine design. Recent work in this area has attempted to define the antigen specificity of the anti-influenza virus cross-reactive CTLs. Initial studies employing reassorted influenza A viruses identified subpopulations of CTLs reactive with a polymerase gene product (Bennick *et al.*, 1982), HA (Braciale *et al.*, 1984), and the nucleoprotein (NP) (Townsend and Skehel, 1984). However, this approach was unable to define the cross-reactive T-cell determinants. This question was addressed through the genetic engineering of mouse cell lines to express individual influenza gene products for use as targets in CTL assays. Townsend *et al.* (1984) constructed mammalian cell expression plasmids in which cDNA clones of either the HA gene or the NP gene were placed under the transcriptional control of the SV40 early or HSV *tk* promoters. These plasmids were transfected into mouse L cells, and the resultant cell clones expressing the respective proteins were used as target cells in standard CTL chromium-release experiments. Such studies revealed NP, but not HA, to be the major target for cross-reactive CTLs. Similar results were obtained by Yewdell *et al.* (1985), using an alternative approach to individual gene expression. They inserted the NP gene into vaccinia virus downstream of the 7.5k gene promoter. The recombinant virus was used as a vector to create NP target cells. The T-cell determinants in the NP protein have been defined further to specific amino acids by constructing target cell lines expressing a series of NP deletion polypeptides (Townsend *et al.*, 1985), and using synthetic peptides (Townsend *et al.*, 1986b). Although these results indicate that the NP protein is a major antigen recognized by cross-reactive CTLs, studies continue on the CTL recognition of other virus proteins (Townsend *et al.*, 1986a;

Bennink *et al.*, 1987; Gotch *et al.*, 1987). The importance of the NP protein, from the perspective of a vaccine, has been demonstrated by the ability of purified NP to induce high levels of cross-reactive CTLs (Wraith and Askonas, 1985), and confer substantial protection of mice from a lethal challenge with a heterologous influenza A virus (Wraith *et al.*, 1987). In this regard, it is noteworthy that the NP protein has been expressed to high levels in *E. coli* under P_R promoter control (Jones and Brownlee, 1985), and appears to have assembly properties analogous to the authentic viral protein (Kingsbury *et al.*, 1987).

The antigen specificity for CTLs has also been investigated for respiratory syncytial (RS) virus. Cell-mediated immunity has been implicated in protection against RS virus infection. Most directly, adoptive transfer of RS virus-primed T cells can clear an otherwise persistent RS virus infection in a mouse model system (cited in Bangham *et al.*, 1986). However, the cellular immune response has also been implicated in disease exacerbation (McIntosh and Fishaut, 1980). Therefore, it is important to define both protective and harmful T-cell specificities to RS virus. To investigate the viral antigens recognized by RS virus-specific CTLS, recombinant vaccinia viruses possessing individual RS virus genes were constructed and used to infect either human or mouse cell lines, creating specific target cells for evaluation of either human or murine CTLs (Bangham and McMichael, 1986; Bangham *et al.*, 1986). The results indicated that the viral nucleoprotein (N) and fusion glycoprotein (F) were recognized by CTLs, but not the major viral glycoprotein G or structural protein 1A. The roles (either positive or negative) of these specific CTL activities in RS virus infection remain to be determined.

The antigenic specificities of measles virus-specific CTLs have also been examined. Not only were the surface hemagglutinin and fusion proteins recognized, but the internal viral antigens (nucleocapsid and membrane proteins) also elicited a strong CTL response (Jacobson *et al.*, 1987). As a final example, the nucleocapsid protein of VSV also serves as a major target for cross-reactive anti-VSV CTLs (Yewdell *et al.*, 1986).

What becomes apparent from the above examples is that important immunologic determinants may reside on components other than "surface" antigens of the pathogen. Nonstructural proteins and non-glycosylated "internal" proteins may be involved in the cellular and protective immune response. This revelation offers exciting potential for biosynthetic subunit vaccines. By their very nature, these proteins would be expected to be less heterogeneous, or more highly conserved, among pathogen serotypes, as compared to surface antigens. Incorporation of these proteins, or select determinants thereof, into subunit vaccines may result in a more broadly protective (cross-reactive or group-specific) immunogen. These considerations also suggest that the failure to include these nonstructural and internal antigens in subunit vaccines may, in part, explain the often observed reduced immunogenic potency of such vaccines. The clear indication is that efficacious subunit vaccines should be composed of multiple components selected so as to elicit a broad-based immunologic response, and that these components not be limited to traditional "surface antigens".

C. NEGATIVE IMMUNOLOGIC REACTIONS

In addition to assessments of positive immune responses elicited by candidate subunits, one must consider also potential negative immunologic reactions that may be evoked by the immunogens. "A good vaccine should cause no harm." The killed RS virus vaccine of the 1960s tended to exacerbate the disease on subsequent exposure to natural infection (Kim *et al.*, 1969). Administration of killed virus vaccine followed by virus challenge enhanced tissue damage in Aleutian disease virus infection of mink (Porter *et al.*, 1972), bluetongue virus disease of cattle (Stott *et al.*, 1984), and caprine arthritis–encephalitis virus-induced arthritis in goats (McGuire *et al.*, 1986). Mechanistic explanations for these observations remain obscure. However, the concept that immune responses to certain components of a pathogen can potentiate infection or disease bears consideration.

The idea that antiviral antibodies might potentiate viral infection and disease stems largely from observations of dengue virus infection in man (Halstead, 1970). Antibody-dependent enhancement (ADE) of infection has been observed either *in vitro* or *in vivo* with members from at least four different RNA and two different DNA virus families (Halstead, 1982; Porterfield, 1982) and with malaria (cited in L. H. Miller *et al.*, 1986). Efforts to identify antigenic and immunoreactive viral determinants mediating ADE are making use of monoclonal antibodies. Generally, enhancement is associated with antibodies that react with the surface of the virus, but can occur independently of phenomena such as neutralization and hemagglutation inhibition. However, examples of ADE exist in which monoclonal antibodies to nonenvelope components potentiate infection (Legrain *et al.*, 1986; Morens *et al.*, 1987). Although more critical information is required for the understanding of this complicated phenomenon before genetic engineers can delete enhancement determinants from their subunit vaccines, an awareness is encouraged; particularly in cases in which

Fc receptor-bearing cells are permissive for virus replication and may also serve as reservoirs for chronic, persistent, or latent infection (e.g., HIV, bovine viral diarrhea virus).

Vaccine subunit components should not evoke autoimmune responses. This problem is exemplified classically in attempts to develop streptococcal vaccines, discussed previously. If an autoimmune response were directed toward components of the immune system, immunosuppression might result. This potential has been suggested in the case of HIV. As discussed earlier, a vaccine directed against the *gag* proteins might overcome the problem of genetic drift of the viral envelope determinants. However, antibodies to a region of homology between HIV p17 and thymosin $\alpha 1$, although virus-neutralizing, might initiate an autoimmune process leading to inactivation of the hormone or damage to the hormone-producing cells of the thymus (Sarin *et al.*, 1986). Similarly, an immune response to the sequence homology noted between the HIV *env* gp41 protein and interleukin 2 (IL-2) might itself be immunosuppressive (Reiher *et al.*, 1986; Weigent *et al.*, 1986). Additional concerns of *env*-mediated autoimmune responses from vaccination or post-infection immunization have been voiced (Bicker, 1986; Ellrodt and Le Bras, 1987).

Additional immunologic phenomena for consideration in subunit vaccine design, include the potential for an immunogen to: (1) generate "blocking antibodies" (Massey and Schochetman, 1981); (2) include or expose "suppressor determinants" (Turkin and Sercarz, 1977; Jennings *et al.*, 1987); and (3) elicit restricted responses that promote the generation of "escape variants."

D. Immunogen Form and Presentation

The above dissertation alludes to the selection the proper immunogenic determinants, and the exclusion of deleterious ones, for subunit vaccines. However, without question, even the "correct" subunit determinants, in isolated form, differ significantly from those represented in the intact pathogen. This difference may be extended further when the immunogens are produced in a heterologous cell expression system. Therefore, it is not unexpected that the immunologic properties of subunit components differ from those of the whole agent. Unfortunately, the difference is usually that of reduced immunogenic potency. And even if the correct determinants have been identified and produced in unlimited quantities in engineered bioproduction systems, the age-old maxim remains: The efficiency of immunization depends on the correct *presentation* to the immune system of the correct immunologic determinants. The concepts of immunogen form, context, and presentation are not new. Examples of the importance of the physical form of immunogens relevant to bacterial and viral vaccines are numerous, and many were reviewed some time ago (Neurath and Rubin, 1971). "The ideas outlined here may comfort those who have not succeeded in producing 'subunit' vaccines effective against a given viral disease, since they offer an explanation for the failure and, perhaps, also a way to achieve future success" (Neurath and Rubin, 1971). Exploring the means by which the various bioproduction systems may be engineered to yield expressed antigens of higher-order structure and the impact this may have on their immunogenic potency remain important areas for investigation in the future of biosynthetic subunit vaccines.

Thus may be attributed the success of two vaccines discussed earlier. Expression of pilin protein of the fastidious *B. nodosus* in *E. coli* yielded abundant quantities of monomeric subunits. However, the requirement of pilus structural integrity for elicitation of protective immunity had been established earlier (Emery *et al.*, 1984), and bioproduction at any expression level of this pilus protein in *E. coli* would be futile for vaccine purposes. Solution was found in a host cell system (*P. aeurginosa*) that was capable of assembling into pili the *B. nodosus* pilin monomers.

An important feature contributing to the success of the recombinant HBV vaccine work lies in the inherent propensity of the expressed viral proteins to assemble into stable, highly immunogenic structures. Indeed, the immunogenicity of HBV 22-nm particles is dependent on the association of the HBsAgs; dissociated HBsAgs were 1000-fold less immunogenic (Cabral *et al.*, 1978). Critical disulfide bridges between the proteins are required for antigenicity, pHSA receptor activity, and the ability to evoke a virus-neutralizing response (Waters *et al.*, 1986).

Due to the auto-assembly characteristic and resultant immunogenic success of the recombinant-produced HBV antigens, attempts have been made to exploit this system for the presentation of other viral antigens. As the pre-S2 region is exposed on the surface of particles (pHSA receptor), but is not required for particle assembly, Valenzuela and co-workers (1985b) chose this region for the insertion of a portion of the HSV gD1 gene. Sequences encoding 300 of the 369 amino acids of the mature gD protein were inserted in phase into the pre-S2 region of their yeast HBsAg expression vector. They found yeast cells expressing this gene fusion assembled the hybrid antigen into particles very similar in size and shape to those previously observed with HBsAg. Unfortunately, immunogenicity data were not reported. Delpeyroux *et al.* (1986) chose a slightly different tack in that they inserted a synthetic DNA fragment encoding a 13-amino-acid poliovirus neutralization epitope into the S gene of an HBV mammalian cell expression vector. They found that transfected mammalian cells expressing the modified S gene secreted hybrid particles closely resembling authentic 22-nm HBsAg particles. However, mice immunized with these HBs-polio-Ag particles responded only weekly to HBsAg and produced only low-titer poliovirus neutralizing antibodies.

Isolated parvovirus capsid proteins (Molitor *et al.*, 1983), or bacterially produced analogs (author's unpublished data) are capable of eliciting neutralizing antibodies, but do so much less efficiently than do intact whole virus particles or empty capsids. The engineered expression of parvovirus structural protein genes in mammalian cells, employing BPV-derived plasmid vectors, resulted in the production of spontaneously self-assembled empty capsid-like particles (Pintel *et al.*, 1984; T. Miller; C. Parrish, personal communications, 1986). Evaluation of the immunogenicity of these particles is underway.

Apparently, as in the examples above (HBV, parvovirus), assembly can on occasion occur in the absence of other viral gene products or the viral genome. In other situations, proteolytic processing by a virus-specific protease may be required to generate multiple mature subunits necessary for auto-morphogenesis. In this context, it is relevant that the *gag* gene protease of Rous sarcoma virus expressed in *E. coli* (Mermer *et al.*, 1983), and of HIV expressed in *E. coli* (Farmerie *et al.*, 1987), yeast (Kramer *et al.*, 1986), and baculovirus (Madisen *et al.*, 1987) systems, are functional. Expression of the poliovirus (Hanecak *et al.*, 1984) and FMDV (Klump *et al.*, 1984) protease gene in *E. coli* also yielded active enzymes. Naturally, all of these viral proteases are functional when expressed in mammalian cells. The idea here is that appropriate choice and manipulation of the expression (vector–host cell) system may allow for the bioproduction of assembled, stable, and highly immunogenic structures. It is essential that efforts in this area be pursued.

In certain situations, post-production assembly of structural immunogens may be applicable for creating more highly immunogenic materials. For example, the VP1 capsid protein of the polyoma papovavirus has been expressed at high levels under the control of the tac promoter in *E. coli* (Leavitt *et al.*, 1985). The purified protein was found to be present as a pentamer, and could readily associate to form capsid-like structures simply by adjustment of ionic strength (Salunke *et al.*, 1986).

In the case of enveloped virus glycoprotein immunogens, aggregated forms of these amphiphilic antigens, either as protein micelles, liposo-mal complexes (virosomes), or "immunostimulating complexes" (is-coms) have been shown to be much more immunogenic than mono-meric forms (Rouse, 1982; Morein and Simons, 1985; Mougin et al., 1987). In fact, immunization with glycoprotein monomers may have an immunosuppressive effect (Morein et al., 1983).

E. ADJUVANTS AND DELIVERY TECHNOLOGY

Two final considerations for the future of biosynthetic subunit vaccines are merely mentioned here: the development of useful, potent adjuvants and the advancement of vaccine delivery technologies. Some propose that the greatest advance in biosynthetic subunit vaccines will come from the development of a safe, effective adjuvant, and that this may be as important as the choice of the immunizing antigens. Of particular interest here will be engineering the coupled bioproduction of immunogen and immunopotentiating components. Although fre-quently stated as an important and required parameter of protective immunity in most bacterial and viral diseases, mucosal immunity is often neglected during subunit immunogen development. Greater consideration (e.g., measurement) of this critical immune response and development of mechanisms for the delivery of appropriate immuno-gens to sites that will elicit strong secretory immune responses must be incorporated into biosynthetic subunit vaccine strategies.

In conclusion, the infant field of modern biosynthetic vaccine devel-opment has already evolved through several phases. First came molecular cloning and expression systems for gene identification and protein mass production. This was followed by a humble appreciation for the complexities of protein immunogenicity and the vivid reminder of the importance of antigen quality, not quantity. Currently, defini-tion of host protective immune responses, the antigen specificities involved, and immunogen form and presentation are paramount. The new technologies have not allowed us to circumvent the need for detailed basic understanding of microbial pathogenesis and immunol-ogy. In fact, they have served to accentuate the complexities involved. And yet they have also provided the genetic engineer and immunolo-gist the methodologies, heretofore lacking, to analyze and dissect these areas. As progress in the definition of "good" and "bad" immunogenic determinants continues, and their presentation requirements are elucidated in the context of the "protective" response, modern vaccinol-ogists will be able more fully to exploit the current expression systems for the efficient bioproduction of unquestionably safe *and* highly efficacious vaccines.

ACKNOWLEDGMENTS

I would like to thank the handful of colleagues who responded to my inquires. The comments, suggestions, and efforts in the review of this work by Paul Anderson and Joel M. Dalrymple are greatly appreciated and respected. Expert manuscript preparation by Kit Wojcik and Sherri Pierson is acknowledged.

REFERENCES

Ada, G. L., Leung, K. -N., and Ertl, H. (1981). *Immunol. Rev.* **58,** 5–24.

Allshire, R. C., and Bostock, C. J. (1986). *Virus Res.* **6,** 141–154.

Amann, E., Brosius, J., and Ptashne, M. (1983). *Gene* **25,** 167–178.

Amann, E., Broker, M., and Wurm, F. (1984). *Gene* **32,** 203–215.

Anderson, B. J., Bills, M. M., Egerton, J. R., and Mattick, J. S. (1984). *J. Bacteriol* **160,** 748–754.

Arciniega, J. L., Burns, D. L., Garcia-Ortigoza, E., and Manclark, C. R. (1987). *Infect. Immun.* **55,** 1132–1136.

Ashley, R., Mertz, G., Clark, H., Schick, M., Salter, D., and Corey, L. (1985). *J. Virol.* **56,** 475–481.

Ashley, R., Mertz, G., and Corey, L. (1987). *J. Virol.* **61,** 264–268.

Bacchetti, S., and Graham, F. L. (1977). *Proc. Natl. Acad. Sci. U. S. A.* **74,** 1590–1594.

Bachrach, H. L. (1985). *Adv. Vet. Sci. Comp. Med.* **30,** 1–38.

Bachrach, H. L., Moore, D. M., McKercher, P. D., and Polatnick, J. (1975). *J. Immunol.* **115,** 1636–1641.

Baer, R., Bankier, A. T., Biggin, M. D., Deininger, P. L., Farrell, P. J., Gibson, T. J., Hatfull, G., Hudson, G. S., Stachwell, S. C., Seguin, C., Tuffnell, P. S., and Barrell, B. G. (1984). *Nature (London)* **310,** 207–211.

Bagdasarian, M. M., Lurz, R., Ruckert, B., Franklin, F. C. H., Bagdasarian, M. M., Frey, J., and Timmis, K. N. (1981). *Gene* **16,** 237–247.

Bagdasarian, M. M., Amann, E., Lurz, R., Ruckert, B., and Bagdasarian, M. (1983). *Gene* **26,** 273–282.

Balachandran, N., Bacchetti, S., and Rawls, W. E. (1982). *Infect. Immun.* **37,** 1132–1137.

Bangham, C. R. M., and McMichael, A. J. (1986). *Proc. Natl. Acad. Sci. U. S. A.* **83,** 9183–9187.

Bangham, C. R. M., Openshaw, P. J. M., Ball, L. A., King, A. M. Q., Wertz, G. W., and Askonas, B. A. (1986). *J. Immunol.* **137,** 3973–3977.

Barbieri, J. T., Rappuoli, R., and Collier, R. J. (1987). *Infect. Immun.* **55,** 1321–1323.

Barr, P. J., Power, M. D., Lee-Ng, C. T., Gibson, H. L., and Luciw, P. A. (1987a). *Bio/Technology* **5,** 486–489.

Barr, P. J., Steimer, K., Sabin, E., Parkes, D., George-Nascimento, C., Stephens, J., Powers, M., Gyenes, A., Van Nest, G., Miller, E., Higgins, K., and Luciw, P. (1987b). *Vaccine* **5,** 90–101.

Barrett, A. D. T., and Gould, E. A. (1986). *J. Gen. Virol.* **67,** 2539–2542.

Beachey, E. H., Tartar, A., Seyer, J. M., and Chédid, L. (1984). *Proc. Natl. Acad. Sci. U. S. A.* **81,** 2203–2207.

Beef (1985). October, p. 51.

Beisel, C., Tanner, J., Matsuo, T., Thorley-Lawson, D., Kezdy, F., and Kieff, E. (1985). *J. Virol.* **54,** 665–674.

Bennett, L. M., Timmins, J. G., Thomsen, D. R., and Post, L. E. (1986). *Virology* **155,** 707–715.

Bennink, J. R., Yewdell, J. W., and Gerhard, W. (1982). *Nature (London)* **296,** 75–76.

Bennink, J. R., Yewdell, J. W., Smith, G. L., and Moss, B. (1987). *J. Virol.* **61**, 1098–1102.

Berkner, K. L., Schaffhausen, B. S., Roberts, T. M., and Sharp, P. A. (1987). *J. Virol.* **61**, 1213–1220.

Berman, P. W., Dowbenko, D., Lasky, L. A., and Simonsen, C. C. (1983). *Science* **222**, 524–527.

Bernard, H. U., Krammer, G., and Rowekamp, W. G. (1985). *Exp. Cell Res.* **158**, 237–243.

Bicker, U. (1986). *Nature (London)* **324**, 307.

Biggin, M., Farrell, P., and Barrell, B. (1984). *EMBO J.* **3**, 1083–1090.

Bittle, J. L., Houghten, R. A., Alexander, H., Shinnick, T. M., Sutcliffe, J. G., Lerner, R. A., Rowlands, D. J., and Brown, F. (1982). *Nature (London)* **298**, 30–33.

Blacklaws, B. A., Nash, A. A., and Darby, G. (1987). *J. Gen. Virol.* **68**, 1103–1114.

Blake, M. S., and Gotschlich, E. C. (1983). *Prog. Allergy* **33**, 298–313.

Boere, W. A. M., Benaissa-Trouw, B. J., Harmsen, N. T., Erich, T., Kraaijeveld, C. A., and Snippe, H. (1985). *J. Virol.* **54**, 546–5551.

Boothroyd, J. C., Harris, T. J. R., Rowlands, D. J., and Lowe, P. A. (1982). *Gene* **17**, 153–161.

Boshart, M., Weber, F., Jahn, G., Dorsch-Hasler, K., Fleckenstein, B., and Schaffner, W. (1985). *Cell (Cambridge, Mass.)* **41**, 521–530.

Braciale, T. J., Braciale, V. L., Henkel, T. J., Sambrook, J., and Gething, M. J. (1984). *J. Exp. Med.* **159**, 341–354.

Brandriss, M. W., Schlesinger, J. J., Walsh, E. E., and Briselli, M. (1986). *J. Gen. Virol.* **67**, 229–234.

Broekhuijsen, M. P., Blom, T., van Rijn, J., Pouwels, P. H., Klasen, E. A., Fasbender, M. J., and Enger-Valk, B. E. (1986). *Gene* **49**, 189–197.

Brown, D. R., and Parker, C. D. (1987). *Infect. Immun.* **55**, 154–161.

Brown, F. (1982). *In* "Viral Diseases in South-East Asia and the Western Pacific" (J. S. Mackenzie, ed.), pp. 628–633. Academic Press, Sydney, Australia.

Buchanan, T. M., Nomaguchi, H., Anderson, D. C., Young, R. A., Gillis, T. P., Britton, W. J., Ivanyi, J., Kolk, A. H. J., Closs, O., Bloom, B., and Mehra, V. (1987). *Infect. Immun.* **55**, 1000–1003.

Buell, G. N., and Panayotatos, N. (1986). *In* "Maximizing Gene Expression" (W. Reznikoff and L. Gold, eds.), pp. 345–364. Butterworth, Boston, Massachusetts.

Buell, G. N., Schulz, M. F., Selzer, G., Chollet, A., Movva, N. R., Semon, D., Escanez, S., and Kawashima, E. (1985). *Nucleic Acids Res.* **13**, 1923–1938.

Burrell, C. J., Mackay, P., Greenway, P. J., Hofschneider, P. H., and Murray, K. (1979). *Nature (London)* **279**, 43–47.

Butters, T. D., Hughes, R. C., and Vischer, P. (1981). *Biochim. Biophys. Acta* **640**, 672–686.

Cabral, G. A., Marciano-Cabral, F., Funk, G. A., Sanchez, Y., Hollinger, F. B., Melnick, J. L., and Dreesman, G. R. (1978). *J. Gen. Virol.* **38**, 339–350.

Cartier, M., Chang, M., and Stanners, C. P. (1987). *Mol. Cell. Biol.* **7**, 1623–1628.

Cepko, C. L., Roberts, B. E., and Mulligan, R. C. (1984). *Cell (Cambridge, Mass.)* **37**, 1053–1062.

Chang, N. T., Chanda, P. K., Barone, A. D., McKinney, S., Rhodes, D. P., Tam, S. H., Shearman, C. W., Huang, J., Chang, T. W., Gallo, R. C., and Wong-Staal, F. (1985a). *Science* **228**, 93–96.

Chang, N. T., Huang, J., Ghrayeb, J., McKinney, S., Chanda, P. K., Chang, T. W., Putney, S., Sarngadharan, M. G., Wong-Staal, F., and Gallo, R. C. (1985b). *Nature (London)* **315**, 151–154.

Cheers, C. (1983). *Dev. Biol. Stand.* **56**, 237–246.

Clark-Curtiss, J., Jacobs, W. R., Docherty, M. A., Ritchie, L. R., and Curtiss, R. (1985). *J. Bacteriol.* **161**, 1093–1102.

Coffin, J., Haase, A. T., Levy, J. A., Montagnier, L., Oroszlan, S., Teich, N., Temin, H., Toyoshima, K., Varmus, J., Vogt, P., and Weiss, R. (1986). *Science* **232**, 697.

Cohen, B. J., and Richmond, J. E. (1982). *Nature (London)* **296**, 677–678.

Cohen, J. I., Ticehurst, J. R., Purcell, R. H., Buckler-White, A., and Baroudy, B. M. (1987a). *J. Virol.* **61**, 50–59.

Cohen, J. I., Rosenblum, B., Ticehurst, J. R., Daemer, R. J., Feinston, S. M., and Purcell, R. H. (1987b). *Proc. Natl. Acad. Sci. U. S. A.* **84**, 2497–2501.

Colbere-Garapin, F., Horodniceanu, F., Kourilsky, P., and Garapin, A. C. (1981). *J. Mol. Biol.* **150**, 1–14.

Collins, F. M. (1984). *In* "Bacterial Vaccines" (R. Germanier, ed.), pp. 373–417. Academic Press, New York.

Cregg, J. M., Tschopp, J. F., Stillman, C., Siegel, R., Akong, M., Craig, W. S., Buckholz, R. G., Madden, K. R., Kellaris, P. A., Davis, G. R., Smiley, B. L., Cruze, J., Torregrossa, R., Velicelebi, G., and Thill, G. P. (1987). *Bio/Technology* **5**, 479–485.

Crowl, R., Ganguly, K., Gordon, M., Conroy, R., Schaber, M., Kramer, R., Shaw, G., Wong-Staal, F., and Reddy, E. P. (1985). *Cell (Cambridge, Mass.)* **41**, 979–986.

Crowley, C. W., Liu, C. -C., and Levinson, A. D. (1983). *Mol. Cell. Biol.* **3**, 44–55.

Dale, J. B., and Beachey, E. H. (1982). *J. Exp. Med.* **156**, 1165–1176.

Dallas, W. S., and Falkow, S. (1980). *Nature (London)* **288**, 499–500.

Dallas, W. S., Ray, P. H., Leong, J., Benedict, C. D., Stamm, L. V., and Bassford, P. J. (1987). *Infect. Immun.* **55**, 1106–1115.

Das, R. C., and Schultz, J. L. (1987). *Biotechnol. Prog.* **3**, 43–48.

Davidson, D., and Hassell, J. A. (1987). *J. Virol.* **61**, 1226–1239.

Davison, A. J., and Scott, J. E. (1986). *J. Gen. Virol.* **67**, 1759–1816.

Davison, A. J., and Wilkie, N. M. (1983). *J. Gen. Virol.* **64**, 1927–1942.

deBoer, H. A., and Kastelein, R. A. (1986). *In* "Maximizing Gene Expression" (W. Reznikoff and L. Gold, eds.), pp. 225–286. Butterworth, Boston, Massachusetts.

deBoer, H. A., Comstock, L. J., and Vasser, M. (1983). *Proc. Natl. Acad. Sci. U. S. A.* **80**, 21–25.

de Graaf, F. K., Wientjes, F. B., and Klaasen-Boor, P. (1980). *Infect. Immun.* **27**, 216–221.

Dehoux, P., Ribes, V., Sobczak, E., and Streeck, R. E. (1986). *Gene* **48**, 155–163.

Della-Porta, A. J. (1983). *Aust. Vet. J.* **60**, 129–135.

Delpeyroux, F., Chenciner, N., Lim, A., Malpiece, Y., Blondel, B., Crainic, R., van der Werf, S., and Streeck, R. E. (1986). *Science* **223**, 472–475.

Deuschle, U., Kammerer, W., Gentz, R., and Bujard, H. (1986). *EMBO J.* **5**, 2987–2994.

DiMarchi, R., Brooke, G., Gale, C., Cracknell, V., Doel T., and Mowat, N. (1986). *Science* **232**, 639–641.

Donkersloot, J. A., Cisar, J. O., Wax, M. E., Harr, R. J., and Chassy, B. M. (1985). *J. Bacteriol.* **162**, 1075–1078.

Dorner, F., and McDonel, J. L. (1985). *Vaccine* **3**, 94–102.

Dowbenko, D. J., Bell, J. R., Benton, C. V., Groopman, J. E., Nguyen, H., Vetterlein, D., Capon, D., and Lasky, L. A. (1985). *Proc. Natl. Acad. Sci. U. S. A.* **82**, 7748–7752.

Dreano, M., Brochot, J., Myers, A., Cheng-Meyer, C., Rungger, D., Voellmy, R., and Bromley, P. (1986). *Gene* **49**, 1–8.

Dubois, M. -F., Pourcel, C., Rousset, S., Chany, C., and Tiollais, P. (1980). *Proc. Natl. Acad. Sci. U. S. A.* **77**, 4549–4553.

Dubray, G., and Bezard, G. (1980). *Ann. Rech. Vet.* **11**, 367–373.

Edman, J. C., Hallewell, R., Valenzuela, P., Goodman, H. M., and Rutter, W. J. (1981). *Nature (London)* **291**, 503–506.

Elder, J. T., Spritz, R. A., and Weissman, S. M. (1981). *Annu. Rev. Genet.* **15**, 295–340.

Elleman, T. C., Hoyne, P. A., Emery, D. L., Stewart, D. J., and Clark, B. L. (1984). *FEBS Lett.* **173**, 103–107.

Elleman, T. C., Hoyne, P. A., Emery, D. L., Stewart, D. J., and Clark, B. L. (1986a). *Infect. Immun.* **51**, 187–192.

Elleman, T. C., Hoyne, P. A., McKern, N. M., and Stewart, D. J. (1986b). *J. Bacteriol.* **167**, 234–250.

Elleman, T. C., Hoyne, P. A., Stewart, D. J., McKern, N. M., and Peterson, J. E. (1986c). *J. Bacteriol.* **168**, 574–580.

Ellrodt, A., and Le Bras, P. (1987). *Nature (London)* **325**, 765.

Emery, D. L., Stewart, D. J., and Clark, B. L. (1984). *Aust. Vet. J.* **61**, 237–238.

Emmrich, F., and Kaufman, S. H. E. (1986). *Infect. Immun.* **51**, 879–883.

Emmrich, F., Thole, J., Van Embden, J., and Kaufman, S. H. E. (1986). *J. Exp. Med.* **163**, 1024–1029.

Enger, H. D., Bloom, B. R., Mehra, V., Britton, W., Buchanan, T. M., Khanolkar, S. K., Young, D. B., Closs, O., Gillis, T., Harboe, M., Ivanyi, J., Kolk, A. H. J., and Shepard, C. C. (1985). *Infect. Immun.* **48**, 603–605.

Epstein, M. A., Morgan, A. J., Finerty, S., Randle, B. J., and Kirkwood, J. K. (1985). *Nature (London)* **318**, 287–289.

Epstein, M. A., Randle, B. J., Finerty, S., and Kirkwood, J. K. (1986). *Clin. Exp. Immunol.* **63**, 485–490.

Ernst, J. F. (1986). *DNA* **5**, 483–491.

Farmerie, W. G., Loeb, D. D., Casavant, N. C., Hutchison, C. A., Edgell, M. H., and Swanstrom, R. (1987). *Science* **236**, 305–308.

Fauci, A. S. (1986). *Proc. Natl. Acad. Sci. U. S. A.* **83**, 9278–9283.

Fehniger, T. E., Walfield, A. M., Cunningham, T. M., Radoff, J. D., Miller, J. N., and Lovett, M. A. (1984). *Infect. Immun.* **46**, 598–607.

Fehniger, T. E., Radolf, J. D., and Lovett, M. A. (1986). *J. Bacteriol.* **165**, 732–739.

Fives-Taylor, P. M., Macrina, F. L., Pritchard, T. J., and Peene, S. S. (1987). *Infect. Immun.* **55**, 123–128.

Foecking, M. K., and Hofstetter, H. (1986). *Gene* **45**, 101–105.

Fox, J. L. (1987a). *ASM News* **53**, 80–81.

Fox, J. L. (1987b). *ASM News* **53**, 134–137.

Francis, D. P. (1983). *Infect. Dis. Rev.* **5**, 322–335.

Franzon, V. L., and Manning, P. A. (1986). *Infect. Immun.* **52**, 279–284.

Friesen, P. D., and Miller, L. K. (1985). *J. Virol.* **54**, 392–400.

Fujisawa, Y., Ito, Y., Sasada, R., Ono, Y., Igarashi, K., Marumoto, R., Kikuchi, M., and Sugino, Y. (1983). *Nucleic Acids Res.* **11**, 3581–3591.

Fujisawa, Y., Ito, Y., Ikeyama, S., and Kikuchi, M. (1985). *Gene* **40**, 23–29.

Gentz, R., Langner, A., Chang, A. C. Y., Cohen, S. N., and Bujard, H. (1981). *Proc. Natl. Acad. Sci. U. S. A.* **78**, 4936–4940.

Germanier, R., ed. (1984). "Bacterial Vaccines." Academic Press, New York.

Gluzman, Y. (1981). *Cell (Cambridge, Mass.)* **23**, 175–182.

Gluzman, Y. (1982). "Eukaryotic Viral Vectors." Cold Spring Harbor Lab., Cold Spring Harbor, New York.

Goff, S. A., and Goldberg, A. L. (1985). *Cell (Cambridge, Mass.)* **41**, 587–595.

Goldberg, A. L., and Goff, S. A. (1986). *In* "Maximizing Gene Expression" (W. Reznikoff and L. Gold, eds.), pp. 287–314. Butterworth, Boston, Massachusetts.

Gong, M., Ooka, T., Matsuo, T., and Kieff, E. (1987). *J. Virol.* **61,** 499–508.

Gotch, F., Rothbard, J., Howland, K., Townsend, A., and McMichael, A. (1987). *Nature (London)* **326,** 881–882.

Gotschlich, E. C. (1984). *In* "Bacterial Vaccines" (R. Germanier, ed.), pp. 353–371. Academic Press, New York.

Gould, E. A., Buckley, A., Barrett, D. T., and Cammack, N. (1986). *J. Gen. Virol.* **67,** 591–595.

Guarente, L., Lauer, G., Roberts, T. M., and Ptashne, M. (1980). *Cell (Cambridge, Mass.)* **20,** 543–553.

Guifang, R., Li, R., Yiming, Z., Lihua, P., Yanxiang, X., Chun, Z., and Jiming, Z. (1984). *Acta Microbiol. Sin. (Engl. Transl.)* **24,** 326–334.

Haase, A. T. (1986). *Nature (London)* **322,** 130–136.

Hall, M. J., and Katrak, K. (1986). *Vaccine* **4,** 138–150.

Halstead, S. B. (1970). *Yale J. Biol. Med.* **42,** 350–362.

Halstead, S. B. (1982). *Prog. Allergy* **31,** 301–364.

Halstead, S. B., Venkateshan, C. N., Gentry, M. K., and Larsen, L. K. (1984). *J. Immunol.* **132,** 1529–1532.

Halter, R., Pohlner, J., and Meyer, T. F. (1984). *EMBO J.* **3,** 1595–1601.

Hambleton, P., Carman, J. A., and Melling, J. (1984). *Vaccine* **2,** 125–132.

Hamer, D. H., and Walling, M. J. (1982). *J. Mol. Appl. Genet.* **1,** 273–288.

Hampl, H., Ben-Porat, T., Enrlicher, L., Habermechl, K. -O., and Kaplan, A. S. (1984). *J. Virol.* **52,** 583–590.

Hanecak, R., Semler, B. L., Ariga, H., Anderson, C. W., and Wimmer, E. (1984). *Cell (Cambridge, Mass.)* **37,** 1063–1073.

Hansen, E. B., Pedersen, P. E., Schouls, L. M., Severin, E., and van Embden, J. D. A. (1985). *J. Bacteriol.* **162,** 1227–1237.

Hardy, K., Stahl, S., and Kupper, H. (1981). *Nature (London)* **293,** 481–483.

Hirschman, S. Z., Price, P., Garfinkel, E., Christman, J., and Acs, G. (1980). *Proc. Natl. Acad. Sci. U. S. A.* **77,** 5507–5511.

Hollingshead, S. K., Fischetti, V. A., and Scott, J. R. (1986). *J. Biol. Chem.* **261,** 1677–1686.

Holmgren, J. (1981). *Nature (London)* **292,** 413–417.

Holt, R. G., Abiko, Y., Saito, S., Smorawinska, M., Hansen, J. B., and Curtiss, R. (1982). *Infect. Immun.* **38,** 147–156.

Honjo, M., Akaoka, A., Nakayama, A., Shimada, H., and Furutani, Y. (1985). *J. Biotechnol.* **3,** 73–84.

Houghten, R. A., Engert, R. F., Ostresh, J. M., Hoffman, S. R., and Klipstein, F. A. (1985). *Infect. Immun.* **48,** 735–740.

Hu, W. -S., and Dodge, T. C. (1985). *Biotechnol. Prog.* **1,** 209–215.

Hu, W. -S., Giard, D. J., and Wang, D. I. C. (1985). *Biotechnol. Bioeng.* **27,** 1466–1476.

Huang, A. L., Ostrowski, M. C., Berard, D., and Hager, G. L. (1981). *Cell (Cambridge, Mass.)* **27,** 245–265.

Hughes, J. V., Stanton, L. W., Tomassini, J. E., Long, W. J., and Scolnick, E. M. (1984). *J. Virol.* **52,** 465–473.

Hummel, M., Thorley-Lawson, D., and Kieff, E. (1984). *J. Virol.* **49,** 413–417.

Husson, R. N., and Young, R. A. (1987). *Proc. Natl. Acad. Sci. U. S. A.* **84,** 1679–1683.

Itoh, Y., Takai, E., Ohnuma, H., Kitajima, K., Tsuda, F., Machida, A., Mishiro, S., Nakamura, T., Miyakawa, Y., and Mayumi, M. (1986a). *Proc. Natl. Acad. Sci. U. S. A.* **83,** 9174–9178.

Itoh, Y., Hayakawa, T., and Fujisawa, Y. (1986b). *Biochem. Biophys. Res. Commun.* **138,** 268–274.

Ivins, B. E., and Welkos, S. L. (1986). *Infect. Immun.* **54,** 537–542.

Iwarson, S., Tabor, E., Thomas, H. C., Snoy, P., and Gerety, R. J. (1985). *Gastroenterology* **88,** 763–767.

Jacob, C. O., Pines, M., and Arnon, R. (1984). *EMBO J.* **3,** 2889–2893.

Jacobson, S., Rose, J. W., Flerlage, M. L., Mingioli, E. E., McFarlin, D. E., and McFarland, H. F. (1987). In "The Biology of Negative Strand Viruses" (B. Mahy and D. Kolakofsky, eds.), pp. 283–289. Elsevier, Amsterdam.

Jahn, G., Kouzarides, T., Mach, M., Scholl, B. -C., Plachter, B., Traupe, B., Preddie, E., Satchwell, S. C., Fleckenstein, B., and Barrell, B. G. (1987). *J. Virol.* **61,** 1358–1367.

Javier, R. T., Sedarati, F., and Stevens, J. G. (1986). *Science* **234,** 746–748.

Jeang, K. -T., Holmgren-Konig, M., and Khoury, G. (1987). *J. Virol.* **61,** 1761–1764.

Jennings, R., Pemberton, R. M., Smith, T. L., Amin, T., and Potter, C. W. (1987). *J. Gen. Virol.* **68,** 441–450.

Jilg, W., Lorbeer, B., Schmidt, M., Wilske, B., Zoulek, G., and Deinhardt, F. (1984). *Lancet* **2,** 1174–1175.

Jones, I. M., and Brownlee, G. G. (1985). *Gene* **35,** 333–342.

Karin, M., Cathala, G., and Nguyen-Huu, M. C. (1983). *Proc. Natl. Acad. Sci. U. S. A.* **80,** 4040–4044.

Kauffman, P. E. (1981). *Appl. Environ. Microbiol.* **42,** 611–614.

Kaufman, R. J. (1985). *Proc. Natl. Acad. Aci. U. S. A.* **82,** 689–693.

Kaufman, R. J., and Sharp, P. A. (1982). *Mol. Cell. Biol.* **2,** 1304–1319.

Kaufman, R. J., Murtha, P., Ingolia, D. E., Yeung, C. -Y., and Kellems, R. E. (1986). *Proc. Natl. Acad. Sci. U. S. A.* **83,** 3136–3140.

Kaufman, R. J., Murtha, P., and Davies, M. V. (1987). *EMBO J.* **6,** 187–193.

Kawamura, F., and Doi, R. H. (1984). *J. Bacteriol.* **160,** 442–444.

Kehoe, M., and Timmis, K. N. (1984). *Infect. Immun.* **43,** 804–810.

Kehoe, M., Winther, M., and Dougan, G. (1983). *J. Bacteriol.* **155,** 1071–1077.

Kehoe, M. A., Piorier, T. P., Beachey, E. H., and Timmis, K. N. (1985). *Infect. Immun.* **48,** 190–197.

Kelly, D. C. (1982). *J. Gen. Virol.* **63,** 1–13.

Kennedy-Stoskopf, S., and Narayan, O. (1986). *J. Virol.* **59,** 37–44.

Kern, F. G., and Basilico, C. (1986). *Gene* **43,** 237–245.

Khoury, G., and Gruss, P. (1983). *Cell (Cambridge, Mass.)* **33,** 313–314.

Kieser, T., Moss, M. T., Dale, J. W., and Hopwood, D. A. (1986). *J. Bacteriol.* **168,** 72–80.

Kim, H. W., Canchola, J. G., Brandt, C. D., Pyles, G., Chanock, R. M., Jensen, K., and Parrott, R. H. (1969). *Am. J. Epidemiol.* **89,** 422–434.

Kingsbury, D. W., Jones, I. M., and Murti, K. G. (1987). *Virology* **156,** 396–403.

Kingsman, S. M., Kingsman, A. J., Dobson, M. J., Mellor, J., and Roberts, N. A. (1985). *Biotechnol. Genet. Eng. Rev.* **3,** 337.

Kleid, D. G., Yansura, D., Small, B., Dowbenko, D., Moore, D., Grubman, J., Morgan, D., Roberston, B., and Bachrach, H. (1981). *Science* **214,** 1125–1128.

Klipstein, F. A., and Engert, R. F. (1981). *Infect. Immun.* **31,** 144–150.

Klipstein, F. A., Engert, R. F., and Clements, J. D. (1981). *Infect. Immun.* **34,** 637–639.

Klipstein, F. A., Engert, R. F., Clements, J. D., and Houghten, R. A. (1984). *Infect. Immun.* **43,** 811–816.

Klipstein, F. A., Engert, R. F., and Houghten, R. A. (1986). *Lancet* **1,** 471–473.

Klump, W., Marquardt, O., and Hofschneider, P. H. (1984). *Proc. Natl. Acad. Sci. U. S. A.* **81,** 3351–3355.

Kniskern, P. J., Hagopian, A., Montgomery, D. L., Burke, P., Dunn, N. R., Hofmann, K. J., Miller, W. J., and Ellis, R. W. (1986). *Gene*

Knowlton, R. G. (1986). *In* "Maximizing Gene Expression" (W. Reznikoff and L. Gold, eds.), pp. 171–194. Butterworth, Boston, Massachusetts.

Koomey, J. M., Gill, R. E., and Falkow, S. (1982). *Proc. Natl. Acad. Sci. U. S. A.* **79,** 7881–7885.

Kornfeld, R., and Kornfeld, S. (1985). *Annu. Rev. Biochem.* **54,** 631–664.

Kramer, R. A., Schaber, M. D., Skalka, A. M., Ganguly, K., Wong-Staal, F., and Reddy, E. P. (1986). *Science* **231,** 1580–1584.

Kupper, H., Keller, W., Kurz, C., Forss, S., Schaller, M., Franze, R., Strohmaier, K., Marquardt, O., Zaslavsky, V. G., and Hofschneider, P. M. (1981). *Nature (London)* **289,** 555–559.

Lagrange, P. H. (1984). *In* "The Mycobacteria: A Source Book, Part B" (G. P. Kubica and G. W. Lawrence, eds.), p. 682. Dekker, New York.

Laporte, J., Grosclaude, J., Wantyghem, J., Bernard, S., and Rouze, P. (1973). *C. R. Hebd. Seances Acad. Sci.* **276,** 3399–3401.

Lasky, L. A., Dowbenko, D., Simonsen, C. C., and Berman, P. W. (1984). *Bio/Technology* **2,** 527–532.

Lasky, L. A., Groopman, J. E., Fennie, C. W., Benz, P. M., Capon, D. J., Dowbenko, D. J., Nakamura, G. R., Nunes, W. M., Renz, M. E., and Berman, P. W. (1986). *Science* **233,** 209–212.

Laub, O., Rall, L. B., Truett, M., Shaul, Y., Standring, D. N., Valenzuela, P., and Rutter, W. J. (1983). *J. Virol.* **48,** 271–280.

Leavitt, A. D., Roberts, T. M., and Garcea, R. L. (1985). *J. Biol. Chem.* **260,** 12803–12809.

Lee, F., Mulligan, R., Berg, P., and Ringold, G. (1981). *Nature (London)* **294,** 228–232.

Legrain, P., Goud, B., and Buttin, G. (1986). *J. Virol.* **60,** 1141–1144.

Levine, M. M. (1984). *In* "Bacterial Vaccines" (R. Germanier, ed.), pp. 187–235. Academic Press, New York.

Levine, M. M., Kaper, J. B., Block, R. E., and Clements, M. L. (1983). *Microbiol. Rev.* **47,** 510–550.

Little, S. F., and Knudson, G. B. (1986). *Infect. Immun.* **52,** 509–512.

Locht, C., and Keith, J. M. (1986). *Science* **232,** 1258–1264.

Locht, C., Barstad, P. A., Coligan, J. E., Mayer, L., Munoz, J. J., Smith, S. G., and Keith, J. M. (1986). *Nucleic Acids Res.* **14,** 3251–3261.

Lubbert, H., and Doerfler, W. (1984). *J. Virol.* **50,** 497–506.

Lukacher, A. E., Braciale, V. L., and Braciale, T. J. (1984). *J. Exp. Med.* **160,** 814–826.

Lukehart, S. A. (1985). *J. Infect. Dis.* **7,** 305–313.

Lusky, M., and Botchan, M. (1981). *Nature (London)* **293,** 79–81.

McAleer, W. J., Buynak, E. B., Maigetter, R. Z., Wampler, D. E., Miller, W. J., and Hilleman, M. R. (1984). *Nature (London)* **307,** 178–180.

McGuire, T. C., Adams, D. S., Johnson, G. C., Klevjer-Anderson, P., Barbee, D. D., and Gorham, J. R. (1986). *Am. J. Vet. Res.* **47,** 537–540.

Machida, A., Kishimoto, S., Ohnuma, H., Miyamoto, H., Baba, K., Oda, K., Nakamura, T., Miyakawa, Y., and Mayumi, M. (1983). *Gastroenterology* **85,** 268–274.

McIntosh, K., and Fishaut, J. M. (1980). *Prog. Med. Virol.* **26,** 94–118.

Mackay, P., Pasek, M., Magazin, M., Kovacic, R. T., Allet, B., Athal, S., Gilbert, W., Schaller, H., Bruce, S. A., and Murray K. (1981). *Proc. Natl. Acad. Sci. U. S. A.* **78,** 4510–4514.

Mackett, M., and Smith, G. L. (1986). *J. Gen. Virol.* **67,** 2067–2082.

Mackett, M., Smith, G. L., and Moss, B. (1982). *Proc. Natl. Acad. Sci. U. S. A.* **79,** 7415–7419.

McLaughlan, A., Milich, D. R., Raney, A. K., Riggs, M. R., Hughes, J. L., Sorge, J., and Chisari, F. V. (1987). *J. Virol.* **61,** 683–692.

Macrina, F. L. (1984). *Annu. Rev. Microbiol.* **38**, 193–219.

Madisen, L., Travis, B., Hu, S. -L., and Purchio, A. F. (1987). *Virology* **158**, 248–250.

Maniatis, T., Fritsch, E. F., and Sambrook, J. (1982). "Molecular Cloning, A Laboratory Manual." Cold Spring Harbor Lab., Cold Spring Harbor, New York.

Manning, P. A. (1987). *Vaccine* **5**, 83–87.

Manning, P. A., Heuzenroeder, M. W., Yeadon, J., Leavesley, D. I., Reeves, P. R., and Rowley, D. (1986). *Infect. Immun.* **53**, 272–277.

Marrs, C. F., Schoolnik, G., Koomey, J. M., Hardy, J., Rothbard, J., and Falkow, S. (1985). *J. Bacteriol.* **163**, 132–139.

Massey, R. J., and Schochetman, G. (1981). *Science* **213**, 447–449.

Mathews, J. H., and Roehrig, J. T. (1982). *J. Immunol.* **129**, 2763–2767.

Matsuura, Y., Possee, R. D., Overton, H. A., and Bishop, D. H. L. (1987). *J. Gen. Virol.* **68**, 1233–1250.

Matthews, T. J., Langlois, A. J., Robey, W. G., Chang, N. T., Gallo, R. C., Fischinger, P. J., and Bolognesi, D. P. (1986). *Proc. Natl. Acad. Sci. U. S. A.* **83**, 9709–9713.

Mattick, J. S., Bills, M. M., Anderson, B. J., Dalrymple, B., Mott, M. R., and Egerton, J. R. (1987). *J. Bacteriol.* **169**, 33–41.

Mehra, V., Sweetser, D., and Young, R. A. (1986). *Proc. Natl. Acad. Sci. U. S. A.* **83**, 7013–7017.

Mellor, J., Dobson, M. J., Roberts, N. A., Tuite, M. F., Emtage, J. S., White, S., Lowe, P. A., Patel, T., Kingsman, A. J., and Kingsman, S. M. (1983). *Gene* **24**, 1–14.

Mellor, J., Dobson, M. J., Roberts, N. A., Kingsman, A. J., and Kingsman, S. M. (1985). *Gene* **33**, 215–226.

Meloen, R. H., and Barteling, S. J. (1986). *Virology* **149**, 55–63.

Mermer, B., Malamy, M., and Coffin, J. M. (1983). *Mol. Cell. Biol.* **3**, 1746–1758.

Mertz, G. J., Peterman, G., Ashley, R., Jourden, J. L., Salter, D., Morrison, L., McLean, A., and Corey, L. (1984). *J. Infect. Dis.* **150**, 242–249.

Mettenleiter, T. C., Lakacs, N., and Rziha, H. -J. (1985). *J. Virol.* **53**, 52–57.

Meyer, T. F., Mlawer, M., and So, M. (1982). *Cell (Cambridge, Mass.)* **30**, 45–52.

Michel, M. -L., Sobczak, E., Malpiece, Y., Tiollais, P., and Streeck, R. E. (1985). *Bio/Technology* **3**, 561–566.

Milich, D. R., Thorton, G. B., Neurath, A. R., Kent, S. B., Michel, M. -L., Tiollais, P., and Chisari, F. V. (1985). *Science* **228**, 1195–1198.

Miller, D. W., Safer, P., and Miller, L. K. (1986). *Genet. Eng.* **8**, 277–298.

Miller, L. H., Howard, R. J., Carter, R., Good, M. F., Nussenzweig, V., and Nussenzweig, R. S. (1986). *Science* **234**, 1349–1356.

Miller, L. K. (1981). *In* "Genetic Engineering in the Plant Sciences" (N. Panopoulous, ed.). Praeger, New York.

Miller, L. K., Lingg, A. J., and Bulla, L. A. (1983). *Science* **219**, 715–721.

Miller, T. J., Peetz, R., Reed, A. P., Kost, T., Brown, A. L., Auerbach, J., and Rosenberg, M. (1985). *In* "Vaccines '85" (R. A. Lerner, R. M. Chanock, and F. Brown, eds.), pp. 95–99. Cold Spring Harbor Lab., Cold Spring Harbor, New York.

Miyanohara, A., Toh-e, A., Nozaki, C., Hamada, F., Ohtomo, N., and Matsubara, K. (1983). *Proc. Natl. Acad. Sci. U. S. A.* **80**, 1–5.

Molitor, T. W., Joo, H. S., and Collett, M. S. (1983). *J. Virol.* **45**, 842–854.

Montaraz, J. A., and Winter, A. J. (1986). *Infect. Immun.* **53**, 245–251.

Montaraz, J. A., Winter, A. J., Hunter, D. M., Sowa, B. A., Wu, A. M., and Adams, L. G. (1986). *Infect. Immun.* **51**, 961–963.

Morein, B., and Simons, K. (1985). *Vaccine* **3**, 83–93.

Morein, B., Sharp, M., Sundquist, B., and Simons, K. (1983). *J. Gen. Virol.* **64**, 1557–1569.

Morens, D. M., Venkateshan, C. N., and Halstead, S. B. (1987). *J. Gen. Virol.* **68,** 91–98.
Moriarty, A. M., Hoyer, B. H., Shih, J. W. -K., Gerin, J. L., and Hamer, D. H. (1981). *Proc. Natl. Acad. Sci. U. S. A.* **78,** 2606–2610.
Morrissey, P., Dougan, G., Russell, R. R. B., and Gilpin, M. (1985). *In* "Vaccines '85" (R. A. Lerner, R. M. Chanock, and F. Brown, eds.), pp. 117–124. Cold Spring Harbor Lab., Cold Spring Harbor, New York.
Motz, M., Deby, G., Jilg, W., and Wolf, H. (1986). *Gene* **44,** 353–359.
Mougin, B., Giraudon, P., Bakouche, O., and Wild, T. F. (1987). *In* "The Biology of Negative Strand Viruses" (B. Mahy and D. Kolakofsky, eds.), pp. 316–320. Elsevier, Amsterdam.
Mulks, M. H., and Knapp, J. S. (1987). *Infect. Immun.* **55,** 931–936.
Mulligan, R. C., and Berg, P. (1980). *Science* **209,** 1422–1427.
Mulligan, R. C., and Berg, P. (1981). *Proc. Natl. Acad. Sci. U. S. A.* **78,** 2072–2076.
Munoz, J. J., Arai, H., and Cole, R. L. (1981). *Infect. Immun.* **32,** 243–250.
Murray, K., Bruce, S., Hinnen, A., Wingfield, P., van Erd, P. C. M. A., de Reus, A., and Schellekens, H. (1984). *EMBO J.* **3,** 645–650.
Murray, M. J., Kaufman, R. J., Latt, S. A., and Weinberg, R. A. (1983). *Mol. Cell. Biol.* **3,** 32–43.
Mustafa, A. S., Gill, H. K., Nerland, A., Britton, W. J., Mehra, V., Bloom, B. R., Young, R. A., and Godal, T. (1986). *Nature (London)* **319,** 63–66.
Naylor, P. H., Naylor, C. W., Badamchian, M., Wada, S., Goldstein, A. L., Wang, S. -S., Sun, D. K., Thornton, A. H., and Sarin, P. S. (1987). *Proc. Natl. Acad. Sci. U. S. A.* **84,** 2951–2955.
Neurath, A. R., and Rubin, B. A. (1971). *Monogr. Virol.* **4,** 1–87.
Neurath, A. R., Kent, S. B. H., Parker, K., Prince, A. M., Strick, N., Brotman, B., and Sproul, P. (1986). *Vaccine* **4,** 35–37.
Nicosia, A., Perugini, M., Franzini, C., Casagli, M. C., Borri, M. G., Antoni, G., Almoni, M., Neri, P., Ratti, G., and Rappuoli, R. (1986). *Proc. Natl. Acad. Sci. U. S. A.* **83,** 4631–4635.
Nicosia, A., Bartoloni, A., Perugini, M., and Rappuoli, R. (1987). *Infect. Immun.* **55,** 963–967.
Nilsson, J., and Skogman, S. G. (1986). *Bio/Technology* **4,** 901–903.
Norgard, M. V., and Miller, J. N. (1983). *Infect. Immun.* **42,** 435–445.
Norgard, M. V., Chamberlain, N. R., Swancutt, M. A., and Goldberg, M. S. (1986). *Infect. Immun.* **54,** 500–506.
Norrild, B. (1980). *Curr. Top. Microbiol. Immunol.* **90,** 67–106.
Oda, M., Cowell, J. L., Burstyn, D. G., and Manclark, C. R. (1984). *J. Infect. Dis.* **150,** 823–833.
Oftung, F., Mustafa, A. S., Husson, R., Young, R. A., and Godal, T. (1987). *J. Immunol.* **138,** 927–931.
Orndorff, P. E., Spears, P. A., Schauer, D., and Falkow, S. (1985). *J. Bacteriol.* **164,** 321–330.
Ottenhoff, T. H. M., Klatser, P. R., Ivanyi, J., Elferink, D. G., de Wit, M. Y. L., and de Vries, R. R. P. (1986). *Nature (London)* **319,** 66–68.
Ottow, J. C. G. (1975). *Annu. Rev. Microbiol.* **29,** 79–108.
Ou, J. -H., and Rutter, W. J. (1987). *J. Virol.* **61,** 782–786.
Overton, H. A., Ihara, T., and Bishop, D. H. L. (1987). *Virology* **157,** 338–350.
Pachl, C., Burke, R. L., Stuve, L. L., Sanchez-Pescador, L., Van Nest, G., Masiarz, F., and Dina, D. (1987). *J. Virol.* **61,** 315–325.
Palva, I., Lehtovaara, P., Kaariainen, L., Sibakov, M., Cantell, K., Schein, C. H., Kashiwagi, K., and Weissman, C. (1983). *Gene* **22,** 229–235.

Panicali, D., and Paoletti, E. (1982). *Proc. Natl. Acad. Sci. U. S. A.* **79,** 4927–4931.

Paton, J. C., Berry, A. M., Lock, R. A., Hansman, D., and Manning, P. A. (1986). *Infect. Immun.* **54,** 50–55.

Persing, D. H., Varmus, H. E., and Ganem, D. (1986). *Science* **234,** 1388–1392.

Petrovskis, E. A., Timmins, J. G., Armentrout, M. A., Marchioli, C. C. Yancey, R. J., and Post, L. E. (1986a). *J. Virol.* **59,** 216–223.

Petrovskis, E. A., Timmins, J. G., and Post, L. E. (1986b). *J. Virol.* **60,** 185–193.

Pintel, D., Merchlinsky, M. J., and Ward, D. C. (1984). *J. Virol.* **52,** 320–327.

Pohlner, J., Halter, R., Beyreuther, K., and Meyer, T. F. (1987). *Nature (London)* **325,** 458–462.

Poirier, T. P., Kehoe, M. A., Dale, J. B., Timmis, K. N., and Beachey, E. H. (1985). *Infect. Immun.* **48,** 198–203.

Polisky, B. (1986). In "Maximizing Gene Expression" (W. Reznikoff and L. Gold, eds.), pp. 143–170. Butterworth, Boston, Massachusetts.

Portela, A., de la Luna, S., Melero, J. A., Vara, J., Jimenez, A., and Orten, J. (1985). *Nucleic Acids Res.* **13,** 7913–7927.

Porter, D. D., Austen, A. E., and Porter, H. G. (1972). *J. Immunol.* **109,** 1–7.

Porterfield, J. S. (1982). *J. Hyg.* **89,** 355–364.

Pucci, M. J., and Macrina, F. L. (1985). *Infect. Immun.* **48,** 704–712.

Pullen, K. F., Johnson, M. D., Phillips, A. W., Ball, G. D., and Finter, N. B. (1985). *Dev. Biol. Stand.* **60,** 175–177.

Pumpen, P., Kozlovskaya, T. M., Borisova, G. P., Bichko, V. V., Dishler, A., Kalis, J., Kukaine, R. A., and Gren, E. J. (1984). *Gene* **30,** 201–210.

Purcell, B. K., and Clegg, S. (1983). *Infect. Immun.* **39,** 1122–1127.

Putney, S. D., Matthews, T. J., Robey, W. G., Lynn, D. L., Robert-Guroff, M., Mueller, T., Langlois, A. J., Ghrayeb, J., Petteway, S. R., Weinhold, K. J., Fischinger, P. J., Wong-Staal, F., Gallo, R. C., and Bolognesi, D. P. (1986). *Science* **234,** 1392–1395.

Radolf, J. D., Borenstein, L. A., Kim, J. Y., Fehniger, T. E., and Lovett, M. A. (1987). *J. Bacteriol.* **169,** 1365–1371.

Rager-Zisman, B., Quan, P. -C., Rosner, M., Moller, J. R., and Bloomn, B. R. (1987). *J. Immunol.* **138,** 884–888.

Rea, T. J., Timmis, J. G., Long, G. W., and Post, L. E. (1985). *J. Virol.* **54,** 21–29.

Reiher, W. E., Blalock, J. E., and Brunck, T. K. (1986). *Proc. Natl. Acad. Sci. U. S. A.* **83,** 9188–9192.

Reiss, C. S., and Schulman, J. L. (1980). *J. Immunol.* **125,** 2182–2188.

Remaut, E., Stanssens, P., and Fiers, M. (1981). *Gene* **15,** 81–93.

Reznikoff, W., and Gold, L., eds. (1986). "Maximizing Gene Expression." Butterworth, Boston, Massachusetts.

Reznikoff, W., and McClure, W. R. (1986). In "Maximizing Gene Expression" (W. Reznikoff and L. Gold, eds.), pp. 1–34. Butterworth, Boston, Massachusetts.

Riedel, H., Kondor-Koch, C., and Garoff, H. (1984). *EMBO J.* **3,** 1477–1483.

Rio, D. C., Clark, S. G., and Tjian, R. (1985). *Science* **227,** 23–28.

Ristroph, J. D., and Ivins, B. E. (1983). *Infect. Immun.* **39,** 483–486.

Robbins, A. K., Weis, J. H., Enquist, L. W., and Watson, R. J. (1984). *J. Mol. Appl. Genet.* **2,** 485–496.

Robbins, A. K., Gold, C., Enquist, L. W., Whealy, M. E., and Watson, R. J. (1985). *Abstr. Int. Herpesvirus Worshop, 10th* p. 130.

Robbins, A. K., Watson, R. J., Whealy, M. E., Hays, W. W., and Enquist, L. W. (1986). *J. Virol.* **58,** 339–347.

Robertson, D. L., and Leppla, S. H. (1986). *Gene* **44,** 71–78.

Robeson, J. P., Barletta, R. G., and Curtiss, R. (1983). *J. Bacteriol.* **153**, 211–221.

Robey, W. G., Arthur, L. O., Matthews, T. J., Langlois, A., Copeland, T. D., Lerche, N. W., Oroszlan, S., Bolognesi, D. P., Gilden, R. V., and Fischinger, P. J. (1986). *Proc. Natl. Acad. Sci. U. S. A.* **83**, 7023–7027.

Robinson, A., Irons, L. I., and Ashworth, L. A. E. (1985). *Vaccine* **3**, 11–22.

Robinson, E. N., McGee, Z. A., Buchanan, T. M., Blake, M. S., and Hitchcock, P. J. (1987). *Infect. Immun.* **55**, 1190–1197.

Rose, J., and Bergman, J. (1982). *Cell (Cambridge, Mass.)* **30**, 753–762.

Rothbard, J. B., and Schoolnik, G. K. (1985). *In* "Vaccines '85" (R. A. Lerner, R. M. Chanock, and F. Brown, eds.), pp. 85–90. Cold Spring Harbor Lab., Cold Spring Harbor, New York.

Rouse, B. T. (1982). *J. Am. Vet. Med. Assoc.* **181**, 988–991.

Ruppen, M., Band, L., and Henner, D. J. (1986). *In* "Bacillus Molecular Genetics and Biotechnology Applications" (A. T. Ganesan and J. A. Hoch, eds.), pp. 423–432. Academic Press, New York.

Salunke, D. M., Caspar, D. L. D., and Garcea, R. L. (1986). *Cell (Cambridge, Mass.)* **48**, 895–904.

Sarin, P. S., Sun, D. K., Thornton, A. H., Naylor, P. H., and Goldstein, A. L. (1986). *Science* **232**, 1135–1137.

Sarver, N., Gruss, P., Law, M. -F., Khoury, G., and Howley, P. M. (1981). *Mol. Cell. Biol.* **1**, 486–496.

Sarver, N., Byrne, J. C., and Howley, P. M. (1982). *Proc. Natl. Acad. Sci. U. S. A.* **79**, 7147–7151.

Sato, Y., Izumiya, K., Sato, H., Cowell, J. L., and Manclark, C. R. (1981). *Infect. Immun.* **31**, 1223–1231.

Sato, Y., Kimura, M., and Fukumi, H. (1984). *Lancet* **1**, 122–126.

Schimke, R. T. (1984). *Cell (Cambridge, Mass.)* **37**, 705–713.

Schlesinger, J. J., Brandriss, M. W., and Walsh, E. E. (1985). *J. Immunol.* **135**, 2805–2809.

Schlesinger, J. J., Brandriss, M. W., Cropp, C. B., and Monath, T. P. (1986). *J. Virol.* **60**, 1153–1155.

Schlesinger, J. J., Brandriss, M. W., and Walsh, E. E. (1987). *J. Gen. Virol.* **68**, 853–857.

Schmaljohn, A. L., Johnson, E. D., Dalrymple, J. M., and Cole, G. A. (1982). *Nature (London)* **297**, 70–72.

Schoolnik, G. K., Tai, J. Y., and Gotschich, E. C. (1983). *Prog. Allergy* **33**, 314–331.

Schultz, L. D., Hofmann, K., Tanner, J., Emini, E. A., Kieff, E., and Ellis, R. W. (1986). *Int. Herpesvirus Workshop, 11th* p. 261.

Scott, J. R., and Fischetti, V. A. (1983). *Science* **221**, 758–760.

Scott, J. R., Hollingshead, S. K., and Fischetti, V. A. (1986). *Infect. Immun.* **52**, 609–612.

Shareck, F., and Cameron, J. (1984). *J. Bacteriol.* **159**, 780–782.

Shimotohno, K., and Temin, H. M. (1981). *Cell (Cambridge, Mass.)* **26**, 67–77.

Shinnick, T. M. (1987). *J. Bacteriol.* **169**, 1080–1088.

Shiroza, T., Nakazawa, K., Tashiro, N., Yamane, K., Yanagi, K., Yamasaki, M., Tamura, G., Sarto, H., Kawade, Y., and Taniguchi, T. (1985). *Gene* **34**, 1–8.

Shuuring, C. (1982). *Nature (London)* **296**, 792.

Siddiqui, A. (1983). *Mol. Cell. Biol.* **3**, 143–146.

Simonsen, C. C., and Levinson, A. D. (1983). *Proc. Natl. Acad. Sci. U. S. A.* **80**, 2495–2499.

Skogman, G., Nilsson, J., and Gustafsson, P. (1983). *Gene* **23**, 105–115.

Smith, G. E., Fraser, M. J., and Summers, M. D. (1983a). *J. Virol.* **46**, 584–593.

Smith, G. E., Summers, M. D., and Fraser, M. J. (1983b). *Mol. Cell. Biol.* **3,** 2156–2165.

Smith, R. A., Duncan, M. J., and Moir, D. T. (1985). *Science* **229,** 1219–1224.

Southern, P. J., and Berg, P. (1982). *J. Mol. Appl. Genet.* **1,** 327–341.

Spandidos, D. A., and Wilkie, N. M. (1983). *EMBO J.* **2,** 1193–1199.

Spanier, J. G., Jones, S. J. C., and Cleary, P. (1984). *Science* **225,** 935–938.

Spear, P. G. (1985). *In* "The Herpes Viruses" (B. Roizman, ed.), Vol. 3, pp. 315–356. Plenum, New York.

Spencer, J. F. T., and Spencer, D. M. (1983). *Annu. Rev. Microbiol.* **37,** 121–142.

Stahl, S., MacKay, P., Magazin, M., Bruce, S. A., and Murray, K. (1982). *Proc. Natl. Acad. Sci. U. S. A.* **79,** 1606–1610.

Stamm, L. V., Folds, J. D., and Bassford, P. J. (1982). *Infect. Immun.* **36,** 1238–1241.

Stamm, L. V., Kerner, T. C., Bankaitis, V. A., and Bassford, P. J. (1983). *Infect. Immun.* **41,** 709–721.

Stanley, J., Bhaduri, L. M., Narayan, O., and Clements, J. E. (1987). *J. Virol.* **61,** 1019–1028.

Stapleton, J. T., and Lemon, S. M. (1987). *J. Virol.* **61,** 491–498.

Stark, G. R., and Wahl, G. M. (1984). *Annu. Rev. Biochem.* **53,** 447–491.

Steinberg, D. A., Watson, R. J., and Maiese, W. M. (1986). *Gene* **43,** 311–317.

Steitz, J. A. (1979). *In* "Biological Regulation and Development" (R. F. Golberger, ed.), Vol. 1, pp. 349–399. Plenum, New York.

Sterling, J. (1987). *Genet. Eng. News* **7,** 1.

Stevens, C. E., Alter, H. J., Taylor, P. E., Zang, E. A., Harley, E. J., Szmuness, W., and Dialysis Vaccine Trail Study Group. (1984). *N. Engl. J. Med.* **311,** 496–501.

Stewart, D. J., Clark, B. L., Peterson, J. E., Griffiths, D. A., and Smith, E. F. (1982). *Res. Vet. Sci.* **32,** 140–147.

Stewart-Tull, D. E. S. (1984). *Vaccine* **2,** 238–248.

Stormo, G. D. (1986). *In* "Maximizing Gene Expression" (W. Reznikoff and L. Gold, eds.), pp. 195–224. Butterworth, Boston, Massachusetts.

Stott, J. L., Anderson, G. A., Jochim, M. M., Barber, T. L., and Osburn, B. I. (1984). *Proc. Annu. Meet. U. S. Anim. Health Assoc.* **86,** 126–131.

Struhl, K. (1986). *In* "Maximizing Gene Expression" (W. Reznikoff and L. Gold, eds.), pp. 35–78. Butterworth, Boston, Massachusetts.

Struhl, K. (1987). *Cell (Cambridge, Mass.)* **49,** 295–297.

Stuve, L. L., Brown-Shimer, S., Pachl, C., Najarian, R., Dina, D., and Burke, R. L. (1987). *J. Virol.* **61,** 326–335.

Subramani, S., Mulligan, R., and Berg, P. (1981). *Mol. Cell Biol.* **1,** 854–864.

Sveda, M., Markoff, L., and Lai, C. (1982). *Cell (Cambridge, Mass.)* **30,** 649–656.

Swancutt, M. A., Twehous, D. A., and Norgard, M. V. (1986). *Infect. Immun.* **52,** 110–119.

Tabatabai, L. B., and Deyoe, B. L. (1984). *Dev. Biol. Stand.* **56,** 199–211.

Tanese, N., Sodroski, J., Haseltine, W. A., and Goff, S. P. (1986). *J. Virol.* **59,** 743–745.

Taylor, P. M., and Askonas, B. A. (1986). *Immunology* **58,** 417–420.

Tharakan, J. P., and Chau, P. C. (1986). *Biotechnol. Bioeng.* **18,** 329–342.

Thole, J. E. R., Dauwerse, H. G., Das, P. K., Groothuis, D. G., Schouls, L. M., and van Embden, J. D. A. (1985). *Infect. Immun.* **50,** 800–806.

Thole, J. E. R., Keulen, W. J., Kolk, A. H. J., Groothuis, D. G., Berwald, L. G., Tiesjema, R. H., and van Embden, J. D. A. (1987). *Infect. Immun.* **55,** 1466–1475.

Thompson, L. D., and Vasantha, N. (1986). *In* "Bacillus Molecular Genetics and Biotechnology Applications" (A. T. Ganesan and J. A. Hock, eds.), pp. 129–140. Academic Press, New York.

DEVELOPMENT OF BIOSYNTHETIC VACCINES 171

Thomsen, D. R., Marchioli, C. C., Yancey, R. J., and Post, L. E. (1987). *J. Virol.* **61**, 229–232.

Thummel, C. S., Tjian, R., and Grodzicker, T. (1981). *Cell (Cambridge, Mass.)* **23**, 825–836.

Tiollais, P., Pourcel, C., and Dejean, A. (1985). *Nature (London)* **317**, 489–495.

Torseth, J. W., Cohen, G. H., Eisenberg, R. J., Berman, P. W., Lasky, L. A., Cerini, C. P., Heilman, C. J., Kerwar, S., and Merigan, T. C. (1987). *J. Virol.* **61**, 1532–1539.

Townsend, A. R. M., and Skehel, J. J. (1984). *J. Exp. Med.* **160**, 552–563.

Townsend, A. R. M., McMichael, A. J., Carter, N. P., Huddleston, J. A., and Brownlee, G. G. (1984). *Cell (Cambridge, Mass.)* **39**, 13–25.

Townsend, A. R. M., Gotch, F. M., Davey, J. (1985). *Cell (Cambridge, Mass.)* **42**, 457–467.

Townsend, A. R. M., Bastin, J., Gould, K., and Brownlee, G. G. (1986a). *Nature (London)* **324**, 575–577.

Townsend, A. R. M., Rothbard, J., Gotch, F. M., Bahadur, G., Wraith, D., and McMichael, A. J. (1986b). *Cell (Cambridge, Mass)* **44**, 959–968.

Tramont, E. C., and Boslego, J. W. (1985). *Vaccine* **3**, 3–10.

Tuite, M. F., Dobson, M. J., Roberts, N. A., King, R. M., Burke, D. C., Kingsman, S. M., and Kingsman, A. J. (1982). *EMBO J.* **1**, 603–608.

Turkin, D., and Sercarz, E. E. (1977). *Proc. Natl. Acad. Sci. U. S. A.* **74**, 3984–3987.

Uhlin, B. E., Molin, S., Gustafsson, P., and Nordstrom, K. (1979). *Gene* **6**, 91.

Ulmanen, I., Lindstrom, K., Lehtovaara, P., Sarvas, M., Ruohonen, M., and Palva, I. (1985). *J. Bacteriol.* **162**, 176–182.

Valenzuela, P., Medina, A., Rutter, W. J., Ammerer, G., and Hall, B. D. (1982). *Nature (London)* **298**, 347–350.

Valenzuela, P., Coit, D., and Kuo, C. H. (1985a). *Bio/Technology* **3**, 317–320.

Valenzuela, P., Coit, D., Medina-Selby, M. A., Kuo, C. H., Van Nest, G., Burke, R. L., Bull, P., Urdea, M. S., and Graves, P. V. (1985b0. *Bio/Technology* **3**, 323–326.

Van Brunt, J. (1986). *Bio/Technology* **4**, 1057–1062.

Van Brunt, J. (1987). *Bio/Technology* **5**, 103–104.

Van Dongen, W. M. A. M., and de Graaf, F. K. (1986). *J. Gen. Microbiol.* **132**, 2225.

van Drunen Littel-van den Hurk, S., and Babiuk, L. A. (1985). *Virology* **144**, 204–215.

van Drunen Littel-van den Hurk, S., and Babiuk, L. A. (1986). *J. Virol.* **59**, 401–410.

van Drunen Littel-van den Hurk, S., van den Hurk, J. V., Gilchrist, J. E., Misra, V., and Babiuk, L. A. (1984). *Virology* **135**, 466–479.

van Drunen Littel-van den Hurk, S., L'italien, J., Lawman, M., Gifford, G., Zomb, I., Hughes, G., and Babiuk, L. A. (1986). *Abstr. Int. Herpesvirus Workshop, 11th* p. 269.

van Embden, J. D., van der Donk, H. J., van Eijk, R. V., van der Heide, H. G., de Jong, J. A., van Oldersen, M. F., Osterhaus, A. D., and Schouls, L. M. (1983). *Infect. Immun.* **42**, 187–196.

van Verseveld, H. W., Bakker, P., van der Woude, T., Terleth, C., and de Graff, F. K. (1985). *Infect. Immun.* **49**, 159–163.

Veronese, F., Copeland, T., DeVico, A., Rahman, R., Oroszlan, S., Gall, R. C., and Sarngadharan, M. (1986). *Science* **231**, 1289–1291.

Verstreate, D. R., Creasy, M. T., Caveney, N. T., Baldwin, C. L., Blab, M. W., and Winter, A. J. (1982). *Infect. Immun.* **35**, 979–989.

Virji, M., and Heckels, J. E. (1985). *Infect. Immun.* **49**, 621–628.

Vodkin, M. H., and Leppla, S. H. (1983). *Cell (Cambridge, Mass.)* **34**, 693–697.

Walfield, A. M., Hanff, P. A., and Lovett, M. A. (1982). *Science* **216**, 522–523.

Walker, J. A., Allen, R. L., Falmagne, P., Johnson, M. K., and Boulnois, G. J. (1987). *Infect. Immun.* **55**, 1184–1189.

Wasylyk, B. (1986). *In* "Maximizing Gene Expression" (W. Reznikoff and L. Gold, eds.), pp. 79–99. Butterworth, Boston, Massachusetts.

Waters, J., Pignatelli, M., Galpin, S., Ishihara, K., and Thomas, H. C. (1986). *J. Gen. Virol.* **67**, 2467–2473.

Wathen, M. W., and Wathen, L. M. K. (1984). *J. Virol.* **51**, 57–62.

Watson, R. J., Weis, J. H., Salstrom, J. S., and Enquist, L. W. (1982). *Science* **218**, 381–384.

Watson, R. J., Weis, J. H., Salstrom, J. S., and Enquist, L. W. (1984). *J. Invest. Dermatol.* **83**, 102s–111s.

Webster, R. G., and Askonas, B. A. (1980). *Eur. J. Immunol.* **10**, 396–401.

Wei, C. -M., Gibson, M., Spear, P. G., and Scolnick, E. M. (1981). *J. Virol.* **39**, 935–944.

Weigent, D. A., Hoeprich, P. D., Bost, K. L., Brunck, T. K., Reiher, W. E., and Blalock, J. E. (1986). *Biochem. Biophys. Res. Commun.* **139**, 367–374.

Weis, J. H., Enquist, L. W., Salstrom, J. S., and Watson, R. J. (1983). *Nature (London)* **302**, 72–74.

Weiss, R. A., Clapham, P. R., Weber, J. N., Dalgleish, A. G., Lasky, L. A., and Berman, P. W. (1986). *Nature (London)* **324**, 572–575.

Whang, Y., Silberklang, M., Morgan, A., Munshi, S., Lenny, A. B., Ellis, R. W., and Kieff, E. (1987). *J. Virol.* **61**, 1796–1807.

Wigler, M., Silverstein, S., Lee, L. S., Pellicer, A., Cheng, Y., and Axel, R. (1977). *Cell (Cambridge, Mass.)* **11**, 223–232.

Wigler, M., Sweet, R., Sim, G. K., Wold, B., Pellicer, A., Lacy, E., Maniatis, T., Silverstein, S., and Axel, R. (1979). *Cell (Cambridge, Mass.)* **16**, 777–785.

Winter, A. J., Verstreate, D. R., Hall, C. E., Jacobson, R. H., Castleman, W. L., Meredith, M. P., and McLaughlin, C. A. (1983). *Infect. Immun.* **42**, 1159–1167.

Winther, M. D., and Dougan, G. (1984). *Biotechnol. Genet. Eng. Rev.* **2**, 1–39.

Winther, M. D., Pickard, D., and Dougan, G. (1985). *FEMS Microbiol. Lett.* **28**, 193–197.

Wong, S. -L., Kawamura, F., and Doi, R. H. (1986). *J. Bacteriol.* **168**, 1005–1009.

Wraith, D. C., and Askonas, B. A. (1985). *J. Gen. Virol.* **66**, 1327–1331.

Wraith, D. C., Vessey, A. E., and Askonas, B. A. (1987). *J. Gen. Virol.* **68**, 433–440.

Yamamoto, T., Tamura, T., and Yokota, T. (1984). *J. Biol. Chem.* **259**, 5037–5044.

Yaniv, M. (1984). *Cell (Cambridge, Mass.)* **50**, 203–216.

Yap, K. L., Ada, G. L., and McKenzie, I. F. C. (1978). *Nature (London)* **273**, 238–239.

Yewdell, J. W., Bennink, J. R., Smith, G. L., and Moss, B. (1985). *Proc. Natl. Acad. Sci. U. S. A.* **82**, 1785–1789.

Yewdell, J. W., Bennink, J. R., Mackett, M., Lefrançois, L., Lyles, D. S., and Moss, B. (1986). *J. Exp. Med.* **163**, 1529–1538.

Young, R. A., and Davis, R. W. (1983). *Proc. Natl. Acad. Sci. U. S. A.* **80**, 1194–1198.

Young, R. A., and Davis, R. W. (1985). *Genet. Eng.* **7**, 29–41.

Young, R. A., Bloom, B. R., Grosskinsky, C. M., Ivanyi, J., Thomas, D., and Davis, R. W. (1985a). *Proc. Natl. Acad. Sci. U. S. A.* **82**, 2583–2587.

Young, R. A., Mehra, V., Sweetser, D., Buchanan, T., Clark-Curtiss, J., Davis, R. W., and Bloom, B. R. (1985b). *Nature (London)* **316**, 450–452.

Zarling, J. M., Moran, P. A., Burkes, R. L., Pachl, C., Berman, P. W., and Lasky, L. A. (1986a). *J. Immunol.* **136**, 4669–4673.

Zarling, J. M., Morton, W., Moran, P. A., McClure, J., Kosowski, S. G., and Hu, S. -L. (1986b). *Nature (London)* **323**, 344–346.

The Development of Chemically Synthesized Vaccines

F. BROWN

Wellcome Biotechnology, Limited, Beckenham, Kent, England

I. Introduction

It is almost 200 years since the principles involved in vaccination against virus diseases and in the application of the vaccines which are in use today started to be laid down. In 1798 Jenner showed conclusively that the lymph from cattle infected with cowpox would protect man against infection with smallpox, thus confirming the observation that milkmaids were less likely to get smallpox than the rest of the population. Almost 100 years later Pasteur (1885) demonstrated the efficacy of his rabies vaccine in protecting people even after they had been bitten by a rabid animal. However, by the time of the Second World War, only two additional viral vaccines had come into use for man, those developed by Semple (1919) for rabies and by Theiler and Smith (1937) for yellow fever. Jenner's vaccine against smallpox, Pasteur's vaccine against rabies, and Theiler's vaccine against yellow fever were attenuated; their efficacy was based on the multiplication of

173

the weakened agent in the host to induce protective immunity without causing clinical disease. In contrast, Semple's rabies vaccine was inactivated and depended for its activity on the presence of a sufficient number of virus particles to elicit the appropriate immune responses.

In addition to the products that had been accepted for use in man, several vaccines were also being used to protect animals at that time. A comprehensive list is provided by Bittle in the first chapter of this book. These vaccines were prepared from viruses grown in animal tissue or in eggs by inactivation with formalin or phenol. However, it was not until Frenkel (1947) described the large-scale growth of foot and mouth disease virus (FMDV) in bovine tongue epithelial fragments that it became feasible to consider the possibility of vaccines which could be used widely. This development was a direct result of the use of antibiotics and the opportunity they provided for growing tissue culture cells on a large scale without the problem of bacterial contamination.

The early use of tissue culture technology for the production of vaccines to control FMD was particularly appropriate because of the widespread occurrence and economic consequences of that disease. In this chapter, I focus attention on FMD to demonstrate that, although the vaccines in current use have been highly successful in bringing the disease under control in certain parts of the world, it may be essential to provide more stable vaccines based on peptides to overcome the problems encountered in other regions of the world.

Because Frenkel was working in Holland, perhaps it was inevitable that the first comprehensive vaccination program against FMD should be conducted in that country. The results were dramatic, as seen in Fig. 1, and other countries in Western Europe soon followed Holland's lead. The annual number of outbreaks in Europe is now very small. The situation in the rest of the world is less satisfactory, partly because of the more hostile terrain, greater distances involved and higher ambient temperatures, making it difficult to deliver the vaccines in good condition. Consequently, there are many outbreaks despite the vaccination programs in operation in most countries where the disease is endemic.

Added to these practical problems of applying the vaccines is that of antigenic variation. The virus occurs as seven serotypes—A, O, C, SAT1, SAT2, SAT3, and Asia 1. There is no cross-protection between serotypes, so an animal that has been infected with virus from one serotypes is still susceptible to infection with viruses belonging to the other serotypes, although it is resistant to reinfection with the homologous virus. As an additional problem in the preparation of vaccines

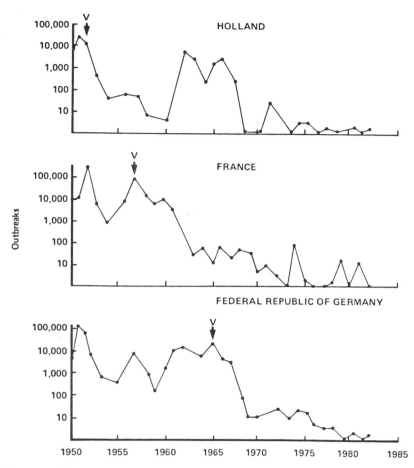

FIG. 1.   Effect of application of comprehensive vaccination against FMD in Holland, France, and West Germany on the number of outbreaks of the disease. V, Start of mass vaccination.

against FMD, there is considerable antigenic variation within sero-types so that a vaccine prepared against one isolate of the virus may not afford adequate protection against other isolates belonging to the same serotype.

These prevailing problems with the current vaccines against FMD have stimulated several groups interested in the molecular aspects of immunization to determine whether other approaches based on mod-ern technology would be useful in providing an entirely new form of vaccine. This chapter illustrates how the emerging understanding at the molecular level of (1) antigenic variation and (2) the features of an antigen that are require to elicit a protective immune response could lead to a synthetic vaccine against the disease. FMDV provides an excellent model for this type of work because there are several experimental animal models in addition to the naturally susceptible hosts. Moreover, there is considerable economic stimulus for the development of a peptide vaccine that would be free from any danger of causing disease.

II. The Concept of Synthetic Vaccines

A. VIRUS SUBUNITS

As long ago as the 1960s, it was shown that several lipid-containing viruses, namely influenza, measles, rabies, and vesicular stomatitis, could be dissected into biologically active fragments by dissolving the lipid membrane. The fragments were separated by a variety of physical methods and their biological activity was studied. The surface projections of the viruses were shown to carry the immunogenic activity, and analysis by polyacrylamide gel electrophoresis showed that this activity was associated with an individual protein. Viruses not possessing a lipid envelope, such as FMDV, required more severe conditions for their dissection, with the consequent greater loss of biological activity. However, it was shown by Laporte *et al.* (1973) that VP1, one of the four capsid proteins of FMDV, would elicit the formation of neutralizing antibody. This observation confirmed the earlier demonstration that the dramatic reduction in infectivity and immunogenicity of the virus particles after treatment with trypsin was due to the cleavage of the same proten *in situ*. The other capsid proteins were unaffected by the treatment (Wild *et al.*, 1969).

The isolated VP1 had very low immunogenic activity compared with that of the virus particle. Thus, at least two injections of 250 μg of the protein were required to achieve the same level of neutralizing antibody as one injection of 10 μg of intact virus particles. Although the production of VP1 in *E. coli* cells by recombinant DNA technology methods was accomplished with high yields, as expected the product was no more immunogenic than the protein isolated from virus particles. Nevertheless, the work acted as a stimulus for the chemical approach which forms the basis for the remainder of this chapter.

B. Epitopes

As the chemical structure of many viruses started to emerge in the 1950s and 1960s, an important advance was described by Anderer (1963) in Germany. He showed that a fragment of the coat protein of tobacco mosaic virus from the carboxyl terminus would elicit the formation of virus-neutralizing antibodies in rabbits. Moreover, the synthetic peptide corresponding to this segment would also elicit neutralizing antibody (Anderer and Schlumberger, 1965). This observation was followed by extensive work on synthetic antigens by Sela and his group in Israel. Of particular significance was the observation that a fragment of 21 amino acids of the coat protein of MS2, an RNA-containing bacteriophage, elicited antibody that reacted with the intact virus particle. Subsequent addition of the anti-species antibody neutralized the infectivity of the virus (Langebeheim et al., 1976). The synthetic peptide corresponding in sequence to this fragment elicited a similar response.

These observations have provided the basis for the subsequent exploration of the concept that small fragments of viral proteins will elicit a protective immune response against infection with viruses that cause diseases in animals and man. Such studies became feasible with many viruses when methods for the sequencing of DNA became available a decade ago (Maxam and Gilbert, 1977; Sanger et al., 1977). The genes coding for the immunogenic proteins of several viruses had already been identified and the availability of nucleic acid sequencing allowed the sequences of the amino acids in these proteins to be derived. Until that time, the number of proteins whose amino acid sequences had been determined was small, but the publication of the nucleic acid sequencing papers opened the floodgates. The remainder of this section describes how active sequences of the coat protein of FMDV were identified.

The virus particle, which sediments at 146S, carries most of the immunogenic activity of virus harvests. It consists of one molecule of single-stranded (ss) RNA, mol. wt. c2.6×10^6 and 60 copies of each of four proteins VP1–VP4. Proteins VP1–VP3 have a mol. wt of c 24×10^3 and VP4 has a mol. wt. of 10×10^3. The virus particle is unstable below pH 7, releasing the RNA in an infectious form, with the protein forming (1) a 12S subunit containing five copies of VP1 to VP3 and (2) an aggregate of VP4. The entire mixture has about 1% of the immunogenic activity of the 146S particle and fractionation studies show that this immunogenicity is associated with the 12S pentameric unit. These observations pointed clearly to the immunogenic activity being correlated with the integrity of the virus particle.

A more compelling piece of evidence was provided by the work, referred to above, that trypsin lowered considerably the infectivity and immunogenicity of a virus of serotype O, although its appearance in the electron microscope was unaltered. Analysis of the proteins of the enzyme-treated virus showed that only VP1 appeared to be altered by the treatment. This protein was cleaved into two fragments whose combined molecular weight was slightly less than that of the molecule in the untreated virus particles.

The trypsin experiment and the more direct approach used by Laporte *et al.* (1973), referred to earlier, focussed attention on the importance of VP1. Two approaches were used to identify potential immunogenic sites. Kaaden *et al.* (1977) and Strohmaier *et al.* (1982) used the direct approach described by Anderer for tobacco mosaic virus and Sela and his colleagues for MS2 bacteriophage. Biologically active fragments were obtained from VP1 of a virus of serotype O either by cyanogen bromide cleavage of the protein which had been isolated from the virus particle or by cleaving it with enzymes *in situ*. The end groups of the separated fragments were determined by classical methods of protein chemistry, thus allowing them to be "placed" on the amino acid map of the complete protein which had been derived from the sequence of that portion of the RNA genome which codes for it (Sangar *et al.*, 1977).

In a second approach, Bittle *et al.* (1982) argued that, in a virus that is highly variable antigenically, the amino acid sequences would vary at the antigenic sites. Nucleic acid sequences corresponding to that part of the virus genome coding for VP1 revealed that although the amino acid sequences were highly conserved between different serotypes, there were three variable regions at positions 42–61, 138–160, and 194–204. The sequence in the 138–160 region was particularly variable.

These predictions were tested directly by measuring the immunogenic activity in guinea pigs of synthetic peptides encompassing the entire sequence of VP1. The virus of serotype O used by Strohmaier *et al.* (1982) was also used in these experiments by Bittle *et al.* (1982). The 141–160 sequence produced high levels of neutralizing antibody, even with one injection, whereas the peptides containing the 194–204 sequence elicited much lower levels and 41–60 produced no neutralizing activity. Moreover, one injection of the 141–160 peptide protected the animals against a severe challenge infection.

Similar experiments showed that peptides corresponding to the sequences of the VP1 of viruses belonging to other serotypes were equally active in eliciting neutralizing activity. Unexpectedly, the anti-peptide sera were less specific in their neutralizing activity than the corresponding anti-virus particle antisera. This observation, which is of considerable importance when considering vaccination against a virus that occurs as several antigenic variants, is discussed in more detail below.

C. PRESENTATION OF THE PEPTIDE

In the early work with peptides as immunogens, it had been assumed that it would be necessary to attach a peptide to a carrier protein to ensure its immunogenicity. Keyhole limpet hemocyanin was a favorite choice with several workers, but other proteins such as tetanus toxoid, which would be more acceptable clinically because it wa already used prophylactically, proved to be as good. None of the methods in general use for the coupling of peptides to proteins could be considered to produce a uniform product in which the location and configuration of the peptide on the carrier protein was known, even approximately. Moreover, the polymerized peptide, in which no carrier protein was used, also proved to be immunogenic, whether it was produced by cross-linking of the peptide molecules with glutaraldehyde or by oxidative linkage via added terminal cysteine residues (Bittle et al., 1984).

It was not surprising therefore that the neutralizing antibody response to the peptide was only about 0.1% of that of an equivalent weight of the sequence when it formed part of the virus particle. Clearly, several factors influenced the response, chief of which was the configuration of the sequence as it exists on the virus particle. An early initiative was to determine the structure of the virus particle by X-ray diffraction and this project is now nearing completion (Fox et al., 1987, and unpublished observations). In the meantime, attempts were made to enhance the response by expressing the peptide as part of a fusion protein with β-galactosidase. By using this approach it was considered that the orientation of the peptide in relation to the carrier protein would be closely defined and the fusion protein would be a much more uniform product. Our own experiments (Winther et al. (1986) and those of Broekhuijsen et al. (1987), which were conducted independently, showed that a fusion protein with the FMDV peptide sequence attached to the amino terminus of the β-galactosidase molecule was no more immunogenic than protein molecules with the peptide attached randomly by chemical methods. This disappointing result emphasized that our knowledge of the presentation of the peptide was at an empirical level and this was further illustrated by the finding of

Broekhuijsen *et al.* (1987) that two or four copies of the peptide, expressed head to tail at the amino terminus of β-galactosidase gave a response in guinea pigs that was several orders of magnitude higher than that obtained with the hybrid containing only one copy of the peptide (Table I). Moreover, one injection of 40 μg of peptide in such a construct protected swine against challenge infection.

Clearly these results are of considerable practical importance because they show that one injection of the peptide can provide protective immunity in a target species. However, the theoretical implications are no less important and it would be very worthwhile to compare the conformation of the peptide in the one-, two- and four-copy constructs.

Since the response to the peptide sequence when it forms part of the virus particle is very high, we have investigated whether multiple copies presented on a particle of the same size range would elicit a greater response than when it is presented as the monomer. It was known that the core protein of hepatitis B virus self-assembles into particles 27 nm in diameter and contains several hundred copies of the molecule. We also knew that a hybrid protein in which a foreign amino acid sequence is expressed at the amino terminal of the hepatitis B core protein would also assemble into core particles (P. E. Highfield, personal communication). In our experiments (Clarke *et al.*, 1987) we have found that an expressed protein consisting of the peptide, six amino acids of pre-core, and the entire core protein can be expressed in vaccinia virus. As little as 2 μg of the expressed hybrid protein, which was separated as a 27-nm particle by sucrose gradient centrifugation, elicited very high levels of neutralizing antibody in guinea pigs. Indeed, the level of neutralizing antibody approached that elicited by an equivalent amount of the peptide when it forms part of the FMDV particle (Table II). This response is by far the highest so far described for the FMDV peptide. Moreover, as little as 0.02 μg of peptide presented in this form, although not eliciting measurable levels of neutralizing antibody, was sufficient to prime guinea pigs so that a second injection of the same amount elicited high levels of neutralizing antibody.

Clearly, the configuration of the peptide presented in this form is approaching that which it takes up on the FMDV particle. However, other factors may be playing a role in the enhanced response. Milich and McLachlan (1986) have shown that the hepatitis B core can induce antibody responses *via* both a T-cell-dependent and a T-cell-independent pathway. Moreover, the core-specific helper T cells can help B cells produce antibody against the hepatitis B envelope antigens even though these antigens are on separate molecules. These

TABLE I

Anti-Peptide Antibody, Neutralizing Antibody, and Protective Immune Response of Guinea-Pigs Inoculated with 200 μg of Fusion Proteins Containing One, Two, or Four Copies of the FMDV Peptide 137–162

No. of copies of peptide	Dose (μg)		Animal number	Peptide antibody titer ($\log_{10}$)		Neutralizing antibody titer ($\log_{10}$ SN$_{50}$)		Protection data[a]
	Fusion protein	VP1 peptide component		28 days	56 days	28 days	56 days	
1	200	5	1	1.0	<1.0	<0.6	<0.6	NP
			2	1.7	2.1	<0.6	<0.6	NP
			3	1.1	1.8	<0.6	<0.6	NP
			4	<1.0	1.4	<0.6	<0.6	NP
2	200	10	1	4.2	4.4	1.9	1.5	P
			2	3.8	4.0	2.0	2.1	P
			3	3.7	3.9	2.2	1.8	P
			4	3.4	3.1	1.8	1.1	P
4	200	20	1	2.3	2.9	1.4	0.9	P
			2	3.1	3.4	2.0	1.7	P
			3	2.9	2.9	0.8	1.2	P
			4	4.2	4.7	1.7	2.4	P
Synthetic peptide 137–160Cys	—	5	1	—	—	<0.6	<0.6	NP
			2	—	—	<0.6	<0.6	NP
			3	—	—	<0.6	<0.6	NP
			4	—	—	<0.6	<0.6	NP

[a] NP, Not protected; P, protected.

TABLE II

COMPARATIVE IMMUNOGENICITY OF INACTIVATED FMDV PARTICLES, SEROTYPE O_1, WITH A
VARIETY OF SYNTHETIC AND BIOSYNTHETIC ANTIGENS

| Test Sample | Dose (μg) | | Days post inoculation | | |
	Total antigen	FMDV VP1 (142–160 sequence)	0	28	42
Inactivated					
FMDV particles	1	0.02	<0.6[a]	1.6	1.7
HBcAg/142–160					
fusion protein	2	0.2	<0.6	2.1	2.9
β-gal/$(137$–$162)_2$					
fusion protein	200	7	<0.6	1.5	1.9
142–160Cys					
peptide	100	100	<0.6	1.8	1.7
137–160Cys					
peptide	120	100	<0.6	2.7	2.2

[a] $\log_{10}$ SN_{50} against 100 $TCID_{50}$ of virus.

properties of the core particles may provide the underlying reason for
the excellent response to the FMDV peptide when it is attached to the
core protein. This finding has important implications for the presentation of peptides to the immune system. Milich *et al.* (1987) have also
shown that a single synthetic T-cell epitope of the core can prime
helper T cells to induce B cells to produce antibody that reacts with
multiple envelope protein antigens.

These relationships between the B- and T-cells responses are now
becoming understood at the molecular level and recent relevant
experiments with the FMDV peptides are described in the next section.

III. Requirements for a Protective Immune Response

In FMD, protection against infection can usually be correlated with
the level of neutralizing antibody in the serum at the time of
challenge. Although there is some disagreement about the validity of
this generally held view, experience over many years has led to its
general acceptance. The current vaccines, based on inactivated tissue
culture harvests of the virus, must meet the requirements of protecting
cattle at 28 days after the inoculation of a single dose of the product.

Such stringent requirements are usually met with the currently available products and 10 μg of inactivated virus particles will provide protection.

The initial efforts to produce a peptide vaccine against FMD suffered from the fact that they were too successful. As little as 100 μg of the 141–160 sequence, linked to keyhole limpet hemocyanin and delivered as one dose, elicited a level of neutralizing antibody in guinea pigs that was higher enough to protect them against challenge infection. However, the neutralizing antibody response in cattle and pigs was lower and not high enough to protect these animals against challenge.

When uncoupled peptide was used, the difference between the responses in guinea pigs and pigs was even greater. The limitation of the host immune response is clearly a problem for vaccine development, but the growing understanding of the importance of the T-cell response and how it functions at the molecular level now allows a rational approach to its study. It has become clear that a peptide will only be immunogenic in those recipients whose histocompatibility proteins recognize it. The requirements for a peptide vaccine, therefore, comprise at least two factors, one recognized by B cells and the second by T cells. Indeed, the helper T cell is the focal point of the immune response because it is necessary for the antibody response and in particular for an anamnestic response. These facts have led us to consider whether the factors that determine the response to the FMDV peptide are related to MHC restriction.

In preliminary experiments, we have studied the response to the uncoupled peptide in a number of well-defined mouse haplotypes. We have found that mice belonging to the H-2^k haplotype respond well to the peptide, whereas H-2^d haplotype mice do not respond (Fig. 2). However, by using a peptide that provides T-cell help in the H-2^d mice in combination with the FMDV peptide, a response was obtained similar to that obtained in the H-2^k mice (Fig. 3). The peptides used were those defined by Berzofsky and Grey and their colleagues (Berkower et al., 1984; Streicher et al., 1984; Shimonkevitz et al., 1984), namely, two sequences from sperm whale myoglobin (SWMI 132–148 and SWMII 105–121) and one sequence from ovalbumin (OVA 323–339). However, the response to the three hybrid peptides differed in one significant respect. Thus, neutralizing antibodies were evoked only in those H-2^d mice receiving the OVA and SWMI sequences. This result suggests that T-helper cell epitopes may control antibody production of specific B-cell clones.

To characterize the nature of the virus, neutralizing and nonneutralizing antibody populations in those mice that had received the hybrid

F. BROWN

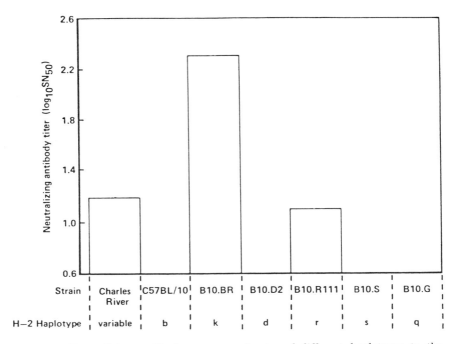

F<small>IG</small>. 2.   Neutralizing antibody response of mice of different haplotypes to the
uncoupled 141–160 peptide of FMDV. The sera were collected 56 days after inoculation
of the uncoupled peptide with Freund's incomplete adjuvant and the neutralizing
activity measured against 100 tissue culture ID_{50} in a microneutralization test.

peptides with the OVA and SWMII T cell sites, the 28 days postinoculation sera were tested with a range of peptides located with the
141–160 sequence of the FMDV peptide. The antibodies to the peptide
with the added OVA T-cell site (i.e., those which neutralize the virus)
recognized peptides from the 147–156 region, which is critical for the
induction of virus-neutralizing antibody. In contrast, the antibodies to
the peptide with the added SWMII T-cell site reacted only with those
peptides from the amino terminus; i.e., they did not react with those
from the region known to be critical for the induction of neutralizing
antibody.

The hybrid peptides were synthesized so that the B-cell epitope was
amino terminal to the T-cell epitope. However, at this stage of the
work, it is not known whether this is the best arrangement of the
individual epitopes or even whether it is necessary for them to be
covalently linked.

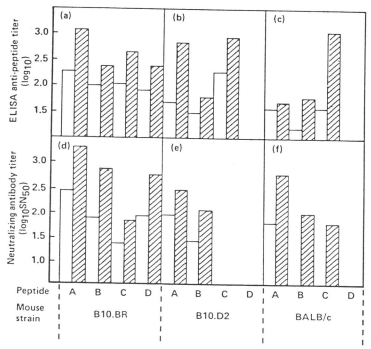

Fig. 3. Anti-peptide and neutralizing antibody response of mice belonging to the H-2^k (B10.BR) and H-2^d (B10.D2 and BALB/c) haplotypes to the 141–160 peptide of FMDV linked at its C terminus to (a) OVA, (b) SWMI, (c) SWMII, or (d) 161–177 from FMDV-VP1 and inoculated with Freund's incomplete adjuvant. The open columns give the values for sera collected 28 days after a single inoculation and the hatched columns give the values 28 days after a second inoculation, 63 days after the first.

IV. The Problem of Antigenic Variation

The occurrence of FMDV as seven serotypes poses severe problems in the control of this disease, because a vaccine prepared from virus belonging to one serotype does not afford protection against infection with viruses of the other serotypes. Moreover, antigenic variation even within a serotype is such that a vaccine may not protect animals against infection with all isolates from the same serotype.

The antigenic relationship between a field isolate and the virus from which a vaccine has been prepared is usually expressed as a ratio (r) between the antibody titers of the anti-vaccine serum against the heterologous and homologous viruses. Values for a group of viruses belonging to serotype O are shown in Table III. Unexpectedly, we found that the r values with an antiserum prepared against the 141–160 peptide were much higher (Ouldridge *et al.*, 1986). The reason for this cross-reactivity may be related to the conserved region of the peptide sequence between amino acids 145 and 151 (Table IV). The viruses that were not neutralized by the anti-peptide antiserum had an amino acid change at position 148. Some of our early work with closely related viruses of serotypes A also showed the importance of the amino acid at this position in determining antigenic specificity (Rowlands *et al.*, 1983).

In preliminary experiments it has been demonstrated that the cross-neutralizing activity of the anti-peptide sera extends to viruses of other serotypes. It seems that if the structural basis for this cross-reactivity can be determined precisely, peptides that will elicit neutralizing antibody against all serotypes can be designed. Of particular interest in this connection is the presence of the sequence Arg-Gly-Asp at positions 145–147. This sequence, first pointed out by Geysen *et al.* (1985), occurs, with one exception, in all the FMDV isolates studied so far. Moreover, a peptide of sequence Asn-Leu-Arg-Gly-Asp-Leu-Glu linked to keyhole limpet hemocyanin elicited antibody that neutralized not only viruses having the same sequence at those positions, but also viruses belonging to other serotypes. These observations indicate that by presenting the Arg-Gly-Asp sequence to the host in different configurations, it may be possible to enhance the cross-reactivity of the response.

TABLE III

CROSS-NEUTRALIZATION TESTS ON ISOLATES OF VIRUSES BELONGING TO FMDV, SEROTYPE O[a]

Serum	Kauf B64	Kauf B7	BFS 1848	BFS 1860	Virus OV1 subtype 6	Hong Kong	Indonesia 7/83	Thailand 1/80
Anti-virus particle BFS 1860	0.2	0.2	0.2	1.0	<0.1	0.5	0.2	0.1
Anti-peptide 141–160	0.9	0.6	1.0	1.0	<0.1	1.0	0.9	0.1

[a] The values are expressed as the ratio: neutralization of heterologous virus/neutralization of homologous virus.

TABLE IV

AMINO ACID SEQUENCES OF THE 141–160 REGION OF VP1 OF SEVERAL ISOLATES OF FMDV, SEROTYPE O

Virus	141									150
Kaufbeuren B64	Val	Pro	Asn	Leu	Arg	Gly	Asp	Leu	Gln	Val
Kaufbeuren B7	.[a]	.	.	.	.	.	.	.	.	.
BFS 1848	.	.	.	.	.	.	.	.	.	.
BFS 1860	.	.	.	.	.	.	.	.	.	.
O-VI (Subtype 6)	.	.	.	Val	.	.	.	Thr	.	.
Hong Kong	Met	Ser	.	Val	.	.	.	.	.	.
Indonesia 7/83	Thr	Thr	.	Val	.	.	.	.	.	.
Thailand 1/80	Leu	Thr	.	Val	.	.	.	Arg	.	.
	151									160
Kaufbeuren B64	Leu	Ala	Gln	Lys	Val	Ala	Arg	Thr	Leu	Pro
Kaufbeuren B7	.	.	.	.	.	.	.	.	.	.
BFS 1848	.	.	.	.	.	.	.	.	.	.
BFS 1860	.	.	.	.	.	.	.	.	.	.
O-VI (Subtype 6)	.	Asp	.	.	.	Ser	.	Ala	.	.
Hong Kong	.	Thr	.	.	Ala	Ser	.	Ala	.	.
Indonesia 7/83	.	.	.	.	Ala	Ala	.	.	.	.
Thailand 1/80	.	.	.	.	Ala	.	.	Pro	.	.

[a] Point signifies no change from Kaufbeuren B64 sequence.

V. The Potential of Peptide Vaccines for Other Diseases

The possibility of developing immunogenic peptides for the control of other diseases, particularly heptatis B and malaria, are also being investigated. The study of these diseases is more difficult than FMD for two main reasons. First, with FMD the target species can be readily used to test potential vaccines for their ability to protect against experimental infection. When the target species is man, as with hepatitis B and malaria, such tests are difficult, if not impossible, to arrange. Consequently, reliance has to be placed on protection tests in experimental animals, with the inherent dangers of extrapolating those results to man. Moreover, for hepatitis B the only suitable experimental animal for protection studies is the chimpanzee, which makes the tests very costly.

Second, the causal agents for these diseases are more complex than that causing FMD. Hepatitis B is caused by a DNA-containing virus, but there are three morphologically distinct structures in the sera of infected patients: (1) 22-nm spherical particles, (2) 22-nm diameter filaments 200–400 nm in length, and (3) the mature 45-nm virus particle. The virion is a double-shelled spherical particle, consisting of a 28-nm core surrounded by a 7-nm lipoprotein coat and surface coat proteins. The surface antigen is found in all three structures. The 22-nm spherical particles are by far the most abundant and can be present in concentrations up to 10^{14}/ml, outnumbering the other structures by more than 1000-fold. Because of their abundance, these particles have served as the basis for vaccine development and the first commerically available vaccines consisted of these particles isolated from the blood of carrier patients. Subsequently, vaccines were prepared from 22-nm particles which had been biosynthesized in yeast cells and the products prepared from both sources are now available commercially.

The 22-nm particles contain 70% protein, 22% lipid, and 8% carhobydrate. The protein consists of a 25,000 mol. wt. molecule, part of which is glycosylated to give a 30,000 mol. wt. molecule and its amino acid sequence has been derived from the base sequence of the gene coding for it. The surface antigen has four serologically defined subtypes, adw, ayw, adr, and ayr, but protection against infection is conferred by antibodies to the group-specific a determinant. However, its location on the sequence and precise definition still remain to be established. For this reason, no synthetic peptide has provided the basis for a totally efficacious vaccine. However, peptides in the 110–150 region of the 226-amino-acid protein elicit antibodies that react with the surface antigen (Harman and Melnick, 1987).

As with the FMDV peptide, presentation of the heptatitis B peptide is important, particularly with respect to the cysteine residues and their involvement in disulfide bonds. Such bonds appear to be important because of the stability and conformation they confer. Reduction of the disulfide bonds followed by alkylation results in the loss of most of the immunogenic activity of the peptide.

The antibody response to the peptide is, without exception, much lower than that obtained with the surface antigen. There could be several reasons for this difference, including the possibility that the immunogen of the surface antigen consists of discontinuous epitopes. Clearly, much remains to be learned about the immunogenic structure of the surface antigen and its presentation to the host.

In addition to the surface antigen, other regions of the virus may be involved in immunogenicity. Work by Neurath *et al.* (1984) indicates that there are important epitopes in the pre-S region of the virus. Moreover, the work of Milich and McLachlan (1986) and Milich *et al.*

(1987) with the core particle of hepatitis B virus indicates that constructions containing amino acid sequences from both the core and surface proteins may provide enhanced activity.

The problems with a peptide vaccine for malaria are even more profound because of the complexity of the life cycle of the agent and its antigenic variability. However, the fact that man can be protected against infection with *Plasmodium falciparum* by vaccination with whole malaria parasites has persuaded several groups to investigate the possibility of engineering a subunit or peptide vaccine.

The development of this approach toward vaccination against malaria requires a knowledge of the complex life cycle of the parasite. Infection is initiated by the bite of the female *Anopheles* mosquito and the injection of sporozoites into the blood of the host. The sporozoites then enter the liver, where they multiply rapidly. One sporozoite gives rise to thousands of merozoites when the hepatocytes rupture. The released merozoites then invade red blood cells and either multiply into asexual stages or mature into the sexual gametocyte stage. Once the gametocytes are ingested by the mosquito, the sexual cycle begins. Following fertilization, the zygotes penetrate the epithelial cells of the gut of the mosquito and transform into oocysts, leading to the development of thousands of thread-like sporozoites. These migrate to the salivary glands and then mature into the infective form.

The possible sources of antigens for vaccines correspond to the three extracellular stages—sporozoites, merozoites, and gametocytes—which could be targets for the immune system. Most attention has been concentrated on the use of sporozoites. Immunization with sporozoites was first described by Mulligan *et al.* (1941). These workers obtained substantial protection, and subsequent work showed that mice could be protected against infection with *P. berghei* with γ-irradiated sporozoites. Similar results were obtained in experiments with primate malaria systems. Sporozoite-induced immunity is stage specific. Mice immunized with sporozoites which are then completely protected against sporozoite challenge are fully susceptible to the inoculation of the blood stages of the same parasite strain.

Anti-sporozoite antibodies have neutralizing activity, suggesting the protective immunity is antibody mediated and that the antigens involved in protective immunity and in the circumsporozoite reactions might be identical. This was proven when it was found that a monoclonal antibody against *Plasmodium berghei* sporozoites had all the properties of a polyclonal sera obtained from vaccinated animals. The monoclonal antibody identified a surface protein of mol. wt. 44×10^3 and its precursors of mol. wt. 56 and 54×10^3. Moreover, passive transfer of the monoclonal antibody afforded complete protection against homologous sporozoite challenge.

Circumsporozoite proteins display an unusual immunological property that is important in the context of developing a peptide vaccine. The Nussenweigs (Zavala *et al.*, 1987) have shown that every monoclonal antibody against the surface membrane of sporozoites appears to binding to the same site, suggesting that there is a single immunodominant region. Moreover, incubation of crude extracts of sporozoites with monoclonal antibody strongly inhibits the subsequent binding of polyclonal anti-sporozoite antibodies.

The gene coding for the circumsporozoite protein of the simian malaria parasite *P. knowlesi* was cloned by Ellis *et al.* (1983). The immunodominant epitope of the protein was found to be a 12-amino-acid sequence Gln-Ala-Gln-Gly-Asp-Gly-Ala-Asn-Ala-Gly-Gln-Pro tandemly repeated 12 times (Godson *et al.*, 1983). This sequence was synthesized and induced sporozoite neutralizing antibodies. Since then, the genes encoding the circumsporozoite proteins of *P. falciparium, P. vivax,* and *P. cynomolgi* have also been cloned. For example, the *P. falciparum* repetitive epitope comprises the tetramer Asn-Ala-Asn-Pro and is identical in sporozoites isolated from widely separated geographic areas and sequential repeats of the tetramer unit linked to a carrier molecule induce anti-sporozoite activity.

As with the other potential peptide vaccines, it is becoming clear that T-cell epitopes are necessary for inducing long-lasting antibody responses that will be boosted by subsequent infections and for overcoming genetic nonresponsiveness. As described above for FMDV, this problem can be overcome by addition of an appropriate T-helper cell epitope to the B-cell epitope. Recent work by Good *et al.* (1987) has shown that by coupling an amphipathic helical sequence corresponding to residues 326–346 of the circumsporozoite protein to the Asn-Ala-Asn-Pro repeat sequence, the nonresponsiveness of mice belonging to the H-2^k haplotype to the repeat sequence alone can be overcome.

VI. What Does the Future Hold?

The concept of a totally synthetic vaccine against FMD, largely unacceptable a few years ago, is now beginning to attract more supporters as the results of a variety of experimental approaches begin to accumulate. The major argument against a peptide vaccine initially was the conceived amount of peptide that would be necessary to evoke a protective immune response. Moreover, the excellent responses to the peptide in guinea pigs appeared not to be reflected in cattle. Two groups of experiments have now shown that these problems can be overcome. First, two or more copies of the peptide linked to the amino terminus of β-galactosidase elicit much higher neutralizing antibody responses than the fusion protein containing only one copy. The reason for this increased activity is not understood and warrants close study. The improved immune response with the hepatitis B core construct is even more dramatic. Milich has provided considerable information on the desirable immunogenic properties of the hepatitis B core particle and this method for presenting peptides may hold the key to the delivery of haptens. More detailed investigations of the T-cell sites of the core particle are proceeding and the results of these are eagerly awaited. It would clearly be of importance to measure the activity of the FMD peptide core construct in cattle and pigs.

The second approach follows from the recognition that to realize their full potential as vaccines, uncoupled peptides must contain domains that react with helper T-cell receptors and Ia antigens in addition to binding sites of anti-protein antibodies. The contrast between the rather disappointing responses in cattle and the encouraging observations in guinea pigs clearly required investigation of the genetic restriction involved. The results of the preliminary experiments in mice, in which it was shown that the genetic restriction in mice of the H-2^d haplotype can be overcome by linking the FMDV peptide to a defined helper T-cell determinant from ovalbumin or sperm whale myoglobin, provide grounds for optimism that the restriction in cattle can be overcome similarly. This rational approach to peptide vaccines based on a detailed knowledge of the immune response should provide the information necessary to design synthetic immunogens with B- and T-cell epitopes that will overcome the "within-species" and "between-species" variations.

In addition to these two approaches, it is becoming apparent that correct targeting of the peptide could lead to enhanced activity. Although many suggestions have been made, this aspect of antigen presentation has only been investigated empirically. As more details of antigen processing become available, there seems to be no reason why this extra dimension in antigen presentation should not become fully understood at the molecular level.

Finally, the vulnerability of the peptide bond clearly needs to be considered when peptide vaccines are under discussion. If we accept that the shape of the epitope is of major importance, there seems to be no reason why the shape of a peptide, which can be established by

direct analysis, should not be mimicked either by peptides consisting of
D-amino acids or even by other invulnerable molecules. Irrespective of
the approach, however, there is the urgent need to understand antigen
processing at the molecular level so that some general rules can be
drawn up.

Even with our largely empirical approach, we have shown that the
activity of the FMDV peptide can be enhanced by several orders of
magnitude. With the refinements outlined in the preceding para-
graphs, there seems to be no reason why potent immunogens based on
amino acid sequences should not emerge as the vaccines of the future.
If, in addition, the structural basis for the cross-reactivity of the
anti-peptide antisera can be elucidated, there will be the added bonus
of a vaccine that can be used against viruses of all serotypes.

REFERENCES

Anderer, F. A. (1963). *Biochim. Biophys. Acta* **71**, 246–248.
Anderer, F. A., and Schlumberger, H. D. (1965). *Biochim. Biophys. Acta* **97**, 503–509.
Berkower, I., Matis, L. A., Buckenmeyer, G. K., Gurd, F. R. N., Longo, D. L., and
    Berzofsky, J. A. (1984). *J. Immunol.* **132**, 1370–1378.
Bittle, J. L., Houghten, R. A., Alexander, H., Shinnick, T. M., Sutcliffe, J. G., Lerner,
    R. A. Rowlands, D. J., and Brown, F. (1982). *Nature (London)* **298**, 30–33.
Bittle, J. L., Worrell, P., Houghten, R. A., Lerner, R. A., Rowlands, D. J., and Brown, R.
    (1984). *In* "Vaccines '84: 'Modern Approaches to Vaccines" (R. M. Chanock and R. A.
    Lerner, eds), pp. 103–107. Cold Spring Harbor Lab., Cold Spring Harbor, New York.
Broekhuijsen, M. P., van Rijn, J. M. M., Blom, A. J. M., Pouwels, P. H., Enger-Valk,
    B. E., Brown, F., and Francis, M. J. (1987). *J. Gen. Virol.* **68**, 3137–3143.
Clarke, B. E., Newton, S. E., Carroll, A. R., Francis, M. J., Appleyard, G., Syred, A. D.,
    Highfield, P. E., Rowlands, D. J., and Brown, F. (1987). *Nature (London)* **330**,
    381–334.
Ellis, J., Ozaki, L. S., Guradz, R. W., Cochrane, A. H., Nussenzweign, V., Nussenzweig,
    R. S., and Godson, G. N. (1983). *Nature (London)* **305**, 536–538.
Fox, G., Stuart, D., Acharya, K. R., Fry, E., Rowlands, D., and Brown, F. (1987). *J. Mol.
    Biol.* **196**, 591–597.
Francis, M. J., Hastings, G. Z., Syred, A. D., McGinn, B., Brown, F., and Rowlands, D. J.
    (1987). *Nature (London)* **330**, 168–170.
Frenkel, H. S. (1947). *Bull. Off. Int. Epizoot.* **28**, 155–162.
Geysen, H. M., Barteling, S. J., and Meloen, R. H. (1985). *Proc. Natl. Acad. Sci. U.S.A.*
    82, 178–182.
Godson, G. N., Ellis, J., Svec, P., Schlesinger, D. H., and Nussenzweig, V. (1983). *Nature
    (London)* **305**, 29–33.
Good, M. F., Maloy, W. K., Lunde, M. N., Margolit, H., Cornette, J. L., Smith, G. O. O.,
    Moss, B., Miller, L. H., and Berzorfsky, J. A. (1987). *Science* **235**, 1059–1062.
Harman, F. R., and Melnick, J. L. (1987). *In* "Synthetic Vaccines" (R. Arnon, ed.), Vol. 2,
    pp. 31–50. CRC Press, Boca Raton, Florida.
Jenner, E. (1798). "An inquiry into the Uses and Effects of the Variolae Vaccinae."
    Sampson Low, London.

Kaaden, O. R., Adam, K.-H., and Stromhaier, K. (1977). *J. Gen. Virol.* **34**, 397–400.
Langebeheim, H., Arnon, R., and Sela, M. (1976). *Proc. Natl. Acad. Sci. U.S.A.* **73**, 4636–4640.
Laporte, J., Grosclaude, J., Wantyghem, J., Bernard, S., and Rouze, P. (1973). *C. R. Hebid. Seances Acad. Sci. D* **276**, 3399–3401.
Maxam, A. M., and Gilbert, W. (1977). *Proc. Natl. Acad. Sci. U.S.A.* **74**, 560–564.
Milich, D. R., and McLachlan, A. (1986). *Science* **234**, 1398–1401.
Milich, D. R., McLachlan, A., Thornton, G. B., and Hughes, J. L. (1987). *Nature (London)* **329**, 547–549.
Mulligan, H. W., Russell, P. F., and Mohan, B. M. (1941). *J. Malar. Inst. India* **4**, 125.
Neurath, A. R., Kent, S., and Strick, N. (1984). *Science* **224**, 392–395.
Ouldridge, E. J., Parry, N. R., Barnett, P. V., Bolwell, C., Rowlands, D. J., Brown, F., Bittle, J. L., Houghten, R. A., and Lerner, R. A. (1986). *In* "Vaccines '86" (F. Brown, R. M. Chanock, and R. A. Lerner, eds.), pp. 45–49. Cold Spring Harbor Lab., Cold Spring Harbor, New York.
Pasteur, L. (1885). *C. R. itebd. Seances Acad. Sci.* **101**, 765.
Rowlands, D. J., Clarke, B. E., Carroll, A. R., Brown, F., Nicholson, B. H., Bittle, J. L., Houghten, R. A., and Lerner, R. A. (1983). *Nature (London)* **306**, 694–697.
Sangar, D. V., Black, D. N., Rowlands, D. J., and Brown, F. (1977). *J. Gen. Virol.* **35**, 281–297.
Sanger, F., Nicklen, S., and Coulson, A. R. (1977). *Proc. Natl. Acad. Sci. U.S.A.* **74**, 5463–5467.
Semple, D. (1919). *Br. Med. J.* **2**, 333–371.
Shimonkevitz, R., Colon, S., Kappler, J. W., Marrack, P., and Grey, H. (1984). *J. Immunol.* **133**, 2067–2074.
Streicher, H. Z., Berkower, I. J., Busch, M., Gurd, F. R. N., and Berzofsky, J. A. (1984). *Proc. Natl. Acad. Sci. U.S.A.* **81**, 6831–6835.
Stromhmaier, K., Franze, R., and Adam, K.-H. (1982). *J. Gen. Virol.* **59**, 295–306.
Theiler, M., and Smith, H. H. (1937). *J. Exp. Med.* **65**, 767–786.
Wild, T. F., Burroughs, J. N., and Brown, F. (1969). *J. Gen. Virol.* **4**, 313–320.
Winther, M. D., Allen, G., Bomford, R. H., and Brown, F. (1986). *J. Immunol.* **136**, 1835–1840.
Zavala, F., Cochrane, A. H., and Nussenzweig, V. (1987). *In* "Synthetic Vaccines" (R. Arnon, ed.), Vol. 2, pp. 149–159. CRC Press, Boca Raton, Florida.

Infectious Recombinant Vectored Virus Vaccines

JOSEPH J. ESPOSITO AND FREDERICK A. MURPHY

Division of Viral Diseases, Center for Infectious Diseases, Centers for Disease Control, Atlanta, Georgia

195

I. Introduction

A. HISTORICAL PERSPECTIVE

Live-virus immunization was practiced as early as the tenth century in China and India; pustular fluid from a patient with smallpox was inoculated into previously uninfected persons. The practice, which we now call variolation, caused disease of varying severity and 1–2% mortality, in contrast to the 25% mortality of natural smallpox infection. By the mid-1700s, the practice had become widespread in many parts of the world. Later in that century, the English country physician, Edward Jenner, observed that variolation did not "take" in persons who previously had been infected with the pox from the teats of cows. In 1796, Jenner inoculated an 8-year-old boy with pustular fluid from a milkmaid's pox lesion. Within a few days an erythematous lesion appeared at the inoculation site and then regressed. Six weeks later Jenner challenged the boy with smallpox pustular fluid; a lesion developed but no disease followed. Jenner successfully repeated the experiment and further showed that the protective element in pus could be maintained by arm-to-arm passage. For almost 200 years the practice (originally called "cowpoxing") spread throughout the world, eventually confirming Jenner's prediction that smallpox could be eliminated. In 1840, Adelchi Negri, in Italy, began maintaining the cowpoxing inoculum in calves. In 1881, Louis Pasteur proposed the term "vaccination" instead of "inoculation," honoring Jenner's discovery; hence, the inoculum became known as vaccinia virus.

From the experiments of Jenner through the development of live-virus vaccines against yellow fever (Theiler and Smith, 1937), poliomyelitis (Sabin, 1955), measles (Enders *et al.*, 1960), and other diseases, vaccine viruses have been derived empirically, usually by repeated passages in animals, embryonating eggs, or cell cultures. The results represent great success stories—the live-virus vaccines have had excellent records of efficacy, reasonable safety, and modest cost. Generally, live-virus vaccines have provided long-lasting protection. Even when immunity levels have fallen with time, natural subclinical reinfections have served as harmless boosters. Inherently, both cell-mediated and humoral immunity have usually been stimulated by live-virus vaccines, just as in natural infections. Despite these and other qualities, live-virus vaccines do have disadvantages, and in many cases some researchers believe that a point of diminishing returns has been reached in regard to new developments. Some also believe that other approaches must be tried if we are to make significant further improvements in viral vaccines.

In the past two decades, technologies for biochemical characterization and genetic manipulation of viruses have led to the development of novel mutant and recombinant viruses. For example, novel deletion mutants of pseudorabies virus, derived by genetic engineering, have proven to be nonpathogenic yet effective in protecting swine from wild-type virus challenge (Kit *et al.,* 1987; Quint *et al.,* 1987). The overall promise of deletion mutants seems limited, however, especially relative to the promise of insertion mutants. In some ways one particular gene insertion strategy, that of heterologous gene insertion into infectious viruses which are then used as vectors, seems most promising of all.

B. The General Context for Vectored Virus Vaccines

Two classes of viral vectors may be differentiated. One class comprises replication-defective vector viruses that produce infectious progeny only via complementation by specifically transformed cells (SV40, adenoviruses) or by helper-virus superinfection (retroviruses). The second class comprises replication-competent viruses. Herpesviruses, adenoviruses, and poxviruses are the most notable examples of viruses that can serve as vectors for heterologous genes while maintaining full infectivity. Studies involving both classes of altered viruses have increased our insight into genomic structure, gene regulation, and transcription and translation, and have furthered our understanding of disease mechanisms and host defenses.

Experimental immunizations with infectious virus vectors carrying one or more heterologous genes for immunogenic proteins have been remarkably successful in experimental animals systems. Such immunizations have enabled the presentation of immunogenic proteins to the host immune system in an authentic way, mimicking closely the way antigens are presented in natural infections. Such successes have vaulted infectious virus vectors into consideration as vaccines for humans and animals.

Clearly, however, the use of poxviruses, herpesviruses, and adenoviruses as candidate vectors is not without problems. They all have complex *in vivo* replication demands, less-than-perfect virulence characteristics, and some undesirable host range traits. They all require further research to define and optimize these characteristics. For example, the persistence of adenoviruses in lymphatic tissues and herpesviruses in neural tissues and the progressive course of vaccinia virus infection in immunocompromised individuals must be studied further. We must better understand the consequences of specific deletion mutations in these vector viruses, such as those caused during the insertion of heterologous DNA. Such mutations may affect virulence, tropism, and host range, as well as immunogenicity.

In considering development and use of infectious vectored virus vaccines, we must be aware of the differences between human and veterinary vaccine use. In the case of human vaccines, the central focus is upon safety. Not only are adverse vaccine reactions objectionable, but they can be the basis for legal liability claims that influence all other aspects of vaccine development and use. In the case of veterinary vaccines, the central focus is upon cost-effectiveness in the context of an overall production–economy equation. There is much less regulatory control over the manufacturing and the quality assurance of animal vaccines as compared to human vaccines. The regulatory infrastructure for human vaccines enjoys a credible national and international reputation with leadership provided through the activities of the U.S. Food and Drug Administration (FDA) and the World Health Organization (WHO).

This chapter highlights aspects of infectious vectored viruses for human and animal vaccines, using the vaccinia virus system as the principal example. Several reviews of this subject have recently been published (Moss *et al.*, 1983; Smith and Moss, 1984; Smith *et al.*, 1984a,b; Quinnan, 1985; Mackett *et al.*, 1985a; Paoletti *et al.*, 1985a,b; Fenner, 1985a; Mackett and Smith, 1986; Moss and Flexner, 1987; Piccini and Paoletti, 1986, 1988; Beaud *et al.*, 1987). The initial success with vaccinia virus as a gene expression vector has now also begun to be extended to other poxviruses, notably fowlpox. Because licensing and use of such vaccines will require rigorous evaluation and efficacy and safety requiring new testing procedures and new regulations, we have approached the subject accordingly. We describe the biological, molecular, and immunological characteristics of vaccinia virus and other viruses in regard to their use as vectored viral vaccines, and we summarize the technology of heterologous gene transfer into vaccinia virus. We describe the nature of the infection caused in humans and animals by standard vaccinia virus, as the basis for study of infections caused in experimental animals by vectored vaccinia virus vaccine candidates. We note areas in need of further research and further policy development. All in all, we try to point out the great promise of this vaccine technology in advancing our capability for controlling diseases of humans and animals in the future.

II. Characteristics of Poxviruses as Vectors

A. POXVIRUSES WITH POTENTIAL FOR USE AS VECTORS

Over many years much experience has been gained with vaccines against human and animal poxvirus diseases. A massive amount of information on vaccinia virus (smallpox) vaccine in humans was gathered during the WHO Smallpox Eradication Programme; this included information on clinical, laboratory, and epidemiological aspects of vaccine usage. In veterinary medicine, poxvirus vaccines have been used to protect many species of animals and birds. These include vaccinia or ectromelia viruses to prevent mousepox and vaccinia virus to prevent rabbitpox and other orthopoxvirus infections of captive and domestic animals. Attenuated fowlpox virus vaccines have been used to protect poultry. Attenuated autologous viruses have been used for vaccinating against goatpox, sheeppox, and lumpy skin diseases. Attenuated myxoma and fibroma virus vaccines have been developed for domestic rabbits. Also, over many years, vaccines have been made from lesions of naturally infected animals (for use similar to variolation in humans) to prevent camelpox and contagious ecthyma (orf) of sheep. Mild to severe infections of animal handlers have been related to the use of such contagious ecthyma "vaccines" (Fenner et al., 1987; Tripathy et al., 1981).

Any poxvirus can be considered as a potential vector for heterologous genes, depending upon particular valuable characteristics, such as a wanted host range. For example, a raccoon poxvirus, recovered from the lungs of healthy raccoons (Alexander et al., 1972), has been used recently as a vector for the rabies virus glycoprotein gene (Esposito et al., 1987, 1988). This vector was developed for use as an oral, bait-delivered vaccine to combat the raccoon rabies outbreak that spread throughout the mid-Atlantic area of the United States during the 1980s (Jenkins and Winkler, 1987; Centers for Disease Control, 1987). Captive raccoons, fed the infectious recombinant virus in bait, have produced high levels of rabies-neutralizing antibodies and were protected against a lethal virus challenge. Safety and further efficacy studies are being planned to pursue field trials.

B. LESSONS FROM THE SMALLPOX ERADICATION PROGRAMME

The major factor in the success of the WHO Smallpox Eradication Programme was the development of a unique international infrastructure, which served as the focus for cooperative clinical, laboratory, and epidemiological research, as well as for vaccine delivery worldwide. Nevertheless, the WHO Programme could not have been successful if it were not for particular characteristics of the etiologic agent, variola virus, and of the disease, smallpox:

1. Smallpox was greatly feared, fostering universal interest and support for the use of a vaccine.
2. Smallpox was easily diagnosed clinically, allowing a focused use of the vaccine.
3. Variola virus did not persist in infected individuals nor in the environment, allowing a one-time sweep by vaccinators without concern for covering individuals missed or born later.
4. Variola virus was transmitted only by relatively close contact, allowing vaccinators to keep up with virus movement and allowing quarantine to be used in certain settings.
5. Variola virus was not transmitted by arthropods, allowing the use of "ring-vaccination" selective containment protocols in the late stages of the WHO Programme.
6. Variola virus had no animal reservoir and no capacity to persist in a zoonotic cycle.

C. Advantages of Vaccinia Virus as a Vaccine and as a Vector

In addition to those characteristics of variola virus and the disease smallpox that favored eradication, several attributes of vaccinia virus vaccine itself contributed to the success of the WHO Programme, particularly in developing countries:

1. Vaccinia virus vaccine is easily administered in a single-dose regimen.
2. Vaccinia virus vaccine is simple to manufacture and inexpensive to test. This is crucial—much of the cost of a vaccine is related to the complexity of production and related costs of quality assurance and safety testing.
3. Vaccinia virus vaccine is very stable. This is an outstanding quality of the virus itself (freeze-dried vaccine withstands 37°C for 30 days).
4. Vaccinia virus vaccine induces a relatively long-lived immunity.

These properties (see also Fenner, 1985a; Henderson and Arita, 1985) of vaccinia virus vaccine also can be taken as a list of advantages for using vaccinia virus and other poxviruses as vectors for human and animal vaccines. Of course certain poxviruses, such as avian poxviruses and myxoma virus, which are arthropod-borne in nature, would be subject to particular additional constraints.

Vaccinia virus vaccine had been very acceptable to people throughout the world because of its great reputation for having brought about the eradication of one of the great plagues of mankind, smallpox. Certainly, the equation of benefit : cost : risk was balanced in favor of its use to achieve smallpox eradication. It might be envisioned that there would be no preconceived bias against its use for another purpose in humans or animals. In many places, however, it has been years since vaccinia virus has been used, thus population re-education might be a significant factor. In some cases where conventional human or animal vaccines have proven inefficacious or too expensive, vaccinia virus-vectored vaccines might be assessed most favorably. The fact that a single vector can be designed to carry several heterologous genes for immunizing against several diseases might further influence public acceptance.

D. Disadvantages of Vaccinia Virus as a Vaccine and as a Vector

Vaccinia vaccination is not without its disadvantages in humans (see Table I) (Arita and Fenner, 1985).

E. Safety of Vaccinia Vaccines

Historically, trial and error guided the selection of the safest strains of vaccinia virus for vaccine production. In recent years, only a few strains have been used: Lister Institute (Lister), New York Board of Health (NYBH), Tian Tan, and Padwadangar. Because of the consideration of vaccinia virus as a vector, Arita and Fenner (1985) re-examined earlier data on the frequency of complications following smallpox vaccination. They collated rates of CNS complications and other adverse effects in seven European countries and the United States during different periods. They found that vaccines originating from either the NYBH or Lister strains produced the lowest rates of complications. Both of these strains were used extensively in developing countries, but little information is available about adverse effects in such settings. In the United States, England, and Wales (where these viruses were used widely) adverse effects occurred at low rates (Table II).

Criticism has occurred concerning the rigor used in confirming the

TABLE I

ADVERSE REACTIONS FOLLOWING VACCINIA VACCINATION IN HUMANS

Reaction	Cause	Occurrence	Mortality rate
Exanthematous disease	Progressive vaccinia resulting from compromised cell-mediated immunity	Mostly in children; very rare	High
	Eczema vaccinatum occurring in individuals vaccinated while having eczema	Very rare	High
	Generalized vaccinia following hematogenous spread of virus with postules on many parts of body	Rare	No mortality
	Accidental infection of conjunctiva or other parts of body after scratching primary vaccination lesion	Transmission can occur by same means with same results	Very low
Central Nervous System (CNS) disease	Vaccinia encephalitis occurring unpredictably resulting in cerebral impairment, hemiplegia, convulsions, coma	Very rare	High
Other complications	Fetal vaccinia infection	Very rare	Varying severity; some mortality

etiology of these adverse effects. Progressive vaccinia infection and eczema vaccinatum are easily diagnosed clinically, but background intercurrent CNS disease is not clinically distinguishable, and specific etiologic confirming tests were not used. Therefore, it is likely that these data overestimate the risk of CNS disease caused by vaccinia virus.

TABLE II

Frequency of Serious Complications of Vaccination in the United States, England, and Wales, Using New York Board of Health and Lister Vaccines

Complication	Cases/million primary vaccinations[a]	
	Age <1 year	Age >1 year
CNS disease	7–14	2.4–11.0
Progressive vaccinia	0–3	0.2–2.0
Eczema vaccinatum	4–8	6.0–10.0
Death	5–13	0.6–1.7

[a] Complications were much less frequent after revaccination. [From Fenner (1985a), reproduced with permission.]

Vaccinia virus, nonetheless, is associated with CNS complications. When Lister strain vaccine replaced other vaccine strains such as Hamburg, Berne, and Copenhagen in three European countries in the 1960s, the incidence of postvaccinal CNS disease dropped markedly (Arita and Fenner, 1985).

If vectored vaccinia virus vaccines are to be introduced for human use, a substantial reduction of adverse effects could be achieved with appropriate prevaccination screening. The Advisory Committee on Immunization Practices of the U.S. Public Health Service has recommended against vaccinating concurrently with other live-virus vaccines and against vaccinating high-risk individuals, such as persons with acute infections, eczema or other chronic dermatitides, pregnant women, children younger than 1 year of age, and immunocompromised persons. The latter includes persons with congenital or acquired defects in cell-mediated immunity such as severe combined immunodeficiency (dysgammaglobulinemia, Hodgkin's diseae, or acquired immunodeficiency syndrome (AIDS)), and persons receiving immunosuppressive drugs (alkylating agents, radiation, steroids, etc.). Even though today there is no reason for smallpox vaccination of general populations, these recommendations would serve well if infectious vectored vaccinia virus vaccines were to be introduced.

Veterinary use of vectored vaccinia virus vaccines would, of course, involve a minimum risk of human adverse effects. The principal risk would be from accidental inoculation, which would be of little consequence if vaccinators were prescreened and vaccinated accordingly. Also, deep intramuscular injection of animals instead of intradermal scarification might be useful in limiting virus transmission. Each vectored recombinant to be considered as a vaccine candidate would have to be evaluated separately in regard to the risk it would pose to vaccinators and other animal handlers, however, no novel untoward effects would be expected.

F. Origins of NYBH and Lister Strains of Vaccinia Virus

Because the NYBH and Lister vaccinia virus strains have caused the lowest rates of adverse effects, they and possibly certain derivatives should be considered primary candidates for human and animal vectored virus vaccines. For this reason, a brief history of these viruses is presented.

The origin of vaccinia virus itself is obscure; it is not thought to be a naturally occurring virus, but rather a recombinant between variola virus and Jenner's cowpoxing virus or a descendant of a now-extinct poxvirus of horses that caused "grease" in Jenner's time. The lineage of Jenner's virus became further obscured as the virus was distributed worldwide via arm-to-arm passage and via passage in calves, sheep, and other animals. Often the inoculum would lose potency when it was mixed with variola pustular material. This practice continued into the early 1900s. Despite this history, vaccinia virus strains are remarkably similar; their DNA restriction profiles are quite similar and distinct from other orthopoxviruses (Esposito *et al.,* 1978, 1985; Esposito and Knight, 1985; Mackett and Archard, 1979).

The NYBH strain of vaccinia virus was established in 1856 from a British vaccine that originated before calf passage had replaced human arm-to-arm passage. It is regarded as one of the most direct descendants of Jenner's vaccine. At the New York City Board of Health laboratories, the virus was maintained by passage in the skin of rabbits and calves and occasionally by intradermal passage in humans. Passage in rabbit testes was practiced to decrease microbial contamination and revitalize potency. The NYBH strain was used for vaccine production by many manufacturers, including Wyeth Laboratories, Inc. This company has passaged the virus in calves since 1929, in later years producing the lyophilized product "Dryvax calf-lymph." Others using the NYBH strain as starting material were Connaught Laboratories, Inc., Lederle Laboratories, Inc., the Massachusetts Department of Health, and national laboratories in many countries.

The Lister strain is said to have been isolated in 1870 during the Franco–Prussian war from a Prussian soldier with smallpox. The strain, first produced at the Lister Institute at Elstree, has been used in Great Britain since 1892. This strain has probably had the widest distribution of any in the world under many synonyms, including

Liverpool, Elstree, Merieux-37, and Nigeria. The Padwadangar strain, used widely in India, is known to have been derived from a mixture of Lister strain and a strain of unknown origin (Ray, 1973; Marennikova *et al.*, 1969). Further information on vaccinia virus strains can be found in papers by Wokatsch (1972), Fenner (1958), Briody (1959), Ghendon and Chernos (1964), Quinnan (1985), and the proceedings of two symposia (Gusic, 1969; Regamy and Cohen, 1973).

In keeping with the modern "seed-virus" concept, standards for good manufacturing practices (GMPs), and U.S. Food and Drug Administration quality assurance provisions for live-virus vaccines (Code of Federal Regulations, Title 21), two laboratories involved in vectored vaccinia virus development have rederived Lister and NYBH vaccine strains from manufacturers' seed viruses (B. Moss and J. Dalrymple, personal communications).

III. General Characteristics of Poxviruses

In the following sections we consider poxvirus virion structure, virion morphogenesis, genome structure, gene expression, biological (phenotypic) markers, and immunobiology, since these characteristics relate to the use of poxviruses as vectors. Reviews of these subjects have been published (White and Fenner, 1986; Fenner *et al.*, 1987, 1988; Fenner and Nakano, 1988; Nakano and Esposito, 1988; Dumbell and Huq, 1986; Moss, 1985; Tripathy *et al.*, 1981; Moss *et al.*, 1983; Holowczak, 1982, 1983; Cole and Blanden, 1982; Wittek, 1982; McFadden and Dales, 1982; Fenner, 1985b; Dales and Pogo, 1981; Cho and Wenner, 1973; Briody, 1959).

A. Poxvirus Virion Structure

Poxvirus virions are structurally complex, brick-shaped, and approximately 300 × 240 × 100 nm in size (except for parapoxviruses, which are ovoid, 260 × 160 nm). Virions have four major components: a dumbell-shaped *core* that contains the DNA genome, *lateral bodies* lying in the concavities of the core, an *outer membrane,* and a surrounding *envelope* (Fenner *et al.*, 1987, 1988; Dales and Pogo, 1981). Two types of infectious virus particles have been recognized during growth of poxviruses: extracellular enveloped virions (EEVs) and intracytoplasmic naked virions (INVs).

EEVs, studied especially in vaccinia and cowpox virus infections, are composed of all four components. They are spontaneously released from infected cells and, depending on virus strain and cell type, may constitute up to 10% of the virus produced (Boulter and Appleyard, 1973). EEVs are antigenically distinctive because of the composition of the envelope, which is derived from modified plasma membrane. Vaccinia virus EEV envelopes contain a 37-kilodalton (kD) palmitate-binding protein that constitutes 7% of the EEV protein mass and nine viral glycoproteins including an 85-kD protein component of the hemagglutinin (Hirt *et al.,* 1986; Payne, 1979, 1986; Shida, 1986a). The poxvirus hemagglutinin is separate from virions; it consists of virus-modified cell membranes. EEVs are involved in virus dissemination *in vivo* (Payne, 1980; Payne and Kristensson, 1985), and therefore are important considering the use of vaccinia virus for infectious vectored virus vaccines. To illustrate, it has been suggested that the distinctive antigenicity of the envelope of EEVs directs tissue tropism, pathogenicity, immunogenicity of the envelope of EEVs directs tissue tropism, pathogenicity, immunogenicity, and possibly host range properties. Therefore, insertion of heterologous proteins into the envelope of EEVs present in vectored vaccinia virus vaccines might alter vaccine properties in deleterious ways. This has not yet been shown with vaccine candidates, but the nature and effect of heterologous proteins present in the envelope of recombinant poxvirus virions must be examined.

INVs, the bulk of infectious particles produced in infected cells, are composed of a core, lateral bodies, and an outer membrane. INVs are released *in vivo* by cytolysis and in the laboratory by mechanical cell disruption. The location in the virion and the functional role (e.g., in absorption, penetration, fusion, etc.) of many vaccinia virus INV outer membrane and core proteins have been determined (Oie and Ichihashi, 1987; Ichihashi and Oie, 1980; Dales and Pogo, 1981; Moss, 1985; Fenner *et al.,* 1987). The genes for some of these proteins have also been mapped and sequences determined (Earl and Moss, 1987; McGeoch *et al.,* 1987; Rodriguez *et al.,* 1987). INVs of some poxviruses (cowpox, ectromelia, raccoon poxvirus, fowlpox) can become occluded in and protected by intracytoplasmic type A inclusion bodies. Since inclusion bodies might affect the stability and transmissibility of vectored poxviruses, their presence and effect should be studied further. Nonspecific entrapment of foreign gene products during maturation of vaccinia virus also must be studied further (Franke and Hruby, 1987).

B. Poxvirus Replication

Poxvirus virion adsorption and penetration occur directly via plasma membrane fusion or indirectly via endophagocytosis. Virion outer membrane fusion and uncoating then occur concomitantly and the virion core is released into the cytoplasm. Virion cores carry a complete transcription system that, during early stages of infection, produce mRNAs for at least 100 proteins, including the viral DNA polymerase and transcription enzymes. Soon after infection, a shutdown of cellular protein synthesis occurs, mediated in part by viral protein(s) and/or by production of 100- to 300-base polyadenylated nontranslated viral RNAs that affect ribosome function (Bablanian and Banerjee, 1986). Although vaccinia virus can replicate in enucleated cells (Villarreal *et al.*, 1984), its distinctive multisubunit RNA polymerase appears to contain host cell RNA polymerase II large-fragment activity (Morrison and Moyer, 1986; Broyles and Moss, 1986; Wilton and Dales, 1986).

Poxvirus replication can be divided into distinctive early and late stages that flank the peak of viral DNA replication. As viral DNA accumulates, transcriptional switch-over occurs and, in late stages, about 100 proteins, primarily virion structural proteins, are synthesized. Altogether, vaccinia virus encodes about 280 proteins, of which about 100 are structural (Carrasco and Bravo, 1986; Essani and Dales, 1979).

Poxvirus replication occurs in intracytoplasmic sites, termed "virus factories" (type B inclusion bodies). Virion morphogenesis becomes visible after the peak of DNA synthesis. Lipoprotein crescents (precursors of virion outer membrane structures) are formed, and these surround condensing viral genomes to form immature virions. Upon maturation, some virions migrate to the cell surface, undergoing a complex process of envelopment (Payne and Kristensson, 1985; Tsutsui *et al.*, 1983) and release as EEVs, but most remain as INVs until cytolysis occurs.

C. The Poxvirus Genome

The genomic DNA of poxviruses is a very large, linear molecule; it ranges in size from 110 to 150 kbp (parapoxviruses, capripoxviruses) to 165 to 210 kbp (orthopoxviruses) to 280 kbp (avipoxviruses). On the basis of DNA endonuclease studies, researchers know that cleavage sites within poxvirus genera are highly conserved among orthopoxviruses (Mackett and Archard, 1979; Esposito and Knight, 1985) and capripoxviruses (Black *et al.*, 1986), less so among leporipoxviruses (Block *et al.*, 1985), molluscipoxviruses (Porter and Archard, 1987), and yatapoxviruses (Esposito, unpublished data), and least so among parapoxviruses (Mercer *et al.*, 1987; Robinson *et al.*, 1987; Gassmann *et al.*, 1985) although there is considerable cross-hybridization within genera.

Both ends of poxvirus DNA are covalently closed, forming hairpin loops. In vaccinia and myxoma viruses, the loops are incompletely base-paired and exist in two equimolar isomeric forms that are inverted and complementary to each other (Upton *et al.,* 1987; Baroudy *et al.,* 1983; Pickup *et al.,* 1983). Extending from 1 to 40 kbp from the hairpin ends, depending on the virus strain, the terminal regions comprise inverted terminal repetitions (ITRs). Within vaccinia virus ITRs, 200 bp from each end, are tandem repetitions arrayed in adjacent sets (about 1 kbp each) that are separated by short intervening sequences (about 400 bp). DNA from highly passaged vaccinia virus strains and vaccinia vaccine stocks exhibits extensive terminal-length heterogeneity; this is caused by multiple recombinations that generate varying numbers and sizes of sets of tandem repeats (Wittek, 1982; DeLange and McFadden, 1987; Pickup *et al.,* 1982).

Significant mutational events, such as deletions, insertions, duplicative rearrangements of terminal regions (ITR copy transpositions), and various recombinatorial effects (e.g., nonhomologous crossover, random nonreciprocal transfer of controlling and/or coding sequences), occur spontaneously during poxvirus DNA replication (Pickup *et al.,* 1984; Moyer *et al.,* 1980; Esposito *et al.,* 1981; Archard *et al.,* 1984; Macaulay *et al.,* 1987). Such genomic rearrangements could generate undesirable novel strains and variants of recombinant viruses used for vectored vaccines; more genome stability would be advantageous to maintain homogeneity of a master seed. Toward this end, Ball (1987) has begun examining intramolecular recombination mechanisms that might be manipulated to control the genome stability of vaccine candidate virus strains.

Topographical similarities and conserved sequences in the DNA of different poxviruses suggest that they evolved from a common ancestor (Drillien *et al.,* 1987). All temperature-sensitive mutants of vaccinia virus map to the central region of the genome, indicating the location of most genes essential for productive infection (Thompson and Condit, 1986). Hypervariability of the ITRs suggests that this region contains most nonessential genes (nonessential at least for cell culture infection). Terminal region mutability seems likely to be the key to virus adaptation. In this regard, several viable terminal region deletion mutants of vaccinia virus have been isolated for possible use as vectors (Perkus *et al.,* 1986; Panicali *et al.,* 1981; Moss *et al.,* 1981). Although DNA structural analysis has been performed on attenuated derivatives of Lister strain virus (Sugimoto *et al.,* 1985), the efficacy and safety of such strains for vectored viral vaccines remain to be determined.

D. POXVIRUS GENE EXPRESSION

Poxvirus DNA is not infectious nor transcribed by cellular RNA polymerase. Both strands of DNA are transcribed via a distinctive RNA polymerase and other RNA-processing enzymes (for capping, polyadenylation, etc.); genes are spaced tightly along the poxvirus genome. Transcripts can be classified into three temporal classes: early, late, and early + late, relative to viral DNA replication (Moss, 1985). Annealing of RNAs from opposite DNA strands occurs very late in infection.

Leader sequences (30–100 bases) of vaccinia virus and early mRNAs appear to be different from each other and from prokaryotic eukaryotic mRNA leaders. Early mRNAs are of relatively uniform size, but late mRNAs, many for abundant proteins, vary in size. For example, the mRNAs for cowpox virus A-type inclusion protein and vaccinia virus structural 11-kD protein (both late proteins) have variable (5–35 bases) A-rich leader sequences (Bertholet et al., 1987; Schwer et al., 1987; Patel and Pickup, 1987). Evidence shows that the variable-sized A-rich leaders result from an inefficient RNA polymerase transcript initiation called "stuttering" (D. Pickup, personal communcation). Late mRNAs contain conserved UAA*AUG* sequences at the translation start codon that represent a conserved transcriptional processing site (Weir and Moss, 1987a; Hanggi et al., 1986; Bertholet et al., 1986). Slight deviations from the conserved sequences markedly diminish translation. The efficiency of translating individual late RNAs within an RNA group that shows varied 5′ ends are yet unresolved.

No genomic template has been found for the 25- to 100-base poly(A) tail on poxvirus mRNAs, but the signla for terminating transcripts at the 3′ end of poxvirus open reading frames appears in the genome as unevenly spaced tandem TTTTTNT sets (Rohrmann et al., 1986; Yuen and Moss, 1986; Upton et al., 1987). Functionally, it appears that viral mRNA capping enzyme plays a major role in terminating early transcripts by recognizing the UUUUUNU signal at the RNA 3′ end (B. Moss, personal communication).

Poxvirus RNA polymerase operates in concert with *cis*-acting promoters (AT-rich sequences immediately upstream of coding sequences). These promoters are distinctive from prokaryotic and eukaryotic promoters. Consensus TATA and AATA promoter sequences, separated by about 25 bp, have been identified for several early and late vaccinia virus genes (Plucienniczak et al., 1985). Minimal promoter units of 15 to 100 bases, upstream of early gene transcription start sites and putative processing sites, have been resolved (Coupar et al., 1987; Wier and

Moss, 1987a,b; Bertholet *et al.,* 1986; Cochran *et al.,* 1985). Interaction between poxvirus RNA polymerase and various promoters results in differential regulated production of mRNAs (Weinrich and Hruby, 1987). This, in turn, regulates the kinetics of protein synthesis. Regulation appears even more complex. For example, production and expression of the vaccinia virus TK, an early allosteric enzyme, may involve (1) feedback inhibition by TK metabolic products, (2) post-translational repression of TK synthesis, and/or (3) shutoff of TK mRNA synthesis by late transcription (Hruby, 1985; Hruby and Ball, 1981a,b; Franke *et al.,* 1985a; Bertholet *et al.,* 1987).

The influence of poxviruses on post-translational modifications of proteins, such as by phosphorylation and glycosylation, are unclear; in the case of simpler viruses, such modifications generally have been shown to be due to host cell enzymatic activities, but with poxviruses this remains to be explained. Some poxvirus proteins are post-translational cleavage products of precursor proteins, but again, whether the proteases carrying out such cleavages are of a host or viral source is not resolved. When proteins expressed by poxvirus vectors have been compared with native proteins, they usually have been found to be processed, transported through the cell, and secreted authentically. For example, influenza virus hemagglutinin, vesicular stomatitis virus glycoprotein, and murine leukemia virus envelope glycoprotein, when expressed by vaccinia recombinants, have been shown to be processed authentically and to migrate to apical or basal plasma membranes of host cells exactly like analogous native proteins (Stephens and Compans, 1986; Stephens *et al.,* 1986; McQueen *et al.,* 1986). An exception is represented by *Plasmodium falciparum* circumsporozoite protein, which when expressed by a vaccine virus vector was processed into two proteins (Smith *et al.,* 1984c). Further, a *Plasmodium* surface protein, when expressed via a vaccinia vector, was secreted from the host cell and thereby was poorly immunogenic; this was corrected by appending coding sequences for the transmembrane anchor domain of IgG to the *Plasmodium* gene (Langford *et al.,* 1986). Human immunodeficiency virus type 1 (HIV-1) envelope protein gp160, expressed via a vaccinia vector, was processed abnormally in HeLa and monkey kidney cell cultures, but was cleaved and glycosylated faithfully when expressed in a lymphocyte cell line (Chakrabarti *et al.,* 1986). Faithful processing of expressed flavivirus proteins also appears problematic (Deubel *et al.,* 1988).

E. Poxvirus Phenotypic Markers

The genetic nature of poxvirus phenotypic variation was first described by Fenner and his colleagues, who first demonstrated the existence of genetic linkage groups in animal viruses (Fenner, 1970, 1979, 1985a). Differentiation of poxvirus phenotypes has depended on detecting differences in many characteristics of virus growth and effects of virus growth in experimental animals, embryonating eggs, and cell cultures. For example, phenotypes have been described in terms of (1) variations in lesions produced by infection in the chorioallantoic membrane (CAM) of embryonating chicken eggs, in the skin of experimentally inoculated animals, and in cells in culture; (2) variations in the degree of virus dissemination and pathogenicity in experimentally inoculated animals; (3) variations in the amount of hemagglutinin and other antigens produced during infection in eggs and cell cultures; (4) variations in virus growth in eggs and cell cultures at restrictive temperatures; and (5) variations in host range in animals and cell cultures.

From the early 1900s, reactogenicity in rabbit skin and in the CAM of embryonating eggs had been regarded as the most reliable indicator of vaccinia vaccine safety and homogeneity. Vaccine stocks producing variable pock size or hemorrhagic pocks on CAMS or ulcerated lesions in rabbit skin were excluded from human use. As smallpox vaccination efforts intensified, exclusions were also based upon reported rates of adverse reactions in human recipients, such as severe local reactogenicity, high frequency of fever, etc. In the 1960s, as the WHO Smallpox Eradication Programme reached its peak, further efforts were made to correlate field reports of adverse reactions with laboratory tests. Still, most laboratory tests measured characteristics of virus replication in eggs and animals (Marennikova et al., 1969; Koller and Zsidai, 1973; Marennikova, 1973). For example, one attempt to grade vaccines involved virus titration by intranasal inoculation of suckling mice; virulence for mice correlated reasonably well with clinical observations of fever and acute illness in vaccinated children (Krag-Andersen, 1969; Polak, 1973). None of these tests, however, could predict the frequency of the most severe, rare complications of vaccination, such as encephalitis. Even today, we are unable to make such predictions on the basis of practical laboratory tests.

Neuro-adapted virus strains (called "neurovaccinia" strains) have been studied extensively in experimental animals, but no study has yet led to a model of the human neurological disease caused rarely by vaccination (Hashizume et al., 1973; Morita et al., 1977; Briody, 1959). If a model were available, it would be used now to evaluate attenuated mutants of vaccinia virus as well as vectored vaccine candidates per se (Morita et al., 1987; Neff, 1985; Hashizume et al., 1985; Mayr et al., 1978).

Today, evaluation of vaccinia virus phenotypic traits, such as neurovirulence, is being approached by genetic analysis. Genes controlling virion structural and functional characteristics are being mapped, including, for example, vaccinia and cowpox virus genes involved in CAM pock morphology and cell culture host range. The product of one vaccinia virus gene, a 29-kD protein, appears to be required for replication in human cell cultures (Gillard *et al.*, 1986). Hemorrhagic CAM pock characteristics, long associated with virulence, appear associated with inhibition of blood coagulation, in part caused by a gene for a 38-kD protein, which resembles mammalian plasma serine protease inhibitors such as antithrombin-III (Pickup *et al.*, 1986). Other genes of poxviruses encode proteins similar in amino acid sequence to host proteins. For example, a gene for a protein similar to mammalian epidermal growth factor (EGF) and transforming growth factor (TGF-α), which are cofactors in wound healing, has been identified (Twardzik *et al.*, 1985; Stroobant *et al.*, 1985; Porter and Archard, 1987; Chang *et al.*, 1987). Genes encoding proteins similar to human and avian cell TK gene products, which affect general cellular replicating activity, have been identified (Bradshaw and Deininger, 1984; Kwoh and Engler, 1984; Weir and Moss, 1983; Hruby *et al.*, 1983; Esposito and Knight, 1984; Boyle *et al.*, 1987). It is hoped that complete analyses of poxvirus genes and their products will help to characterize virus strains most suitable for substrates for producing vectored vaccines.

At least 20 vaccinia virus genes have been analyzed, including the gene for the viral DNA polymerase, which resembles the polymerase genes of herpesviruses and adenoviruses (Earl and Moss, 1987; McGeoch *et al.*, 1987; Earl *et al.*, 1986), and genes for subunits of the viral RNA polymerase, which resemble RNA polymerase genes of yeast, *Escherichia coli,* and *Drosophila* (Broyles and Moss, 1986). Genes for other vaccinia virion proteins, such as the 37-kD major envelope protein (Hirt *et al.*, 1986), the abundant type A inclusion body protein (Patel *et al.*, 1986), and the hemagglutinin protein (Shida, 1986a), have also been analyzed. Relevant to vector virus construction, deletion of the TK gene diminished vaccinia virus virulence in mice, rabbits, and chimpanzees (Buller *et al.*, 1985). The genetic basis of virulence is also being studied by constructing recombinants between vaccinia and ectromelia (mousepox) viruses, which differ in their CAM pock characteristics and pathogenic properties for rabbits and mice (Chernos *et al.*, 1985). None of these studies has brought us to the point of being able to predict vaccinia vaccine characteristics or side effects, but they illustrate a rational approach to the problem.

F. Immune Response to Poxvirus Infection and Vaccination

Under natural conditions, poxviruses are transmitted by the respiratory route and by contact (some are also transmitted by arthropods), and infection is initiated in epithelial cells at the site of virus entry. The same occurs following poxvirus vaccination. The progression of infection is influenced by many factors, such as the virulence of the virus (substantial in the case of smallpox virus infection, minimal in the case of vaccinia virus vaccination), other biologic characteristics of the virus (e.g., tropism, replicating requirements), and innate determinants of the host response (specific and nonspecific cell-mediated immune responses, humoral immune response, age, hormonal effects, and action of interferons). Specific immunity is the principal mechanism for developing resistance against poxviruses; recovery from infection depends in large part upon the development of a cell-mediated immune response to viral proteins.

At sites of infection, virus particles are taken up first by macrophages, where in nonimmune hosts virus replication occurs (replication is abortive in immune hosts). Viral proteins produced via this infection are subsequently presented to induce specific T- and B-cell reactivities. Concomitantly, early NK-cell and cytotoxic T-cell activities are initiated. The cell-mediated immune response continues in infected epidermal (*stratum spinosum epidermidis*) and subcutaneous tissues, as well as other sites of virus replication *in vivo*. In the case of pathogenic poxvirus infections, the race between the virus and the host immune response may be settled in favor of either, but, in the case of vaccination, the race is settled quickly in favor of the host.

The cell-mediated immune response occurs via the production by T cells and specifically activated macrophages of a vast array of soluble mediators that affect virus, infected cells, and the local environment of the infection site. Eventually, these mediators even destroy virus within the pustules of pathogenic infections and the pustule that forms at the site of vaccination. In pathogenic poxvirus infections and in vaccinated individuals, the B-cell response generates non-neutralizing and neutralizing antibodies at about the time dermal vesicles begin to form and resolve into pustules. All of these host response events would be expected to be the same whether or not the infecting poxvirus expressed heterologous proteins. That is, it is most likely that vectored poxviruses will behave generally like their parents. However, similarities and differences must be determined directly with each vectored virus as it is advanced toward vaccine candidacy.

IV. Poxvirus Vector Construction and Applications

A. GENE TRANSFER BY MARKER RESCUE

With smaller viruses, genetic recombination is manipulated in the laboratory via directed DNA ligation, but because of the very large size of the poxvirus genome, the method for inserting foreign genes involves site-directed homologous DNA recombination between the vector virus genome and the heterologous insert. This method works well because genetic recombination occurs readily in poxvirus infections; in mixed poxvirus infections up to 50% of progeny are recombinants. The historical development of infectious recombinant vectored vaccinia virus and a summary of the gene expression method by thymidine kinase insertional inactivation are depicted in Figs. 1 and 2.

Genetic recombination was first studied in poxviruses under the term "nongenetic reactivation." This was done by coinoculation of two inactivated poxviruses into animals, embryonating eggs, or cell cultures (Fenner, 1970, 1979). Specifically, this phenomenon involves rescue of a poxvirus inactivated by heat or urea treatment (protein inactivation) by an homologous or heterologous poxvirus inactivated by ultraviolet light (DNA inactivation). Coinoculation of protein-inactivated virus with an infectious preparation of virus of the same genus produces recombinants with traits of both parents; such coinoculations involving heterologous poxvirus genera effect reactivation of the protein-inactivated virus but produce no recombinants. Reactivation occurs largely because of cross-reactivity of poxvirus core-uncoating enzymes (Pedley and Cooper, 1987) and complementation between poxvirus transcription and gene regulation systems. For example, the fowlpox virus TK gene, with its own promoter, has been expressed after insertion into a TK$^-$ vaccinia virus (Boyle and Coupar, 1986). Similarly, rabies virus G and N coding sequences have been expressed under control of two different vaccinia virus promoters after insertion into raccoon poxvirus (Esposito et al., 1988; W. Bellini, personal communication).

Extending classic studies on "nongenetic reactivation," Sam and Dumbell (1981) reported the recovery of rabbitpox virus when its DNA was transfected into cells that had been infected with ectromelia virus. More importantly, when they transfected DNA restriction fragments of the rabbitpox strain of vaccinia virus into cells already infected with a phenotypically different vaccinia virus, recombinants with rabbitpox and vaccinia virus phenotypic markers were recovered. Although gene insertions and deletions via targeted recombination had been used

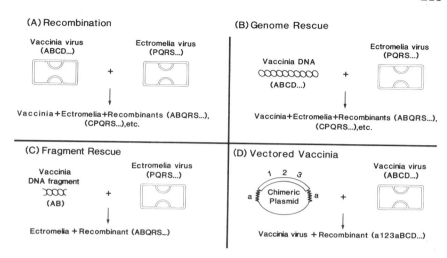

FIG. 1. Steps in the historical development of the use of vaccinia virus as an expression vector for heterologous DNA sequences. (A) Demonstration of recombination between vaccinia and ectromelia viruses by coinfecting cells with both viruses producing vaccinia, ectromelia, and recombinant viruses (Fenner 1970, 1979). (B) Rescue of vaccinia virus genome in cells transfected with intact vaccinia virus DNA and infected with ectromelia virus or temperature-sensitive mutants of vaccinia virus to produce vaccinia, ectromelia, and recombinant viruses (Sam and Dumbell, 1981). Genome rescue is similar to nongenetic reactivation in which cells are coinfected with heat-inactivated poxvirus and live poxvirus of homologous genus (Fenner 1970, 1979). (C) Marker rescue of fragment of vaccinia virus DNA by homologous DNA recombination in cells transfected with vaccinia virus fragment (marker+ DNA) and infected with marker− virus (Sam and Dumbell, 1981; Weir et al., 1982; Nakano et al., 1982; Condit et al., 1983). (D) Targeted insertion of heterologous coding sequences into vaccinia virus genome by homologous DNA recombination. Chimeric plasmid DNA that contains vaccinia virus DNA flanking the heterologous DNA is transfected into cells already infected with vaccinia virus (Mackett et al., 1982; Panicali and Paoletti, 1982). Chimeric plasmid: a, vaccinia virus DNA flanking sequences; 1, vaccinia virus regulatory elements (promoter, RNA start); 2, heterologous DNA coding sequences; 3, vaccinia virus transcript termination elements. [From Fenner (1985a), redrawn with permission.]

earlier in prokaryotic systems (bacterial "homogenotization" and the like; Miller, 1972) and other eukaryotic systems, the experiments of Sam and Dumbell marked the first demonstration of marker rescue for poxviruses. About the same time, Post and Roizman (1981) described a generalized method of selectable marker rescue for inserting or deleting genes at specific loci in eukaryotic cells or viruses. They produced a gene deletion in a TK− herpesvirus mutant by interrupting the functioning gene with TK+ sequences.

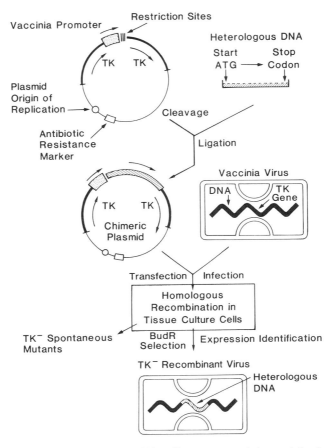

FIG. 2.   Insertion of heterologous DNA coding sequences into vaccinia virus by insertional inactivation of the virus thymidine kinase (TK) gene. A chimeric plasmid is
constructed in such a way that the coding sequences are inserted downstream of a
vaccinia virus transcript start site that follows vaccinia virus promoter sequences; this
cassette interrupts coding sequences for the vaccinia virus TK gene. Cells already infected with vaccinia virus are transfected with the chimeric plasmid before the peak of
viral DNA replication. The infection is then allowed to proceed to completion. Three types
of progeny virus are produced: wild-type TK$^+$, spontaneous TK$^-$ mutants, and TK$^-$ recombinants. TK$^-$ viruses are isolated by plaque purification using TK$^-$ cells (mouse L,
human 143, etc.) that are maintained in overlay medium containing 5-bromo-2'-
deoxyuridine or trifluorothymidine. Recombinants are then differentiated from spontaneous mutants by hybridization and immunological methods using cells infected with
virus from individual virus plaques (Mackett *et al.,* 1985a).

Separately confirming and extending the concept of poxvirus DNA fragment rescue, Condit et al. (1983), Nakano et al. (1982), and Weir et al. (1982) identified physical loci of ts mutations, reconstituted a vaccinia deletion mutant, and mapped the vaccinia TK locus. These studies led immediately to the development, by Panicali and Paoletti (1982) and Mackett et al. (1982), of methods for inserting heterologous coding sequences into vaccinia DNA, thereby producing the first infectious vectored vaccinia virus recombinants. In the studies of Mackett et al. (1982), the selectable system was based on interrupting the vaccinia TK gene; in these studies it was first noted that distinctive cis-acting vaccinia virus promoters were required for regulating foreign gene expression. This approach has been developed into a detailed protocol for selecting recombinants via insertional inactivation of the vaccinia TK locus, followed by plaque purifying the recombinants in TK⁻ cells under medium containing bromodeoxyuridine (Mackett et al., 1985a).

The original methods for producing vectored vaccinia viruses involved targeted recombination between vaccinia virus genomic DNA and chimeric plasmids that contained a specific vaccinia DNA segment into which a heterologous DNA segment had been inserted. Briefly, such chimeric plasmids are constructed so that the flanking DNA correctly provides promoter and transcript leader sequences upstream of the heterologous DNA. All of the sequences must be in the proper reading frame, with the stop codon appropriately followed by a poxvirus transcript terminator. The poxvirus portions of the insert can be a contiguous part of the flanking DNA or include poxvirus regulatory elements translocated by genetic engineering from distal regions of the genome. The chimeric plasmid usually is transfected into cell cultures just after infection by the virus that is to serve as the vector. After a complete cycle of virus replication, recombinants are identified by differential plaque selection procedures using hybridization, immunofluorescence, or other tests. Selection of recombinants also has been accomplished by use of a restrictive temperature to rescue vectored ts mutants (Kieny et al., 1984) and by use of coexpression of bacterial β-galactosidase (Chakrabarti et al., 1985; Panicali et al., 1986), neomycin phosphotransferase (Franke et al., 1985b; Beaud et al., 1987), or herpesvirus TK (Panicali and Paoletti, 1982; Mackett et al., 1982; Al'tshtein et al., 1986). A novel system has been described in which cells are coinfected with two vaccinia-vectored recombinants, one expressing T7 phage RNA polymerase and the second containing the desired heterologous gene fused between a T7 strong promoter and transcript terminator (Fuerst et al., 1987). Vaccinia genome loci, such as those for hemagglutinin protein (Shida, 1986a,b), rifampicin resistance (Baldrick and Moss, 1987; Tartaglia *et al.,* 1986), and isatin-β-thiosemicarbizone dependents (Fathi *et al.,* 1986), have also been used to select recombinants.

B. APPLICATIONS OF VACCINIA VIRUS VECTORING IN VACCINE DEVELOPMENT

During the past few years, many genes coding for important proteins of viruses and other microorganisms have been inserted into vaccinia virus. Such recombinants have been used in basic studies of gene expression, transcription, protein processing, transport, secretion, etc. They have also been used in immunological studies, particularly for the generation of target cells expressing epitopes on their surfaces for use as cell-mediated immune reaction targets (Walker *et al.,* 1987), and, most importantly, in the development of infectious vectored vaccines. Several reviews and symposia have dealt with the application of vaccinia virus vectoring to vaccine development, some including partial listings of experimental products (Piccini and Paoletti, 1988; Moss and Flexner, 1987; Quinnan, 1985; Chanock *et al.,* 1988) Table III represents an overview of experimental products known to the authors. The listing illustrates the diversity of experimental vaccine development but is not comprehensive because many recombinants discussed informally have not been reported in the literature. In addition, a few examples of vectored vaccinia virus experimental vaccines are described below to illustrate particular advantages and disadvantages of the approach.

1. Vaccinia : Rabies Vaccines

The surface spike glycoprotein (G) gene of the ERA strain of rabies virus was expressed after insertion into the TK region of Copenhagen vaccinia virus (Wiktor *et al.,* 1984, 1988; Kieny *et al.,*1984). Mice, rabbits, skunks, raccoons, foxes, and cattle inoculated intradermally (ID) with this recombinant produced neutralizing antibodies and were protected (except cattle, not challenged; Koprowski *et al.,* 1987) against an otherwise lethal rabies virus challenge (Rupprecht *et al,* 1986; Blancou *et al.,* 1986; Wiktor *et al.,* 1988). Raccoons and foxes, but not dogs or skunks, were fully protected via the oral (PO) vaccination route. Lymphocytes from vaccinated mice were found to be primed for a secondary specific anti-rabies cytotoxic T-lymphocyte response. Because the Copenhagen strain, when used before the 1960s as a smallpox vaccine, had been associated with a high incidence of encephalitic complications (Polak, 1973; Krag-Andersen, 1969), six recombinants of the less

TABLE III

VACCINIA VIRUS VECTORED VACCINE CANDIDATES

Disease	Etiologic agent/gene product	Vaccine application	Reference
Human			
Herpes genital disease	Herpes simplex virus types 1 and 2/gB, gD, gG	Universal vaccine	Sullivan and Smith (1987); Cremer *et al.* (1985); Paoletti *et al.* (1984)
Infectious mononucleosis	Epstein-Barr virus/gp340	Universal vaccine	Mackett and Arrand (1985)
Cytomegalovirus disease	Human cytomegalovirus/gB	Universal vaccine	Cranage *et al.* (1986)
Hepatitis B	Hepatitis B virus/S, MS, LS, Core	Vaccine for high-risk groups in developed countries, universal vaccine for developing countries	Cheng and Moss (1987); Clarke *et al.* (1988)
AIDS	Human immunodeficiency virus/gp 160, gp 120, gp41, gag, 3'ORF	Vaccine for high-risk groups, perhaps vaccine for highly endemic areas	Chakrabarti *et al.* (1986); Zarling *et al.* (1987); Zagury *et al.* (1987)
Respiratory syncytial disease	Respiratory syncytial virus/G, F, N	Universal vaccine	Olmstead *et al.* (1988); King *et al.* (1987)
Parainfluenza	Human parainfluenza 3/F, HN	Universal vaccine	Spriggs *et al.* (1987)
Influenza	Influenza virus/PB1, PB2, PA, HA, NA, NS1, NS2, NP, M1, M2	Universal vaccine, and vaccine for high-risk groups	Smith *et al.* (1987); M. Shaw, personal communication
Rotavirus gastroenteritis	Rotavirus SA-11/VP7	Universal vaccine for developing countries, vaccine for high-risk groups in developed countries	Andrew *et al.* (1987)
Rabies	Rabies virus/G, N	Preexposure vaccine for high-risk groups, universal vaccine in some endemic areas	Esposito *et al.* (1987, 1988) and unpublished; Wiktor *et al.* (1988)

(continued)

TABLE III (*Continued*)

Disease	Etiologic agent/gene product	Vaccine application	Reference
Lassa fever	Lassa fever virus/G1, G2, N	Universal vaccine for endemic areas	Auperin *et al.* (1987, 1988) and unpublished; Clegg and Lloyd (1987)
Hemorrhagic fever with renal syndrome	Hantaan virus/G1, G2, N	Universal vaccine for endemic areas	Pensiero *et al.* (1988)
Argentine hemorrhagic fever	Junin virus/G1, G2, N	Universal vaccine for endemic areas	[a]
Dengue fever	Dengue virus/C, NS1, prM/M, E	Universal vaccine for endemic areas	Zhao *et al.* (1987); Deubel *et al.* (1988)
Malaria	*Plasmodium falciparum* and others/CSP, merozoite S, RESA	Universal vaccine for endemic areas	Langford *et al.* (1988); Vijaya *et al.* (1988); Smith *et al.* (1986)
Tumor immunotherapy	Human melanoma-associated p97	Universal vaccine for high-risk groups	McKenzie *et al.* (1988); Estin *et al.* (1988)
Veterinary			
Rift Valley fever	Rift Valley fever virus/G1, G2	Vaccine for sheep in endemic areas of Africa, and vaccine for stockpiling in case of introduction into other continents	Collett *et al.* (1987)
Foot-and-mouth disease	Foot-and-mouth disease viruses/VP1	Vaccine for cattle in endemic areas, and vaccine for stockpiling in case of introduction into nonendemic countries	Clarke *et al.* (1988)
Rabies	Rabies virus/G, N	Preexposure vaccine for cattle, dogs, and wildlife species in endemic areas	Esposito *et al.* (1987, 1988), and unpublished; Wiktor *et al.* (1988)

Venezuelan equine encephalitis	Venezuelan equine encephalitis virus/capsid, E1-3, 6 kD	Vaccine for horses	Kinney et al. (1989)
Vesicular stomatitis	Vesicular stomatitis viruses/G, N	Vaccine for cattle	Mackett et al. (1985b)
Pseudorabies	Pseudorabies virus/gp50, gIII	Vaccine for swine and cattle	E. Jones and D. Panicali, personal communication
Transmissible gastroenteritis of swine	Transmissible gastroenteritis virus/g195	Vaccine for swine	Hu et al. (1985)
Swine influenza	Swine influenza virus H1	Vaccine for swine, cattle, poultry	Boyle et al. (1986)
Equine influenza	Equine influenza virus/H3, H7, N7, N8	Vaccine for horses	B. Cordell, personal communication
Avian influenza	Avian influenza virus/H5	Vaccine for poultry	De et al. (1988)
Avian infectious bronchitis	Infectious bronchitis virus/gp180	Vaccine for poultry	Tomley et al. (1987)
Feline leukemia	Feline leukemia virus/gp70	Vaccine for cats	Gilbert et al. (1987)
Bovine leukemia	Bovine leukemia virus/glycoprotein	Vaccine for cattle	[a]
Avian sarcoma	Avian sarcoma virus Pr ASV-C/env	Vaccine for poultry	[a]
Bluetongue	Bluetongue viruses 1-24/VP2	Vaccine for cattle and sheep	[a]
Murine cytomegalovirus infection	Murine cytomegalovirus/p89	Model for human cytomegalovirus prophylaxis	Koszinowski et al. (1988)
Lymphocytic choriomeningitis	Lymphocytic choriomeningitis virus/G1, G2, N	Model for cell-mediated immunity	[a]
Sindbis virus infection	Sindbis virus/C, PE2, E1, E2	Model for immune prophylaxis	Rice et al. (1985)
Babesiosis	Babesia sp./surface proteins	Vaccine for cattle	[a]
Anaplasmosis	Anaplasma marginale/surface proteins	Vaccine for cattle	[a]

[a] Uncited.

virulent NYBH strain of vaccinia virus (Fenner, 1985a; Krag-Andersen, 1969) that carried the G coding sequences of the CVS strain of rabies virus were produced in a collaborative study between virologists at the Centers for Disease Control and the National Institute of Allergy and Infectious Diseases (Esposito et al., 1987). The six recombinants allowed researchers to compare the expression efficiency of two different promoters, the widely used $P_{7.5}$ (early-late class) promoter and the P_{11} (late class) promoter that had been presumed to be able to regulate higher levels of protein synthesis because it controls production of an abundant structural protein of vaccinia virus. Each of the six recombinants faithfully expressed rabies virus G protein conformational forms GI and GII, and each directed proper transport of this protein to the surface of infected cells. Three of the P_{11}-type recombinants produced in infected cell cultures about 10-fold more G protein than did the $P_{7.5}$-type recombinants. One P_{11}-type recombinant with an altered mRNA leader sequence induced about 100-fold less G protein than those with usual leader sequences. Single ID tail scarification or footpad (FP) inoculation with these vectored viruses induced rabies virus-neutralizing antibodies and protected mice against an otherwise lethal intracranial (IC) or peripheral FP challenge (Table IV). One vaccine candidate inoculated intramuscularly (IM) into dogs protected all recipients against an otherwise lethal rabies virus challenge.

As mentioned above, CVS rabies virus G and N coding sequences have been expressed via raccoon poxvirus. One P_{11}-type and one $P_{7.5}$-type chimeric plasmid that was used for developing vectored NYBH viruses was used again in recombinations to produce vectored raccoon poxviruses because of strong homology of TK sequences observed (Esposito and Knight, 1985) between these two orthopoxviruses. Oral vaccination experiments with raccoon poxvirus: G protein recombinants in animals showed induction of significant rabies virus-neutralizing antibodies in 100% of raccoons, dogs, cotton rats, and bobcats and in 33% of skunks; to date dogs, raccoons, and cotton rats have been challenged and were fully protected (Esposito et al., 1988).

The G sequences of rabies virus also have been expressed after insertion into fowlpox virus using two systems: (1) an abortive infection of mammalian cell cultures and (2) a productive infection of avian cell cultures (J. Taylor, personal communication). Neutralizing antibodies were detected after injecting this recombinant fowlpox virus into rabbits (ID), rats (ID), cats (subcutaneous, SQ), dogs (SQ), cattle (SQ, ID, and IM), and mice (FP). Vaccinated mice were shown to resist challenge. On the basis of these studies, this fowlpox:rabies

TABLE IV

Rabies Virus-Neutralizing Antibodies and Resistance of Mice to Challenge after
Vaccination with Six Different New York Board of Health Vaccinia : Rabies
Glycoprotein Vaccines[a]

| Vaccine | Neutralizing antibody | | Mortality after challenge[b] |
	Median	[Range]	
Intradermal			
A	5,700	[1,400–7,000]	0/11
B	5,700	[1,400–7,000]	0/12
C	1,600	[900–7,000]	0/7
D	2,400	[1,400–6,000]	0/9
E	3,125	[1,400–7,000]	0/11
F	6,200	[1,400–7,000]	0/9
Vaccinia control	<5		11/11
Footpad			
A	1,400	[1,100–1,400]	0/12
B	1,400	[625–1,400]	0/12
C	280	[40–1,800]	0/10
D	1,000	[280–5,100]	0/9
E	1,200	[56–6,300]	0/10
F	1,400	[625–3,125]	0/11
Vaccinia control	<5		10/10

[a] All vaccines used the NYBH strain of vaccinia virus and a recombinant insert derived from the G gene of the CVS strain of rabies virus. In vaccines A–D, the rabies virus gene was expressed under control of the vaccinia promoter P_{11}; A and B were fusion protein versions, C had an altered mRNA leader, and D mimicked the promoter and leader of the naturally occurring 11-kD vaccinia gene. In vaccines E and F, the rabies gene was expressed under the control of the vaccinia promoter $P_{7.5}$; they differed in sequences flanking the translation start codon.

[b] Four-week-old female A/J mice were inoculated with 10^8 PFU of virus. Mice were bled 4 weeks postinoculation, tested for antibody, and challenged 2 weeks later by footpad inoculation of 10 MLD_{50} of street rabies virus (CDC, Mexico dog strain 2699) (Esposito *et al.*, 1987).

vaccine was proposed for use when a vaccinia : rabies vaccine might be unacceptable.

Poxvirus-vectored rabies vaccines could play a significant role in animal and human rabies control programs, but this must be evaluated in regard to risk : benefit, separately, in each of several settings:

1. *Human vaccine in developed countries.* Poxvirus recombinants would have to be compared with presently available, very potent, very safe, inactivated cell culture-derived vaccines. These vaccines are

largely used for postexposure prophylaxis where speed of the immune response, not cost, is most important. In fact, the major disadvantage of presently available vaccines is their very high cost, which surely would be reduced if poxvirus recombinant products were to meet current standards for safety, efficacy, and speed of antibody induction.

2. *Human vaccine in developing countries.*   Poxvirus recombinants would have to be evaluated as above in regard to efficacy, safety, and speed of antibody induction, but against a much poorer standard—the standard set by present rabies vaccines that are derived from neural tissues of animals. The prospect of this is not clear, but the probable low cost and practicality of local production of vectored poxvirus vaccines suggest that further study is worthwhile.

3. *Pet animal vaccines in developed and developing countries.*   Poxvirus recombinants would have to be compared with presently available potent and safe attenuated-live and inactivated rabies vaccines. These vaccines are used only for preexposure prophylaxis, where efficacy, safety, and cost are important. Safety considerations would have to include assessment of risks of transmitting vectored virus from animals to humans. Because of this, the prospect of using poxviruses that cause abortive infection, such as fowlpox virus, appears to warrant further study.

4. *Livestock animals in developed and developing countries.*   Poxvirus recombinants would have to be evaluated against a tradition for very little vaccine usage, even in areas where losses due to rabies are substantial. Because poxvirus-vectored vaccines would have a low cost and would be easily administered, this is an exciting prospect.

5. *Wildlife species in developed countries.*   Poxvirus recombinants would have to be compared with attenuated live-virus vaccines now being used in Canada and a few European countries to immunize some wildlife species via oral bait-delivered vaccine. For wildlife species in which these attenuated-live rabies virus vaccines are not immunogenic by the oral route, vectored vaccines represent a novel approach to a most difficult problem. The possibility of using other viruses as infectious vectors, such as raccoon poxvirus (Esposito *et al.*, 1988) or canine adenovirus (infectious canine hepatitis virus), could add the extra element of host range specificity to such vaccines. All of these approaches offer exciting prospects.

2. *Vaccinia : Lassa Fever Vaccine*

Vaccinia virus recombinants expressing Lassa virus (Josiah strain) glycoproteins (G1 and G2 via cleavage of polyprotein GPC) (Auperin *et al.*, 1987, 1988) or the nucleocapsid protein (N) (Clegg and Lloyd, 1987; D. Auperin, personal communication) have been produced and are being evaluated for use in a candidate human vaccine. When a NYBH vaccinia : Lassa virus GPC recombinant was inoculated intradermally into guinea pigs or rhesus monkeys, it evoked only low levels of nonneutralizing G-specific antibodies. However, all monkeys and most guinea pigs survived lethal challenge. At the time, when standard NYBH virus vaccinated control animals became sick and died, the GPC recombinant vaccinated animals had a brief low-grade viremia and transient fever. No significant protection of rhesus or cynomolgous monkeys was observed with a NYBH : Lassa (Josiah strain) N recombinant virus made at the Centers for Disease Control. The NYBH : N and a Lister vaccinia : Lassa (Nigeria strain) N recombinant, produced at the Public Health Laboratory Service at Porton Down, England, protected guinea pigs. The reasons for these contrasting results have not been resolved. The present results, taken together with those of other studies (J. McCormick, personal communication), have suggested that neutralizing antibodies are not critical in the recovery of inoculated animals or naturally infected humans from Lassa virus infection. Rather, growing evidence shows the importance of a cell-mediated immune response elicited against the virus proteins.

Coupling of two fundamental epidemiological observations makes the need for a human vaccine against Lassa fever most urgent; in West African countries more than 300,000 cases of the disease are estimated to occur annually, and every attempt to date to develop a vaccine by conventional approaches has failed. Inactivated virus vaccines have not been efficacious in damping viremia or in protecting experimental animals, and attempts to use a naturally attenuated variant, Mopeia virus, are stymied because of the inability to predict in animal models the possibility of rare adverse events, such as CNS invasion. In this context, the development of a usable vaccinia : Lassa virus vaccine represents an exciting prospect. In West Africa, this development must include concern for adverse effects of vaccinia virus use in persons immunosuppressed by HIV infection.

3. Vaccinia : Venezuelan Equine Encephalitis Vaccine

Vaccinia virus recombinants carrying the 26S polygene of Venezuelan equine encephalitis (VEE) virus (strains TC-83 or Trinidad donkey) have been produced at the Centers for Disease Control (Kinney et al., 1989). When inoculated into BSC-40 monkey cell cultures, the recombinants faithfully expressed the native polyprotein, which was normally cleaved to form all of the virion structural proteins (map order: capsid, E3, E2, 6 kD, E1). Colony-bred NIH Swiss and inbred A/J and C3H strains of mice were inoculated with the recombinants intradermally (via tail scarification). Mice developed VEE virus-neutralizing antibodies and were protected against an otherwise lethal intraperitoneal challenge with virulent VEE virus (Table V).

Lymphocytes isolated from animals inoculated with TC-83 or the recombinant vaccinia virus vaccine exhibited VEE-specific *in vitro* proliferative responses. Protection was demonstrated against each subtype of VEE. Protection against intranasal challenge, however, was only 10–20% effective. Vaccinated, challenged mice developed very high antibody titers, presumably due to subclinical systemic infection. The recombinants were as effective as the attenuated-live virus TC-83 vaccine in inducing cross-protection against challenge with subtypes of VEE virus isolated from outbreaks. These recombinants are now being developed as candidate vaccines.

The potential value of a vaccinia : VEE recombinant vaccine must be considered against needs as they occur in the face of epizootics/epidemics:

1. *Equine vaccine.* Epizootic VEE has been devastating to equine populations in Central and South America, in areas where agriculture is heavily dependent upon horses and mules. Increasing numbers of infected horses and mules in an outbreak amplify the presence of VEE virus, thereby furthering risks to human populations. The present attenuated live-virus vaccine (strain TC-83) is efficacious but suffers from cold-chain and other logistic problems. To prove its value, a vaccinia virus recombinant product will have to be evaluated in realistic settings in Central or South America; this is an exciting prospect.

2. *Human vaccine.* Laboratory workers and disease control field workers are at high risk of infection and disease; a vaccine is necessary to protect such persons who may contract the disease via insect bite, accidental inoculation, or aerosol. TC-83 vaccine, formulated for human use, appears generally efficacious, but does cause adverse effects in some recipients. An inactivated cell culture-derived vaccine (strain TC-84) is safe but not very potent. A vaccinia virus recombinant product would have to be evaluated against this background; this is an exciting prospect.

4. Vaccinia : Influenza Vaccines

a. *Vaccinia : Avian Influenza (H5) Vaccine.* Avian influenza H5 virus was selected at the Centers for Disease Control for use as a model system to evaluate the feasibility of using a vaccinia virus-vectored vaccine to interrupt rapidly moving epidemics/epizootics, such as those caused by human and avian influenza viruses. The hemagglutinin (HA) of avirulent A/Chicken/Scotland/59 virus was expressed using the

TABLE V

Venezuelan Equine Encephalitis (VEE) Virus Antibodies and Resistance of Mice to Challenge after Vaccination with NYBH Vaccinia : VEE Vaccine[a]

Vaccine	Antibody titer (reciprocal, mean)			Mortality after challenge
	Neutralizing	HI	ELISA	
Vaccinia : VEE				
Prechallenge	1,180	43	2,100	
Postchallenge	55,000	890	86,000	0/8
Vaccinia control	<5	<5	<5	8/8
VEE TC-83				
Prechallenge	51,200	340	Not done	
Postchallenge	56,000	1,560	Not done	0/8

[a] Five-week-old mice were inoculated intradermally (tail scarification) with 10^8 PFU of vaccinia : VEE vaccine or intraperitoneally with 10^4 PFU of TC-83 attenuated-live virus vaccine. Mice were bled 19 days postinoculation, tested for antibodies, and challenged by intraperitoneal inoculation of 100 MLD_{50} of virulent VEE virus (Trinidad donkey strain). Fourteen days later, surviving mice were bled again and tested for antibodies.

NYBH vaccinia virus vector system (De *et al.*, 1988). In human 143 cells, the HA expressed via the NYBH vector was slightly larger by electrophoresis than the influenza virus authentic protein, possibly because of extra glycosylation, otherwise it appeared identical to the native HA. Vaccine was prepared from γ-irradiated vector virus-infected cells by homogenization with Freund's complete adjuvant. Adult chickens, immunized intramuscularly with this preparation, developed H5 influenza virus-neutralizing and hemagglutination-inhibiting (HI) antibodies and were protected against an otherwise lethal challenge with A/Chicken/Scotland/59 or A/Chicken/Pennsylvania/83 virulent influenza viruses (Table VI). Kuroda *et al.* (1986) had previously demonstrated the protective value of an H7 hemagglutinin protein produced in a baculovirus expression system. Taken together, the two experiments suggest the merit of vaccination, rather than slaughter and disinfection, in the face of avian influenza epizootics. By extension, the two experiments suggested the merit of considering similar vaccines for human influenza. It will now be of interest to express H5 and H7 proteins using a vaccine strain of fowlpox virus, thereby adding the advantages of an infectious vectored virus vaccine for poultry.

TABLE VI

AVIAN INFLUENZA ANTIBODIES AND RESISTANCE OF ADULT CHICKENS TO CHALLENGE AFTER VACCINATION WITH AN INACTIVATED VACCINIA : H5 INFLUENZA VIRUS (A/Chicken/ Scotland/59) HEMAGGLUTININ VACCINE[a]

	Antibody titer (reciprocal, mean)		Mortality after challenge
Vaccine	HI	Neutralization	
Vaccinia:			
H5-HA			
Prechallenge	<5	240	
Postchallenge	112	6,400	1/20
Vaccinia control	<5	<5	20/20

[a] Chickens were inoculated subcutaneously with NYBH vaccinia : H5 avian influenza virus hemagglutinin vaccine prepared in chick fibroblast cells. The recombinant vaccine contained $10^{6.2}$ PFU/ml; it contained 0.5 μg of H5-HA protein per dose. The vaccine was inactivated by γ-irradiation and homogenized in Freund's complete adjuvant. At 14 days after vaccination chickens were tested for antibodies and challenged with 10^6 PFU of virulent A/Chicken/Scotland/59 influenza virus. Serum specimens from surviving birds were tested 32 days after challenge.

b. Vaccinia:Influenza B Vaccine. When influenza B viruses are cultivated in embryonating chicken eggs or in cell cultures, antigenically distinct variants are differentially selected (Schild *et al.*, 1983). These variants differ by single amino acid substitutions in a key domain of the hemagglutinin. To decide which host system, eggs or cell cultures, is most suitable for producing the most efficacious vaccine, researchers at the Centers for Disease Control constructed two NYBH vaccinia virus recombinants, one containing the HA gene from B/England/222/83 virus grown in eggs and the other, the same gene from the same virus grown in MDCK cells (Rota *et al.*, 1987). The vaccinia virus recombinants were used to vaccinate groups of mice, which were then separately cross-challenged with B/England/222/82 virus grown in either host system. All mice were protected against challenge. When the sera of the challenged mice were used in cross-absorption tests, however, a much broader neutralizing antibody response was evoked by the vaccinia virus recombinant expressing the HA of the egg-derived virus. Because of uncontrollable mutations continuing during growth of influenza viruses in such experiments, the vaccinia virus recombinants were crucial for stabilizing the respective HA genes in DNA form. In parallel experiments, serum specimens from persons immunized with influenza B vaccine (derived from B/Singapore/222/79 strain virus, grown in eggs) were found to have comparable neutralization titers against influenza B virus grown in eggs or MDCK cells. These findings contribute to proof that the current influenza vaccine manufacturing process, using embryonating eggs, produces vaccines that are broadly efficacious against viruses circulating in nature. Of course, the very broad immunogenicity that is required of influenza vaccines to protect against the different viruses circulating in nature at any given time must be achieved by incorporating into vaccine multiple viruses and by changing these as viruses change in nature.

5. Other Vectored Poxvirus Vaccine Candidates

As illustrated in Table III and with the development of vectored fowlpox and raccoon poxvirus, many choices are available for initial trials (phase 1, 2, and 3 clinical trials in humans, closed and open field trials in livestock animal species) of vectored virus candidate vaccines. Yet no single candidate, for either human or animal use, can be easily identified as being above controversy. The choices for initial trials must be based on analyses of risk : benefit, cost : benefit, alternative product availability, public acceptability, environmental impact, etc. For some candidate vaccines, considerations may be based upon universal factors, but for others, including the examples given in the preceding sections, needs are limited to selected populations in limited geographic areas and considerations are greatly affected by varying views of these needs. Candidate human vaccines against AIDS, respiratory syncytial virus disease, hepatitis B, dengue, and malaria, and candidate animal vaccines against rabies, vesicular stomatitis, and transmissible gastro-enteritis of swine have received much attention. Each of these candidates raises complex questions, as does the concept of infectious vectored virus vaccines in general. As a result, there is a perceived inertia in moving from feasibility experiments in laboratory animal species to clinical and field trials. Although a vaccinia : HIV-1 env-protein vaccine candidate has been used experimentally in humans in Africa (Zagury *et al.*, 1987) and a vaccinia : rabies G is being field-tested in Belgium (WHO Veterinary Public Health Unit, personal communication), one can still ask: "Which should go first, in the context of which vaccine candidate can best meet an immediate need and at the same time best contribute to our understanding of infectious vectored virus vaccines in general?" Clearly, different investigators, research institutions, government agencies, and regulatory authorities will answer these questions differently, but perhaps in ways that overcome the inertia of the day.

V. Other Infectious Vectored Virus Vaccines

A. VECTORED HERPESVIRUS VACCINES

No one virus or family of viruses identified has ideal characteristics for use as the substrate for all infectious vectored virus vaccines. Differences in the desired usage of vaccines are such that different vectors may be envisioned in different circumstances. Hence, the feasibility for using any virus with a large enough genome to carry heterologous genes must be considered. In this regard, the herpesviruses offer several unique advantages, and a few disadvantages.

In general, the herpesviruses evoke very strong cell-mediated immune responses, as well as strong and long-lasting humoral responses. Additionally, the viruses have rather narrowly specific host ranges, which might be considered advantageous in any live-virus vaccine. Particular herpesviruses are also associated with neurologic and neoplastic diseases, however, and all herpesviruses are associated with persistent infection and life-long carriage. These characteristics, unless further defined and absolutely controlled, would be considered unacceptable in any live-virus vaccine.

The biology, molecular biology, and immunobiology of the human and animal herpesviruses have been reviewed (Roizman, 1985; Roizman and Lopez, 1985; Lopez and Roizman, 1986). Herpesviruses contain linear double-stranded DNA (120–250 kbp), which varies in physical structure among genera and encodes 50–80 genes. Purified DNA is infectious. Virus replication takes place in the nucleus and virion maturation, via envelopment, takes place at the nuclear and plasma membranes of the infected cell. Replication requires cellular polymerase II for transcription and expression of viral proteins. Polypeptides arise in a cascade fashion, coordinately regulated and sequentially ordered. For example, immediate-early α-gene products are required for β-gene expression, the products of which in turn effect late γ-genes that code for virion structural proteins.

Methods for the insertion, deletion, and substitution of endogenous and exogenous DNA sequences into herpesviruses, particularly herpes simplex virus, via homologous recombination, have been reviewed (Jenkins and Roizman, 1986; Roizman and Jenkins, 1985; Roizman and Arsenakis, 1985a,b; Dix, 1987). Herpes simplex virus has been used successfully as a vector for expressing hepatitis B virus surface antigen (Shih et al., 1984) and for Epstein Bar virus nuclear antigen 1 (Hummel et al., 1986). An attenuated varicella virus strain (OKA), which has been licensed in some countries for use as a universal vaccine or special-use (in pediatric leukemias, etc.) vaccine, has been used for the expression of EB virus gp350/220 glycoprotein (Lowe et al., 1987).

Unique prototype herpes simplex virus vectors have been developed (Meigner et al., 1988). They consist of herpes simplex type 1 virus from which 15% of the genome has been deleted and into which genes for herpes simplex type 2 virus immunogenic proteins (gG, gD, gI) have been inserted. Because of the extent of the deletions, these viruses have genomic space for the insertion of more than 10 kbp of heterologous DNA. Safety and immunogenicity of these recombinants have been examined in experimental animals. These recombinants do not disseminate from the site of inoculation nor do they cause systemic infection. Neurovirulence has been eliminated; direct intracerebral inoculation of experimental animals does not appear to cause infection. Both recombinants have been shown to protect mice, guinea pigs, rabbits, and two species of primates against challenge with wild-type herpes simplex type 1 and 2 viruses. These recombinants could be configured as a human vectored vaccine against several viral diseases.

Although persistent, life-long infection is usually viewed as an undesirable characteristic in regard to use of herpesviruses as infectious vectored vaccines, it can also be viewed as a unique advantage. The immune system of the person or animal receiving a herpesvirus-vectored vaccine would be continuously or intermittently (via recrudescence) stimulated. Although the genes responsible for the persistence of herpesviruses have not been identified, it is thought that they must be nonessential for basic virus replication, and therefore removable. Proponents of vectored herpesvirus vaccines have indicated that, at least for herpes simplex type 1 and 2 viruses, this is feasible (Roizman and Arsenakis, 1985a,b; Meigner *et al.*, 1988). The counterargument is that we may never know enough about the complex viral characteristics that lead to herpesvirus persistence to warrant the risk involved in vaccination.

Persistence and long-term immunostimulation would be a disadvantage in regard to vectored vaccine usage if one vaccination precluded the effectiveness of subsequent vaccinations. However, evidence shows that (1) individuals with preexisting high-titered antibody to herpes simplex type 1 virus do allow local replication of superinfecting virus and (2) individuals with a strong immune responsiveness to herpes simplex type 1 virus allow infection and replication of type 2 virus. So, it remains to be seen whether multiple vaccination regimens, using different vectored herpesviruses, would be efficacious.

Many attenuated-live virus vaccines for herpesvirus diseases are now being used in livestock, companion animals, and poultry. Each of these can be considered as a potential substrate for vectored vaccines for the host species. Because herpesviruses are such important pathogens of animals and poultry, very large numbers of doses of these attenuated-live virus vaccines are now used. Therefore, it might be anticipated that vectored vaccine products that protected against the homologous substrate virus as well as the agent of the heterologous insert would have a strong marketing base. The value of each vaccine virus chosen for use as a vector would have to be judged independently of its value as an attenuated-live virus vaccine, but it would be the combined homologous and heterologous immunogenicity that would determine vaccine usage. Because of the narrow host specificity of the animal and poultry herpesviruses, the overall environmental risk of use of infectious vectored herpesvirus vaccines would be expected to be limited, but this would have to be proven in closed and open field trials.

B. Vectored Adenovirus Vaccines

Like the herpesviruses, the adenoviruses have advantages and disadvantages in regard to their use as vectors for human and animal vaccines. Adenoviruses are capable of evoking good humoral and cell-mediated immune responses, and in natural respiratory tract infections they evoke good mucosal immune responses. The viruses have narrowly specific host ranges, usually considered an advantage for live-virus vaccines.

Since the 1960s, U.S. military personnel have been vaccinated with a live-virus vaccine to prevent acute respiratory disease, a particular problem in training facilities. Outbreaks of respiratory disease in such settings are most often caused by adenovirus types 3, 4, 7, 14, or 21. The vaccine consists of nonattenuated cell culture-propagated adenovirus types 4 and 7. The vaccine is administered orally via enterically coated capsules, which avoids respiratory tract infection and virus denaturation in the stomach. Infection of the intestinal tract is asymptomatic, but does result in effective immunity against the homologous virus types and lesser, but valuable, immunity against the other virus types that cause disease in these settings. Because of this successful experience, current proposals for the use of adenoviruses as vectors for human vaccines have started with the licensed vaccine viruses and with enterically coated capsules as a delivery system.

The biology, molecular biology, and immunobiology of the adenoviruses have been reviewed (Ginsberg, 1984; Doerfler, 1984). Forty-three human adenovirus types, organized into seven major groups, have been identified. The viruses replicate in the nucleus and are released by cytolysis. Their genome consists of one molecule (36 kbp) of double-stranded DNA with ITRs; the genome encodes 11–15 structural proteins and at least 15 nonstructural proteins. The small size of the adenovirus genome and virion packaging constraints limit the amount of heterologous DNA that may be inserted.

The feasibility of using adenoviruses as infectious vectored vaccines was first explored with human adenovirus type 5, which can be evaluated in a hamster model. Hepatitis B virus surface antigen (HBsAg) coding sequences under control of the adenovirus major late promoter (MLP) was inserted by homologous recombination into the genome of adenovirus, downstream of the promoter for the early E3 region (Morin et al., 1987). This has been done with prototype adenovirus type 5, with an E3-deletion mutant, and with the adenovirus type 7 vaccine strain (Morin et al., 1988). The insert was placed to immediately precede or replace coding sequences for the adenovirus 19-kD glycoprotein, a protein that is apparently unnecessary for viral replication in cell culture. When these recombinants were inoculated intranasally into hamsters, they evoked antibodies to both adenovirus and HBsAg. Other adenovirus recombinants have been developed: one adenovirus type 5 : HBsAg recombinant when inoculated intravenously into chimpanzees produced partial protection against challenge (Ballay *et al.*, 1985; Levrero *et al.*, 1988).

In adenovirus infections, the 19-kD viral glycoprotein may mediate the host cellular immune response; the protein appears to affect the expression on infected cells of class I major histocompatibility antigens that are part of the immune recognition site. This phenomenon may significantly modulate infected cell evasion from immune surveillance (Severinsson *et al.*, 1986; Pettersson, 1984). Adenovirus types 4 and 7 vectors have been of value with an MLP : HBsAg cassette inserted near the right-end ITR, which has provided evaluation of expression of the 19-kD glycoprotein (B. Mason, personal communication).

The prospect for the use of vectored adenovirus vaccines in humans cannot be fully evaluated at this time. The prospect of having vaccines that could be delivered orally is exciting, but the limited heterologous gene carrying capacity of the viruses, their nuclear site of DNA replication, their mRNA splicing capability, their ability to cause transformation in cell cultures and tumors in animals (under highly artificial conditions; Graham, 1984), their ability to form functional hybrids with SV40 virus (Klessig, 1984), and their persistence in lymphoid tissues represent unanswered concerns.

The prospect for the use of vectored adenovirus vaccines in animals seems much more exciting. More than 50 adenoviruses of animals have been identified, some recognized as important pathogens, and some attenuated and used as live-virus vaccines. For example, the insertion of genes for protective epitopes of canine adenovirus type 2 into the attenuated live-virus vaccine strain of canine adenovirus type 1 (infectious canine hepatitis virus) represents a simple approach to a bivalent vaccine. A more far-reaching prospect would be the expression of rabies virus G and N coding sequences by an attenuated live-virus vaccine strain of canine adenovirus type 1. Such a recombinant vaccine with the infectiousness and transmissibility of the parent adenovirus vaccine strain could be used as an oral rabies vaccine for dogs and even for raccoons (also infectable by this adenovirus). Like the parent canine adenovirus vaccine strain, an adenovirus : rabies recombinant might be transmitted naturally from vaccinated animals to other susceptible contact animals, thereby achieving a greater herd immunity than otherwise possible.

VI. Conclusions

In the long term, ideas for better vaccine usage are dominated by the potential of genetically engineered vaccines. The "ideal vaccine" of today is best represented by some of the pediatric attenuated live-virus vaccines. In fact, when we insist that the "ideal vaccine" mimic natural infection in its influence upon the recipient, we set a very high standard, a standard that so far has been most easily attained by attenuated live-virus vaccines. This standard will be difficult to match with any genetically engineered product, unless full attention is paid to cell-mediated and humoral immunogenicity as well as other host responses. Likewise, new vaccines must be evaluated in regard to their capability to evoke maternal immunity that is transferable to the fetus and newborn and their efficacy in the face of prior vaccination or maternal antibodies. New vaccines must also be evaluated appropriately in regard to their thermal stability, that is, their usefulness in areas where the "cold-chain" is not reliable. All in all, it seems clear that there are today too few "ideal vaccines," but it is still too early to judge how infectious vectored virus vaccines will contribute to an overall vaccine armamentarium.

Vectored virus vaccines should be considered model systems in the overall context of safe vaccine use in disease control. For example, small genetic changes in attenuated live-virus vaccine seed stocks can lead to the production of vaccine lots with unacceptable pathogenicity. For this reason, attenuated live-virus vaccines will always have to be proven safe on a lot-by-lot basis. For the vaccine producer, it may well be attractive to eliminate this problem by eliminating all need of working with mutable seed viruses. Recombinant DNA viruses carrying desired genes for heterologous immunogenic proteins would be genetically very stable. They would also allow the rapid production of large amounts of vaccine in a short time, as required in the face of epidemics and epizootics. In such settings, recombinant vaccines need not overburden safety and quality assurance testing, nor other aspects of the regulatory process.

A. Outlook for Infectious Vectored Virus Vaccines for Humans

Member viruses of the three families (Poxviridae, Herpesviridae, Adenoviridae), described here as having potential for use as infectious vectored virus vaccines, have characteristics that lead to a complex judgment as to the overall promise for the practical use of end products in the field. Feasibility seems clear even though, in most cases, questions of stability of recombinants and level of expression of inserted gene products have not been fully answered. Virus vectors now under development have the ability to carry enough heterologous DNA to code for single or multiple genes for immunogenic proteins. Vector systems allow remarkably faithful transcription and translation from inserted genes, as well as proper post-translational processing and transport. Some researchers are optimistic that increased expression will be achieved by the use of better natural or synthetic promoters. Similarly, some are optimistic that increased immunogenicity may be achieved by novel linkages of genes for immunogenic proteins with those for lymphokines and other immunomodulators (Flexner et al., 1988).

At this time, the major concern over the use of infectious vectored virus vaccines for humans is safety. In the face of a substantial rate of disease occurrence and conditions affecting immunocompetence (chemical immunosuppression, AIDS, malnutrition, etc.), the safety of all live-virus vaccines, including infectious vectored vaccines, must be assured. After a U.S. military recruit, who was unknowingly infected with HIV, developed disseminated vaccinia after routine vaccination (Redfield et al., 1987), it was suggested that all research on recombinant vaccinia vaccines be discontinued. Halsey and Henderson (1987) retorted: ". . . it would be extremely unfortunate if routine immunizations were unnecessarily withheld because of over-interpretation of information and speculations [from one case of vaccination complication] . . . ." Further, they noted that available data indicated that several hundred HIV-seropositive military recruits must have received many different immunizations without ill effects before routine screening and exclusion of HIV-positive applicants.

Genetic manipulation of vectored viruses to minimize their pathogenicity is one major response to safety concerns. This approach is based upon understanding of the functions of the many viral genes that contribute to virulence characteristics, such as invasiveness, tropism, escape from nonspecific host defenses, escape from specific host defenses, etc. Although this is a very complex area of research, much progress is being made. However, progress made in the laboratory toward developing candidate vaccines with predictable and stable safety characteristics will only be worthwhile if it is complemented by progress in developing a reasonable public perspective of biotechnology and its products.

Public "informed consent" must involve public interest groups that are critical of biotechnological (genetic engineering) development. Such consent must achieve widespread awareness and agreement that these vaccines are needed and are safe. Certain public interest groups active in this subject area, such as the Foundation on Economic Trends in the United States and the Green Party in the Federal Republic of Germany, have taken the position that all genetic manipulation involves far greater risk than is generally realized and thus must be prohibited (American Society for Microbiology, 1987a). Such groups have taken legal action affecting experimentation per se, the evaluation of experimentation, and the regulation of experimentation and its products (American Society for Microbiology, 1987b). Other groups have sought to dissect the overall subject into its parts, so that separate judgments might be made. In this case, vaccines become quite appealing because of their unique cost-effective value for tackling difficult problems in developed and developing countries. At this point, it seems that the attitude of most scientists and government agencies in most countries, as reflected in extramural research funding and intramural research programs, is very supportive of developmental research but rather cautious in regard to clinical and field trials. In these same countries the attitude of the public is still not clear. In the opinion of the authors, biotechnologically produced products, including vaccines, can be made safe, and public confidence in the safety, efficacy, and value of these products can be gained by full disclosure and informative communication. Important positive elements in this process are contained in the proposal by the U.S. Office of Science and Technology for a "Coordinated Framework for Regulation of Biotechnology," (Federal Register, 1985).

B. OUTLOOK FOR INFECTIOUS VECTORED VIRUS VACCINES FOR ANIMALS

From the first days of the genetic engineering revolution, some researchers believed that vaccines for animal diseases would be the proving ground for human vaccines. It was thought that funding would flow into this research field because demands for vaccine safety and efficacy are less stringent, licensing is simpler, and markets are larger. To some extent this has been the case; according to a survey done for the Center for Veterinary Medicine, U.S. Food and Drug Administration (American Society for Microbiology, 1986), approximately 100 firms have been pursuing at least 200 separate veterinary biotechnology projects in the United States. The largest number of these projects have been for disease management, i.e., diagnostics reagents and kits, therapeutics, and in the largest numbers, vaccines. Nevertheless, the premise that veterinary products represent the brightest area for biotechnology enterprise has partially collapsed, and many of the largest companies are shying away from the animal vaccine market. This disillusionment should be examined—perhaps promises did outdistance reality, but, in view of the most recent developments in the technology and its application, there seems reason for optimism. The promise of vectored virus vaccines should be seen as a specific reason for optimism.

In several livestock industries, especially in the poultry and swine industries, the use of vaccines is considered crucial. In others, such as the cattle industries (cow-calf, feedlot, dairy), most vaccines are used with skepticism and with constant questions of poor cost/benefit ratios. The initial optimism of the new bioengineering companies as they looked at the animal vaccine market was based upon the extraordinarily large numbers of doses of vaccines produced. In 1985, in the United States, total production of all veterinary vaccine formulations was over 17 billion doses, of which about 93% consisted of poultry vaccines, representing about 39% of the total dollar value. The poultry vaccines were used to vaccinate 4.5 billion broilers, 45 million breeders, and 300 million layers. A total of 2.8 billion doses of Marek's disease vaccine were produced.

The initial enthusiasm of the new bioengineering companies waned in the realization that a very large number of doses of produced vaccines support a veterinary biologic industry with sales of only $300–400 million per year, of which about $118 million is in the poultry biologic industry. As an example of this fiscal reality, a common poultry vaccine is sold in a 25-ml vial containing 10,000 doses (delivered in broiler house water supply), which is sold for about $8.00. Of the nonpoultry vaccines, the largest market is that of rabies vaccines for pet animals. So, one question facing bioengineering companies is how to make a profit by expanding markets, not by just redividing them. To date, bioengineered vaccines for animals (and humans) that have reached the marketplace have been priced higher than conventional vaccines (e.g., swine pseudorabies vaccines). Larger markets will be built only if data and perceptions indicate to the farmer, rancher, and poultry producer that new bioengineered vaccines actually represent an improvement in value, that is, an improvement in cost/benefit equations.

The future role of vectored virus vaccines for animal diseases must be viewed in light of these realities. Products will only have value if they meet safety and efficacy demands, as set by government regulatory agencies and the public at large. If this can be achieved, then the great advantage of vectored virus vaccine products could lie in the low cost of manufacturing and ease of delivering them. Setbacks in the development of vectored virus vaccines for animal diseases have been caused by regulatory oversight of some animal experimentation and open field trials, but this will be corrected as regulatory details become clearer and more widely communicated.

In the end, overall benefit : cost : risk equations will determine the use of particular vectored virus vaccines in preventing and controlling animal diseases. In our opinion, these equations will indicate an important role for many specific products that are now in development. The long-term future only promises more and more valuable products.

C. VACCINE TECHNOLOGY TRANSFER FOR DEVELOPING COUNTRIES

Some international agencies have stated that conventional vaccine production infrastructure can be leap-frogged and bioengineered vaccine production can be started from scratch in developing countries. Not everyone agrees. Several problems are: (1) there is too little opportunity (and funding) for training scientists from developing countries in the necessary technology, especially the technology used in manipulating genes and constructing recombinants by marker rescue; (2) most products and processes involving this technology are patented and limited in availability by proprietary ownership; and (3) foreign exchange shortages preclude most cooperative ventures between owners of proprietary products and processes and institutions in developing countries. One major problem is that no central international agency is charged with providing necessary leadership. An important activity of such an agency should be to develop standards. Currently, no standards exist for safety and efficacy. For example, with vectored vaccinia virus vaccines there is a need to monitor mutations in seed stocks as they undergo serial passage.

Several international agencies are funding the construction of vaccine factories in developing countries through various forms of bilateral and consortium agreements. In this context, recombinant DNA technology is proving to be particularly difficult to adapt to these arrangements because the technology demands extremely sophisticated facilities. Vectored poxvirus vaccines, in final form for production, may represent the first technology that is truly transferable to the Third World for local manufacture. Such technology transfer certainly must be tried.

REFERENCES

Alexander, A. D., Flyger, V., Herman, Y. F., McConnell, S. J., Rothstein, N., and Yager, R. H. (1972). *J. Wildl. Dis.* **8**, 119–126.

Al'tshtein, A. D., Andzhaparidze, O. G., Antonova, T. P., Baev, A. A., and Baisar, D. (1986). *Dokl. Akad. Nauk SSSR* **289**, 1493–1496.

American Society for Microbiology. (1986). *Am. Soc. Microbiol. News* **52**, 570.

American Society for Microbiology. (1987a). *Am. Soc. Microbiol. News* **53**, 71–72.

American Society for Microbiology. (1987b). *Am. Soc. Microbiol. News* **53**, 126.

Andrew, M. E., Boyle, D. B., Coupar, B. E., Whitfield, P. L., Both, G. W., and Bellamy, A. R. (1987). *J. Virol.* **61,** 1054–1060.

Archard, L. C., Mackett, M., Barnes, D. E., and Dumbell, K. R. (1984). *J. Gen. Virol.* **65,** 875–886.

Arita, I., and Fenner, F. (1985). *In* "Vaccinia Viruses as Vectors for Vaccine Antigens" (G. V. Quinnan, ed.), pp. 49–60. Elsevier, New York.

Auperin, D. D., Esposito, J. J., Lange, J. V., and McCormick, J. B. (1987). *In* "Vaccines '87: Modern Approaches to New Vaccines" (R. M. Chanock, R. A. Lerner, F. Brown, and H. Ginsberg, eds.), pp. 403–407. Cold Spring Harbor Lab., Cold Spring Harbor, New York.

Auperin, D. D., Esposito, J. J., Lange, J. V., Bauer, S. P., Knight, J. C., Sasso, D. R., and McCormick, J. B. (1988). *Virus Res.* **9,** 233–248.

Bablanian, R., and Banerjee, A. K. (1986). *Proc. Natl. Acad. Sci. U.S.A.* **83,** 1290–1294.

Baldrick, C. J., and Moss, B. (1987). *Virology* **156,** 138–145.

Ball, L. A. (1987). *J. Virol.* **61,** 1788–1795.

Ballay, A., Levrero, M., Buendia, M. A., Tiollais, P., and Perricaudet, M. (1985). *EMBO J.* **4,** 3861–3865.

Baroudy, B. M., Venkatessan, S., and Moss, B. (1983). *Cold Spring Harbor Symp. Quant. Biol.* **47,** 723–729.

Beaud, G., Mars, M., and Vassef, A. (1987). *Dev. Biol. Stand.* **66,** 49–54.

Bertholet, C., Stocco, P., Van Meir, E., and Wittek, R. (1986). *EMBO J.* **5,** 1951–1957.

Bertholet, C., Van Meir, E., ten Heggeler-Bordier, B. and Wittek, R. (1987). *Cell (Cambridge, Mass.)* **50,** 153–162.

Black, D. N., Hammond, J. M., and Kitching, R. P. (1986). *Virus Res.* **5,** 277–292.

Blancou, J., Kieny, M. P., Lathe, R., Lecocq, J. P., Pastoret, P. P., Soulebot, J. P., and Desmettre, P. (1986). *Nature (London)* **322,** 373–375.

Block, W., Upton, C., and McFadden, G. (1985). *Virology* **140,** 113–124.

Boulter, E. A., and Appleyard, G. (1973). *Prog. Med. Virol.* **16,** 86–108.

Boyle, D. B., and Coupar, B. E. (1986). *J. Gen. Virol.* **67,** 1591–1600.

Boyle, D. B., Coupar, B. E., Parsonon, I. M., Bagust, T. J., and Both, G. W. (1986). *Res. Vet. Sci.* **41,** 40–44.

Boyle, D. B., Coupar, B. E., Gibbs, A. J., Seigman, L. J., and Both, G. W. (1987). *Virology* **156,** 355–365.

Bradshaw, H. D., and Deininger, P. L. (1984). *Mol. Cell. Biol.* **4,** 2316–2320.

Briody, B. A. (1959). *Bacteriol. Rev.* **23,** 61–95.

Broyles, S. S., and Moss, B. (1986). *Proc. Natl. Acad. Sci. U.S.A.* **33,** 3141–3145.

Buller, R. M., Smith, G. L., Cremer, K., Notkins, A. L., and Moss, B. (1985). *Nature (London)* **317,** 813–815.

Carrasco, L., and Bravo, R. (1986). *Virology* **58,** 569–577.

Centers for Disease Control. (1987). *Morbid. Mortal. Wkly. Rep.* **36,** Suppl. 3S, 1–27.

Chakrabarti, S., Brechling, K., and Moss, B. (1985). *Mol. Cell. Biol.* **5,** 3403–3409.

Chakrabarti, S., Robert-Guroff, M., Wong-Staal, F., Gallo, R. C., and Moss, B. (1986). *Nature (London)* **320,** 535–537.

Chang, W., Upton, C., Hu, S. L., Puruchio, A. F., and McFadden, G. (1987). *Mol. Cell. Biol.* **7,** 535–540.

Chanock, R. M., Lerner, R. A., Brown, F., and Ginsberg, H., eds. (1988). "Vaccines '88: Modern Approaches to New Vaccines." Cold Spring Harbor Lab., Cold Spring Harbor, New York.

Cheng, K. C., and Moss, B. (1987). *J. Virol.* **61,** 1286–1290.

Chernos, V. I., Antonova, T. P., and Senkevich, T. G. (1985). *J. Gen. Virol.* **66,** 621–626.

Cho, C. T., and Wenner, H. A. (1973). *Bacteriol. Rev.* **37,** 1–18.

Clarke, B. E., Carroll, A. R., Francis, M. J., Appleyard, G., Syred, A. D., Highfield, P. E., Rowlands, D. J., Brown, F., and Newton, S. E. (1988). *In* "Vaccines '88: Modern Approaches to New Vaccines" (R. M. Chanock, R. A. Lerner, F. Brown, and H. Ginsberg, eds.), pp. 127–131. Cold Spring Harbor Lab., Cold Spring Harbor, New York.

Clegg, J. C., and Lloyd, G. (1987). *Lancet* **2**, 186–187.

Cochran, M. A., Puckett, C., and Moss, B. (1985). *J. Virol.* **53**, 30–37.

Cole, G. A., and Blanden, R. V. (1982). *Compr. Immunol.* **9**, 1–19.

Collett, M. S., Keegan, K., Hu, S.-L., Sridar, P., Purchio, A. F., Ennis, W. H., and Dalrymple, J. M. (1987). *In* "The Biology of Negative Strand Viruses" (B. Mahy and D. Kolakofsky, eds.), pp. 321–329. Elsevier, New York.

Condit, R. C., Motyczka, A., and Spizz, G. (1983). *Virology* **128**, 429–443.

Coupar, B. E. H., Boyle, D. B., and Both, G. W. (1987). *J. Gen. Virol.* **68**, 2299–2309.

Cranage, M. P., Kouzarides, T., Bankier, A. T., Satchwell, S., Weston, K., Tomlinson, P., Barrell, B., Hart, H., Bell, S. E., Minson, A. C., *et al.* (1986). *EMBO J.* **5**, 3057–3063.

Cremer, K. J., Mackett, M., Wohlenberg, C., Notkins, A. L., and Moss, B. (1985). *Science* **228**, 737–740.

Dales, S., and Pogo, B. G. T. (1981). *Virol. Monogr.* **18**, 1–109.

De, B. K., Shaw, M. W., Rota, P. A., Harmon, M. W., Esposito, J. J., Rott, R., Cox, N. J., and Kendal, A. P. (1988). *Vaccine* **7**, 257–261.

DeLange, A. M., and McFadden, G. (1987). *J. Virol.* **61**, 1957–1963.

Deubel, V., Kinney, R. M., Esposito, J. J., Cropp, C. B., Vorndam, A. V., Monath, T. P., and Trent, D. W. (1988). *J. Gen. Virol.* **69**, 1921–1929.

Dix, R. D. (1987). *Prog. Med. Virol.* **34**, 89–128.

Doerfler, W. (1984). *Curr. Top. Microbiol. Immunol.* **108**, 79–98.

Drillien, R., Spehner, D., Villeval, D., and Lecocq, J. (1987). *Virology* **160**, 203–209.

Dumbell, K. R., and Huq, F. (1986). *Am. J. Epidemiol.* **123**, 403–415.

Earl, P. L., and Moss, B. (1987). *In* "Genetic Maps 1987" (S. J. O'Brian, ed.), pp. 116–123. Cold Spring Harbor Lab., Cold Spring Harbor, New York.

Earl, P. L., Jones, E. V., and Moss, B. (1986). *Proc. Natl. Acad. Sci. U.S.A.* **83**, 3659–3663.

Enders, J. F., Katz, S. L., Milovanovic, M. V., and Holloway, A. (1960). *N. Engl. J. Med.* **263**, 153–159.

Esposito, J. J., and Knight, J. C. (1984). *Virology* **135**, 561–567.

Esposito, J. J., and Knight, J. C. (1985). *Virology* **143**, 230–251.

Esposito, J. J., Obijeski, J. F., and Nakano, J. H. (1978). *Virology* **89**, 53–66.

Esposito, J. J., Cabradilla, C. D., Nakano, J. H., and Obijeski, J. F. (1981). *Virology* **109**, 231–243.

Esposito, J. J., Nakano, J. H., and Obijeski, J. F. (1985). *Bull. W.H.O.* **63**, 695–703.

Esposito, J. J., Brechling, K., Baer, G., and Moss, B. (1987). *Virus Genes* **1**, 7–21.

Esposito, J. J., Knight, J. C., Shaddock, J. H., Novembre, F. J., and Baer, G. M. (1988). *Virology* **165**, 313–316.

Essani, K., and Dales, S. (1979). *Virology* **95**, 385–394.

Fathi, Z., Sridar, P., Pacha, R. F., and Condit, R. C. (1986). *Virology* **155**, 97–105.

Federal Register (1985). *Fed. Regist.* **50**, 220 (47174–47195).

Fenner, F. (1958). *Virology* **5**, 502–529.

Fenner, F. (1970). *Annu. Rev. Microbiol.* **24**, 297–334.

Fenner, F. (1979). *Intervirology* **11**, 137–157.

Fenner, F. (1985a). *Aust. J. Exp. Biol. Med.* **63**, 607–622.

Fenner, F. (1985b). *In* "Virology" (B. N. Fields, D. M. Knipe, R. M. Chanock, J. L. Melnick, B. Roizman, and R. E. Shope, eds.), pp. 661–684. Raven Press, New York.

Fenner, F., and Nakano, J. H. (1988). In "Laboratory Diagnosis of Infectious Diseases" (E. Lennette, P. Halonen, and F. A. Murphy, eds.), Vol. 2. Springer-Verlag, New York (in press).

Fenner, F., Bachmann, P. A., Gibbs, E. P. J., Murphy, F. A., Studdert, M. J., and White, D. O. (1987). "Veterinary Virology," pp. 387–405. Academic Press, Orlando, Florida.

Fenner, F., Henderson, D. A., Arita, I., Jezek, Z., and Ladnyi, I. D. (1988). "Smallpox and Its Eradication," pp. 69–168. World Health Organization, Geneva.

Flexner, C., Hügin, A., and Moss, B. (1988). In "Vaccines '88: Modern Approaches to New Vaccines" (R. M. Chanock, R. A. Lerner, F. Brown, and H. Ginsberg, eds.), pp. 179–184. Cold Spring Harbor Lab., Cold Spring Harbor, New York.

Franke, C. A., and Hruby, D. E. (1987). Arch. Virol. 94, 347–351.

Franke, C. A., Roseman, N. A., and Hruby, D. E. (1985a). Virus Res. 3, 13–17.

Franke, C. A., Rice, C. M., Strauss, J. H., and Hruby, D. E. (1985b). Mol. Cell. Biol. 5, 1918–1924.

Fuerst, T. R., Earl, P. L., and Moss, B. (1987). Mol. Cell. Biol. 7, 2538–2544.

Gassmann, U., Wyler, R., and Wittek, R. (1985). Arch. Virol. 83, 17–31.

Ghendon, Y. Z., and Chernos, V. I. (1964). Acta Virol. (Engl. Ed. 8, 359–368.

Gilbert, J. H., Pederson, N. C., and Nunberg, J. H. (1987). Virus Res. 7, 49–67.

Gillard, S., Sphener, D., Drillian, R., and Kirn, A. (1986). Proc. Natl. Acad. Sci. U.S.A. 83, 5573–5577.

Ginsberg, H. S., ed. (1984). "The Adenoviruses." Plenum, New York.

Graham, F. L. (1984). In "The Adenoviruses" (H. S. Ginsberg, ed.), pp. 339–398. Plenum, New York.

Gusic, B., ed. (1969). "Smallpox." Yugoslav Acad. Sci. Arts, Zagreb.

Halsey, N. A., and Henderson, D. A. (1987). N. Engl. J. Med. 316, 683–685.

Hanggi, M., Bannwarth, W., and Stunnenberg, H. G. (1986). EMBO J. 5, 1951–1957.

Hashizume, S., Morita, T., Yoshisowa, H., Suzuki, K., Arita, M., Komatsu, T., Amano, H., and Tagaya, I. (1973). Symp. Ser. Immunobiol. Stand. 19, 325–331.

Hashizume, S., Yoshizawa, H., Morita, M., and Suzuki, K. (1985). In "Vaccinia Viruses as Vectors for Vaccine Antigens" (G. V. Quinnan, ed.), pp. 87–99. Elsevier, New York.

Henderson, D. A., and Arita, I. (1985). In "Vaccinia Viruses as Vectors for Vaccine Antigens" (G. V. Quinnan, ed.), pp. 61–67. Elsevier, New York.

Hirt, P., Hiller, G., and Wittek, R. (1986). J. Virol. 58, 757–764.

Holowczak, J. A. (1982). Curr. Top. Microbiol. Immunol. 97, 27–79.

Holowczak, J. A. (1983). In "Replication of Viral and Cellular Genomes" (Y. Becker, ed.), pp. 205–236. Martinus Nijhoff, Boston, Massachusetts.

Hruby, D. E. (1985). Virus Res. 2, 151–156.

Hruby, D. E., and Ball, L. A. (1981a). Virology 113, 594–601.

Hruby, D. E., and Ball, L. A. (1981b). J. Virol. 40, 456–464.

Hruby, D. E., Maki, R. A., Miller, D. B., and Ball, L. A. (1983). Proc. Natl. Acad. Sci. U.S.A. 80, 3411–3415.

Hu, S., Bruszewski, J., Smalling, R., and Browne, J. K. (1985). Adv. Exp. Med. Biol. 185, 63–82.

Hu, S.-L., Estin, C. D., Stevenson, U. S., Plowman, G. D., Hellström, I., and Hellström, K.-E. (1988). In "Vaccines '88: Modern Approaches to New Vaccines" (R. M. Chanock, R. A. Lerner, F. Brown, and H. Ginsberg, eds.), pp. 47–52. Cold Spring Harbor Lab., Cold Spring Harbor, New York.

Hummel, M., Arsenakis, M., Marchini, A., Lee, L., Roizman, B., and Kieff, E. (1986). Virology 148, 337–481.

Ichihashi, Y., and Oie, M. (1980). Virology 101, 50–60.

Jenkins, F. J., and Roizman, B. (1986). *BioEssays* **5**, 244–247.

Jenkins, S. R., and Winkler, W. G. (1987). *Am. J. Epidemiol.* **126**, 429–437.

Kieny, M. P., Lathe, R., Drillien, R., Sphener, D., Skory, S., Schmitt D., Wikor, T., Koprowski, H., and Lecocq, J. P. (1984). *Nature (London)* **312**, 163–166.

King, A. M. Q., Stott, E. J., Langer, S. J., Young, K.-Y., Ball, A., and Wertz, G. W. (1987). *J. Virol.* **61**, 2885–2890.

Kinney, R. M., Esposito, J. J., Mathews, J. H., Roehrig, J. T., Johnson, B. J., Barrett, A. D., and Trent, D. W. (1989). *J. Virol.* (in press).

Kit, S., Sheppard, M., Ichimura, H., and Kit, M. (1987). *Am. J. Vet. Res.* **48**, 780–793.

Klessig, D. F. (1984). *In* "The Adenoviruses" (H. S. Ginsberg, ed.), pp. 399–449. Plenum, New York.

Koller, M., and Zsidai, J. (1973). *Symp. Ser. Immunobiol. Stand.* **19**, 313–318.

Koprowski, H., Celis, E., Curtis, P., Dietzschold, B., Rupprecht, C., Tollis, M., and Wunner, W. (1987). *Nature (London)* **326**, 636.

Koszinowski, U. H., Volkmer, H., Messerle, M., Jonjic, S., and Wittek, R. (1988). *In* "Vaccines '88: Modern Approaches to New Vaccines" (R. M. Chanock, R. A. Lerner, F. Brown, and H. Ginsberg, eds.), pp. 41–45. Cold Spring Harbor Lab., Cold Spring Harbor, New York.

Krag-Andersen, E. (1969). *In* "Smallpox" (B. Gusic, ed.), pp. 53–64. Yugoslav Acad. Sci. Arts, Zagreb.

Kuroda, K., Hauser, C., Rott, R., Klenk, H. D., and Doerfler, W. (1986). *EMBO J.* **5**, 1359–1365.

Kwoh, T. J., and Engler, J. A. (1984). *Nucleic Acids Res.* **12**, 3959–3971.

Langford, C. J., Edwards, S. J., Smith, G. L., Mitchell, G. F., Moss, B., Kemp, D. J., and Anders, R. F. (1986). *Mol. Cell. Biol.* **6**, 3191–3199.

Langford, C. J., Smith, D., Keam, L., Corcoran, L., Peterson, G., McIntyre, P., Kemp, D. J., Anders, R. F. Edwards, S. J., and Pye, D. (1988). *In* "Vaccines '88: Modern Approaches to New Vaccines" (R. M. Chanock, R. A. Lerner, F. Brown, and H. Ginsberg, eds.), pp. 89–94. Cold Spring Harbor Lab., Cold Spring Harbor, New York.

Levrero, M., Ballay, A., Schellekens, H., Tiollais, P., and Perricaudet, M. (1988). *In* "Vaccines '88: Modern Approaches to New Vaccines" (R. M. Chanock, R. A. Lerner, F. Brown, and H. Ginsberg, eds.), p. 384. Cold Spring Harbor Lab., Cold Spring Harbor, New York.

Lopez, C., and Roizman, B., eds. (1986). "Human Herpesvrus Infections: Pathogenesis, Diagnosis, and Treatment." Raven Press, New York.

Lowe, R. S., Keller, P. M., Keech, B. J., Davison, A. J., Whang, Y., Morgan, A. J., Kieff, E., and Ellis, R. W. (1987). *Proc. Natl. Acad. Sci. U.S.A.* **84**, 3896–3900.

Macaulay, C., Upton, C., and McFadden, G. (1987). *Virology* **158**, 381–393.

McFadden, G., and Dales, S. (1982). *In* "Organization and Replication of Viral DNA" (A. S. Kaplan, ed.), pp. 173–190. CRC Press, Boca Raton, Florida.

McGeoch, D. J., Howard, C. R., and Desselberger, U. (1987). *J. Gen. Virol.* **68**, 1501–1524.

McKenzie, S., Destree, A., Gordon, E., Panicali, D., Bernards, R., and Weinberg, R. (1988). *In* "Vaccines '88: Modern Approaches to New Vaccines" (R. M. Chanock, R. A. Lerner, F. Brown, and H. Ginsberg, eds.), pp. 19–23. Cold Spring Harbor Lab., New York.

Mackett, M., and Archard, L. C. (1979). *J. Gen. Virol.* **45**, 683–701.

Mackett, M., and Arrand, J. R. (1985). *EMBO J.* **4**, 3229–3234.

Mackett, M., and Smith, G. L. (1986). *J. Gen. Virol.* **67**, 2067–2082.

Mackett, M., Smith, G. L., and Moss, B. (1982). *Proc. Natl. Acad. Sci. U.S.A.* **79,** 7415–7419.

Mackett, M., Smith, G. L., and Moss, B. (1985a). *In* "DNA Cloning: A Practical Approach" (D. M. Glover, ed.), Vol. 2, pp. 191–211. IRL Press, Washington, D.C.

Mackett, M., Yilma, T., Rose, J., and Moss, B. (1985b). *Science* **227,** 433–435.

McQueen, N., Nayak, D. P., Stephens, E. B., and Compans, R. W. (1986). *Proc. Natl. Acad. Sci. U.S.A.* **83,** 9318–9322.

Marennikova, S. S., Chimishkyan, K. L., Maltseva, N. N., Shelukhina, E. M., and Fedorov, V. V. (1969). *In* "Smallpox" (B. Gusic, ed.). pp. 65–79. Yugoslav Acad. Sci. Arts, Zagreb.

Marennikova, S. S. (1973). *Symp. Ser. Immunobiol. Stand.* **19,** 253–260.

Mayr, A., Stickl, H., Muller, H. K., Danner, K., and Singer, H. (1978). *Zentralbl. Bakteriol., Parasitenkd., Infektionskrankh. Hyg., Abt. 1: Orig., Reihe* **167,** 375–390.

Meigner, B., Longnecker, R., and Roizman, B. (1988). *In* "Vaccines '88: Modern Approaches to New Vaccines" (R. M. Chanock, R. A. Lerner, F. Brown, and H. Ginsberg, eds.). Cold Spring Harbor Lab., Cold Spring Harbor, New York.

Mercer, A. A., Fraser, K., Barns, G., and Robinson, A. J. (1987). *Virology* **157,** 1–12.

Miller, J. H., ed. (1972). *In* "Experiments in Molecular Genetics," pp. 265–268. Cold Spring Harbor Lab., Cold Spring Harbor, New York.

Morin, J. E., Lubeck, M. D., Barton, J. E., Conley, A. J., Davis, A. R., and Hung, P. P. (1987). *Proc. Natl. Acad. Sci. U.S.A.* **84,** 4626–4630.

Morin, J. E., Barton, J., Lubeck, M., Molnar-Kimber, K., Mason, B., Domber, E., Dheer, S., Bhat, B., Conley, A., Davis, A., and Hung, P. (1988). *In* "Vaccines '88: Modern Approaches to New Vaccines" (R. M. Chanock, R. A. Lerner, F. Brown, and H. Ginsberg, eds.), p. 384. Cold Spring Harbor Lab., Cold Spring Harbor, New York.

Morita, M., Aoyama, Y., Arita, M., Amano, H., Yoshisowa, H., Hashizume, S., Komatu, T., and Tagaya, I. (1977). *Arch. Virol.* **53,** 197–208.

Morita, M., Suzuki, K., Yasuda, A., Kojima, A., Sugimoto, M., Watanabe, K., Kobayashi, H., Kajima, K., and Hashizume, S. (1987). *Vaccine* **5,** 65–70.

Morrison, D. K., and Moyer, R. W. (1986). *Cell (Cambridge, Mass.)* **44,** 587–596.

Moss, B. (1985). *In* "Virology" (B. N. Fields, D. M. Knipe, R. M. Chanock, J. L. Melnick, B. Roizman, and R. E. Shope, eds.), pp. 685–703. Raven Press, New York.

Moss, B., and Flexner, C. (1987). *Annu. Rev. Immunol.* **5,** 305–324.

Moss, B., Winters, E., and Cooper, J. A. (1981). *J. Virol.* **40,** 387–395.

Moss, B., Smith, G. L., and Mackett, M. (1983). *In* "Gene Amplification and Analysis" (T. S. Papas, M. Rosenberg, and J. G. Chirikjian, eds.), Vol. 3, pp. 201–214. Elsevier, New York.

Moyer, R. W., Graves, R. L., and Rothe, C. T. (1980). *Cell (Cambridge, Mass.)* **22,** 545–553.

Nakano, E., Panicali, D., and Paoletti, E. (1982). *Proc. Natl. Acad. Sci. U.S.A.* **79,** 1593–1596.

Nakano, J. H., and Esposito, J. J. (1988). *In* "Diagnostic Procedures for Viral, Rickettsial and Chlamydial Infections" (N. J. Schmidt and R. W. Emmons, eds.), 6th ed., pp. 224–265. Am. Public Health Assoc., Washington, D.C.

Neff, J. (1985). *In* "Vaccinia Viruses as Vectors for Vaccine Antigens" (G. V. Quinnan, ed.), pp. 69–75. Am. Elsevier, New York.

Oie, M., and Ichihashi, Y. (1987). *Virology* **157,** 449–459.

Olmstead, R. A., Buller, R. M., Murphy, B. R., Beeler, J. A., Collins, P. L., and London, W. T. (1988). *In* "Vaccines '88: Modern Approaches to New Vaccines" (R. M. Chanock, R. A. Lerner, F. Brown, and H. Ginsberg, eds.), pp. 205–210. Cold Spring Harbor Lab., Cold Spring Harbor, New York.

Panicali, D., and Paoletti, E. (1982). *Proc. Natl. Acad. Sci. U.S.A.* **79,** 4927–4931.

Panicali, D., Davis, S. W., Mercer, S. R., and Paoletti, E. (1981). *J. Virol.* **37,** 1000–1010.

Panicali, D., Grzelecki, A., and Huang, C. (1986). *Gene* **47,** 193–199.

Paoletti, E., Lipinskas, B. R., Samsonoff, C., Mercer, S., and Panicali, D. (1984). *Proc. Natl. Acad. Sci. U.S.A.* **81,** 193–197.

Paoletti, E., Perkus, M., Piccini, A., Wos, S., and Lipinskas, B. R. (1985a). *In* "Medical Virology" (L. M. de la Maza and E. M. Paterson, eds.), Vol. 4, pp. 409–430. Erlbaum, Hillsdale, New Jersey.

Paoletti, E., Perkus, M. E., and Piccini, A. (1985b). *Antiviral Res. Suppl.* **1,** 301–307.

Patel, D. D., and Pickup, D. J. (1987). *EMBO J.* **6,** 3787–3794.

Patel, D. D., Pickup, D. J., and Joklik, W. K. (1986). *Virology* **149,** 174–189.

Payne, L. G. (1979). *J. Virol.* **31,** 147–155.

Payne, L. G. (1980). *J. Gen. Virol.* **50,** 89–100.

Payne, L. G. (1986). *Arch. Virol.* **90,** 125–133.

Payne, L. G., and Kristensson, K. (1985). *J. Gen. Virol.* **66,** 643–646.

Pedley, C. B., and Cooper, R. J. (1987). *J. Gen. Virol.* **68,** 1021–1028.

Pensiero, M. N., Jennings, G. B., Schmaljohn, C. S., and Hay, J. (1988). *J. Virol.* **62,** 696–702.

Perkus, M. E., Panicali, D., Mercer, S., and Paoletti, E. (1986). *Virology* **152,** 285–297.

Pettersson, U. (1984). *In* "The Adenoviruses" (H. S. Ginsberg, ed.), pp. 205–270. Plenum, New York.

Piccini, A., and Paoletti, E. (1986). *BioEssays* **5,** 248–252.

Piccini, A., and Paoletti, E. (1988). *Adv. Virus Res.* **34,** 43–64.

Pickup, D. J., Bastia, D., Stone, H. O., and Joklik, W. K. (1982). *Proc. Natl. Acad. Sci. U.S.A.* **79,** 7112–7116.

Pickup, D. J., Bastia, D., and Joklik, W. K. (1983). *Virology* **124,** 215–217.

Pickup, D. J., Ink, B. S., Parsons, B. L., Hu, W., and Joklik, W. K. (1984). *Proc. Natl. Acad. Sci. U.S.A.* **81,** 6817–6821.

Pickup, D. J., Ink, B. S., Hu, W., Ray, C. A., and Joklik, W. K. (1986). *Proc. Natl. Acad. Sci. U.S.A.* **83,** 7698–7702.

Plucienniczak, A., Schroeder, E., Zettlmeissl, G., and Streek, R. E. (1985). *Nucleic Acids Res.* **13,** 985–998.

Polak, M. F. (1973). *Symp. Ser. Immunobiol. Stand.* **19,** 235–242.

Porter, C. D., and Archard, L. C. (1987). *J. Gen. Virol.* **68,** 673–682.

Post, L., and Roizman, B. (1981). *Cell (Cambridge, Mass.)* **25,** 227–232.

Quinnan, G. V., ed. (1985). "Vaccinia Viruses as Vectors for Vaccine Antigens." Elsevier, New York.

Quint, W., Gielkens, A., Van Oirschot, J., Berns, A., and Cuypers, H. T. (1987). *J. Gen. Virol.* **68,** 523–534.

Ray, S. N. (1973). *Symp. Ser. Immunobiol. Stand.* **19,** 47–51.

Redfield, R. R., Wright, D. C., James, W. D., Jones, T. S., Brown, C., and Burke, D. S. (1987). *N. Engl. J. Med.* **316,** 673–676.

Regamy, R. H., and Cohen, H., eds. (1973). *Symp. Ser. Immunobiol. Stand.* "International Symposium on Smallpox Vaccine," Vol. 19. Karger, Basel.

Rice, C. M., Franke, C. A., Strauss, J. H., and Hruby, D. E. (1985). *J. Virol.* **56,** 227–239.

Robinson, A. J., Barns, G., Freser, K., Carpenter, E., and Mercer, A. A. (1987). *Virology* **157,** 13–23.

Rodriguez, J. F., Paez, E., and Esteban, M. (1987). *J. Virol.* **61,** 395–404.

Rohrmann, G., Yuen, L., and Moss, B. (1986). *Cell (Cambridge, Mass.)* **46,** 1029–1035.

Roizman, B., ed. (1985). "The Herpesviruses," Vols. 1, 2, and 3. Plenum, New York.
Roizman, B., and Arsenakis, M. (1985a). *In* "Vaccinia Viruses as Vectors for Vaccine Antigens" (G. V. Quinnan, ed.), pp. 211–223. Am. Elsevier, New York.
Roizman, B., and Arsenakis, M. (1985b). *In* "Microbiology—1985" (O. Schlessinger, ed.), pp. 233–236. Am. Soc. Microbiol., Washington, D. C.
Roizman, B., and Jenkins, F. J. (1985). *Science* **229,** 1208–1214.
Roizman, B., and Lopez, C., eds. (1985). "The Herpesviruses," Vol. 4. Plenum, New York.
Rota, P., Shaw, M. W., and Kendal, A. P. (1987). *Virology* **161,** 269–275.
Rupprecht, C. E., Wiktor, T. J., Johnston, D. H., Hamir, A. N., Dietzschold, B., Wunner, W. H., Glickman, L. T., and Koprowski, H. (1986). *Proc. Natl. Acad. Sci. U.S.A.* **83,** 7947–7950.
Sabin, A. B. (1955). *Science* **109,** 85–87.
Sam, C. K., and Dumbell, K. R. (1981). *Ann. Virol.* **132E,** 135–150.
Schild, G. C., Oxford, J. S., de Jong, J. C., and Webster, R. W. (1983). *Nature (London)* **303,** 706–709.
Schwer, B., Visca, P., Vos, J. C., and Stunnenberg, H. G. (1987). *Cell (Cambridge, Mass.)* **50,** 163–169.
Severinsson, L., Martens, I., and Peterson, P. A. (1986). *J. Immunol.* **137,** 1003–1009.
Shida, H. (1986a). *Virology* **150,** 451–462.
Shida, H. (1986b). *Uirusu* **36,** 23–33.
Shih, M. F., Arsenakis, M., Tiollais, P., and Roizman, B. (1984). *Proc. Natl. Acad. Sci. U.S.A.* **81,** 5867–5870.
Smith, G. L., and Moss, B. (1984). *BioTechniques* **2,** 306–312.
Smith, G. L., Mackett, M., and Moss, B. (1984a). *Biotechnol. Genet. Eng. Rev.* **2,** 383–407.
Smith, G. L., Mackett, M., Murphy, B. R., and Moss, B. (1984b). *In* "Modern Approaches to Vaccines" (R. Chanock and R. Lerner, eds.), pp. 313–317. Cold Spring Harbor Lab., Cold Spring Harbor, New York.
Smith, G. L., Godson, G. N., Nussenzweig, V., Nussenzweig, R. S., Barnwell, J., and Moss, B. (1984c). *Science* **224,** 397–399.
Smith, G. L., Cheng, K. C., and Moss, B. (1986). *Parasitology* **92,** Suppl. S, 109–117.
Smith, G. L., Levin, J. Z., Palese, P., and Moss, B. (1987). *Virology* **160,** 336–345.
Spriggs, M. K., Murphy, B. R., Prince, G. A., Olmstead, R. A., and Collins, P. L. (1987). *J. Virol.* **61,** 3416–3423.
Stephens, E. B., and Compans, R. W. (1986). *Cell (Cambridge, Mass.)* **47,** 1053–1059.
Stephens, E. B., Compans, R. W., Earl, P., and Moss, B. (1986). *EMBO J.* **5,** 237–245.
Stroobant, P., Rice, A. P., Gullick, W. J., Cheng, D. J., Kerr, I. M., and Waterfield, M. D. (1985). *Cell (Cambridge, Mass.)* **42,** 383–393.
Sugimoto, M., Yasuda, A., Miki, K., Morita, M., Suzuki, K., Uchida, N., and Hashizume, S. (1985). *Microbiol. Immunol.* **29,** 421–428.
Sullivan, V., and Smith, G. L. (1987). *J. Gen. Virol.* **68,** 2587–2598.
Tartaglia, J., Piccini, A., and Paoletti, E. (1986). *Virology* **155,** 45–54.
Theiler, M., and Smith, H. H. (1937). *J. Exp. Med.* **65,** 787–800.
Thompson, C. L., and Condit, R. C. (1986). *Virology* **150,** 10–20.
Tomley, F. M., Mockett, A. P. A., Boursnell, M. E. G., Binns, M. M., Cook, J. K. A., Brown T. D. K., and Smith, G. L. (1987). *J. Gen. Virol.* **68,** 2291–2298.
Tripathy, D. N., Hanson, L. E., and Crandell, R. A. (1981). *In* "Comparative Diagnosis of Viral Diseases" (E. Kurstak and C. Kurstak, eds.), Vol. 3, pp. 267–346. Academic Press, Inc., New York.
Tsutsui, K., Uno, F., Akatsuka, K., and Nii, S. (1983). *Arch. Virol.* **75,** 213–218.
Twardzik, D. R., Brown, J. P., Ranchalis, J. E., Todaro, G. J., and Moss, B. (1985). *Proc. Natl. Acad. Sci. U.S.A.* **82,** 5300–5304.

Upton, C., DeLange, A. M., and McFadden, G. (1987). *Virology* **160,** 20–30.

Vijaya, S., Elango, N., and Moss, B. (1988). *In* "Vaccines '88: Modern Approaches to New Vaccines" (R. M. Chanock, R. A. Lerner, F. Brown, and H. Ginsberg, eds.), pp. 211–214. Cold Spring Harbor Lab., Cold Spring Harbor, New York.

Villarreal, E. C., Roseman, N. A., and Hruby, D. E. (1984). *J. Virol.* **51,** 359–356.

Walker, B. D., Chakrabarti, S., Moss, B., Paradis, T. J., Flynn, T., Durno, A. G., Blumberg, R. S., Kaplan, J. C., Hirsch, M. S., and Schooley, R. T. (1987). *Nature (London)* **328,** 345–348.

Weinrich, S. L., and Hruby, D. E. (1987). *J. Virol.* **61,** 639–645.

Weir, J. P., and Moss, B. (1983). *J. Virol.* **46,** 530–537.

Weir, J. P., and Moss, B. (1987a). *J. Virol.* **61,** 75–80.

Weir, J. P., and Moss, B. (1987b). *Virology* **158,** 206–210.

Weir, J. P., Bajszar, G., and Moss, B. (1982). *Proc. Natl. Acad. Sci. U.S.A.* **79,** 1210–1214.

White, D. O., and Fenner, F. (1986). "Medical Virology," 3rd ed. pp. 433–444. Academic Press, Orlando, Florida.

Wiktor, T. J., Macfarlan, R. I., Reagan, K. J., Dietzschold, B., Curtis, P. J., Wunner, W. H., Kieny, M. P., Lathe, R., Lecocq, J. P., Mackett, M., Moss, B. and Koprowski, H. (1984). *Proc. Natl. Acad. Sci. U.S.A.* **81,** 7194–7198.

Wiktor, T. J., Kieny, M. P., and Lathe, R. (1988). *In* "Applied Virology Research" (E. Kurstak, R. G. Marusyk, F. A. Murphy, and M. H. V. Van Regenmortel, eds.), Vol. 1, pp. 69–90, Plenum, New York.

Wilton, S., and Dales, S. (1986). *Virus Res.* **5,** 323–341.

Wittek, R. (1982). *Experientia* **38,** 285–297.

Wokatsch, R. (1972). *In* "Strains of Human Viruses" (M. Majer and S. A. Plotkin, eds.), pp. 241–257. Karger, Basel.

Yuen, L., and Moss, B. (1986). *J. Virol.* **60,** 320–323.

Zagury, D., Leonard, R., Fouchard, M., Reveil, B., Bernard, J., Ittele, D., Cattan, A., Zirimivabagobo, L., Kalumbu, M., Justin, W., Salaun, J., and Goussard, B. (1987). *Nature (London)* **326,** 249–250.

Zarling, J. M., Eichberg, J. W., Moran, P. A., McClure, J., Sridar, P., and Hu, S. L. (1987). *J. Immunol.* **139,** 988–990.

Zhao, B., Prince, G., Horsewood, R., Eckels, K., Summers, P., Chanock, R., and Lai, C-J. (1987). *J. Virol.* **61,** 4019–4022.

Modern Approaches to Live Virus Vaccines

ERLING NORRBY

Department of Virology, Karolinska Institute, School of Medicine,
Stockholm, Sweden

I. Introduction

In the field of veterinary medicine, as in its human counterpart, the decisive factors in deliberations on vaccine development projects are the burden of the target disease, its relative preventability, and the potential for evaluation of an effective immunoprophylactic product. The possibilities for advances in the field of animal vaccines may be viewed as comparatively more favorable since licensing is simpler and large markets are at hand. For these reasons animal vaccines have been considered as good test cases for products to be used in humans. However, there are limitations to such comparative evaluations, because in the case of animal vaccines the requirements for absence of side-reactions may be less stringent, the need for a durable immunity sometimes may not be as pronounced, and so forth. Another obvious qualitative difference is the economical considerations, which apply conspicuously to all animal vaccines. Thus, even the most effective veterinary vaccine may not come into use if it costs too much to produce.

Recent biotechnological developments have put remarkable tools in

the hands of vaccinologists. The advent of introduction of recombinant DNA technology has opened new opportunities for advances into
unexpected realms, both in the case of live and inactivated vaccines. Furthermore, the use of monoclonal antibodies and peptide
immunoreagents allows unique opportunities for dissection of immunoprotective as well as possibly immunopotentiating epitopes on
different structural components of a virus. The new biotechnology is
widely applied in the modern design of vaccine products. The development of biosynthetic vaccines, defined as a formulation containing a
noninfectious, protective subunit immunogen that is produced by use of
a biologic system, is dealt with in the chapter by Collett. Noninfectious
immunogens in the form of synthetic peptides are also discussed in a
separate chapter by Brown. Finally, the presentation of selected immunogens by use of viral or prokaryotic vectors containing heterologous
genes is considered separately (Murphy-Esposito). The focus of this
chapter, therefore, will be on live vaccine products. However, before the
presentation of different approaches to the development of such products, some general comments will be given on the advantages and
disadvantages of these kinds of immunogens.

II. General Views on the Development and Use of Live
Virus Vaccines

The choice in developments of vaccines stands between products
containing live attenuated virus or nonreplicating immunogens. If basic requirements on a vaccine such as ease of use, harmlessness, and
induction of effective and durable immunoprotection can be achieved by
use of an inactivated vaccine, this product represents the one of choice.
However, often this is not the case and in such situations a live vaccine
may represent an option. One general advantage of a live vaccine is
that potentially it can mobilize all the different arms of the immune
system. Furthermore, when the primary replication of vaccine virus
occurs in a mucosal membrane, attractive conditions for establishment
of a local immunity are obtained. This appreciation has given the
incentive for development of live vaccines to protect against local infections in the respiratory and enteric tracts (Chanock, 1981; Chanock and
Murphy, 1980; Chanock et al., 1988). There are certain situations that
would seem less amenable for exploitation of the use of live vaccines.
This is the case when the vaccine virus genome can integrate into
cellular genomes, possibly leading to alterations in the properties of
cells. This applies to infections with e.g., herpesviruses and retroviruses.

Two contrasting problems are encountered in the development of live vaccines. On one hand the vaccine candidate virus may become overattenuated so that the extent of the generalized or local infection is too limited to induce an immunity of satisfactory duration. On the other hand, the vaccine virus may display genetic instability and, due to regaining its virulent properties, give an extensive infection with unacceptable symptoms. The problem of genetic instability is amplified in situations when the virus can spread from the vaccine to susceptible individuals or animals in the environment.

It has become appreciated that definition of the molecular basis for virus virulence is a complex issue, even in the case of viruses that are relatively simple genetically. Occasionally a single property of a virus may have a dominating influence on its pathogenic potential. One example is the effects relating to the interaction between the viral capsid or envelope and receptors on a potential target cell. Virion variants with an altered surface structure can be selected as escape mutants by propagation of the virus in the presence of neutralizing monoclonal antibodies. Because some of these antibodies can be assumed to react directly with the receptor-seeking structure or other structures in their proximity at the virion surface, altered expression of ligand functions may be anticipated. In studies of reoviruses (Spriggs *et al.*, 1983), paramyxoviruses (Löve *et al.*, 1985), rhabdoviruses (Coulon *et al.*, 1982), and coronaviruses (Dalziel *et al.*, 1986; Fleming *et al.*, 1986), reduction of virulence was observed in some of the mutants selected by this approach.

It is to be expected that attenuation of a virus based on a single mutagenic event will not be stable, except perhaps if the basis for the alteration is a deletion in the genome. Considering the high mutation frequencies of viruses, in particular those with single-stranded genomes (Steinhauer and Holland, 1987), revertants with a regained virulence or pathogenicity will emerge readily. Expectedly, more fruitful approaches to the establishment of genetically stable vaccine candidate strains should encompass multiple genomic alterations. This can be achieved by reassortment in the case of viruses with segmented genomes or production of chimeric virus strains by use of cassette transfer of genetic material between different types of viruses. Recombinant DNA technology allows the latter approach to be taken with DNA viruses, retroviruses, and also with positive-strand RNA viruses. However, it has not been possible as yet to transfer properties of viral cDNA back into functioning negative-strand virus RNA.

Three different approaches to the identification of attenuated virus can be considered for use in the development of live vaccines. Sometimes these approaches can be applied in consort. In the following sections, each of them will be discussed separately.

III. Spontaneously Occurring Attenuated Virus Strains

There are two different sources to spontaneously occurring candidate live vaccine strains. One source is the emergence of nonvirulent virus strains in the natural host. The other source is the potentially attenuated properties of a virus infecting a nonnatural host, be it an animal virus giving a symptomless infection in man or vice versa. Identification of vaccine candidates in the latter situation can be referred to as the Jennerian approach.

There are only few examples of the use of naturally attenuated human viruses. It was observed a long time ago that some strains of poliovirus recovered from healthy individuals exhibited markedly variable neurovirulence when injected intracerebrally or intraspinally in monkeys (Sabin, 1957). About one-fifth of the strains appeared highly attenuated. In fact, the Sabin type 2 vaccine poliovirus was identified by this kind of analysis.

It was appreciated more recently that certain rotaviruses of low virulence are a frequent cause of infection in neonates. It appears that the degree of enterovirulence is not correlated to viral serotype. Recent studies (Flores *et al.*, 1986) demonstrate that the basis for this naturally occurring attenuation is the special features of the fourth gene of rotaviruses. This gene shows a conserved sequence in attenuated nursery strains representing all four serotypes of rotaviruses, but differs from the corresponding gene in various virulent rotaviruses. The fourth gene of rotaviruses directs the synthesis of the outer capsid protein VP3. This protein must be cleaved proteolytically for rotaviruses to become infectious. There are 89 amino acid positions in VP3 that are conserved among rotaviruses causing asymptomatic infections, whereas virulent virus strains show a completely different pattern of conservation in this gene product (Gorziglia *et al.*, 1986). It is of particular interest that some of these amino acid differences of attenuated and virulent strains involve the region of the protein that is subjected to cleavage to give two products of VP3. The absence of any corresponding systematic variation between different other homogeneous gene products in attenuated and virulent strains emphasizes the potential role of VP3 in determining virulence. There are plans to test the potential vaccine use of nursery strains in clinical trials (Chanock *et al.*, 1988).

Spontaneously occurring strains of adenovirus types 3, 4, and 7 are used as a live vaccine in humans in the form of enteric coated capsules (Takafuji *et al.*, 1979). By directing the replication of virus to the gut, there is no development of symptoms, but the local immunity established is transferred to involve the respiratory tract. Interestingly, it has been found that the strain of type 7 selected for inclusion in the vaccine may represent a nonvirulent variant of this type of adenovirus, based on the combined analysis of restriction enzyme patterns of strains and the epidemiological occurrence of infection with these strains (Wadell *et al.*, 1980).

The Jennerian approach has been exploited not only by use of cowpox virus to protect against smallpox in man, but the same virus has also been used to prevent ectromelia in mice. The basis for this kind of approach is that a virus adapted to growth in one species frequently replicates more poorly in a heterologous species. Provided it replicates efficiently enough in the heterologous species, it may give protection in this species against infection with an immunologically related virus. There are many examples of this situation. One of these concerns morbilliviruses. This genus of the family paramyxoviruses includes three closely related viruses—measles virus in man, distemper virus in dogs, and rinderpest virus in cattle. These viruses have two surface glycoproteins which play a dominating role in immune protection. The surface components are the hemagglutinin (H) in measles, and the equivalent component in the other two viruses, which carries responsibility for attachment to cell receptors, and the fusion (F) protein, which as the name implies mediates penetration of nucleocapsids into cells by membrane fusion. Among all the six structural components of morbilliviruses, it appears that the H protein shows the most pronounced evolutionary divergence, whereas the F protein is the most highly conserved component (Norrby *et al.*, 1985; Sheshberadaran *et al.*, 1986; Barrett *et al.*, 1987). The conservation of the amino acid sequence of the F component probably reflects some particular functional constringency of variation in its structure. Rinderpest virus may be the archevirus in the genus Morbilliviruses. It is somewhat more closely related to measles virus than to distemper virus. In general terms, rinderpest and measles virus provide a better protection against distemper virus infection than the other way around (*cf.* Fraser and Martin, 1978). The heterologous cross-protection by rinderpest virus has, for obvious reasons, not been exploited. Nor has the protective effect of measles virus against rinderpest (Plowright, 1962) come into use, probably because of a superior effect of homologous strains of attenuated virus. However, live measles virus is used for immunization of dogs against distemper. An analysis of the antibody response in the immunized animals reveals that the protection is mediated by an antibody response to the F protein (Appel *et al.*, 1984). The protection is not complete, but instead is infection permissive in many cases. It has been observed also in other virus systems such as influenza A virus that an isolated immunity to a single surface glycoprotein, the neuraminidase component, gives an infection-permissive immunity (Kilbourne, 1976). Finally, distemper virus was tried in early experiments for immunization of humans against measles (Adams *et al.*, 1959), but again homologous attenuated virus was soon found to be the preparation of choice.

Human parainfluenza virus type 3, like morbilliviruses, is a paramyxovirus and consequently also has two surface glycoproteins—an attachment protein referred to as the HN component because it carries neuraminidase activity in addition to the hemagglutinating activity and an F component. Monoclonal antibodies against some epitopes in both the HN and the F components provide protection against a parainfluenza 3 virus encephalitis in hamsters when used for passive protection (Rydbeck *et al.*, 1988). Both the HN and the F components have been expressed via a vaccinia virus vector and found to induce protection in cotton rats (Spriggs *et al.*, 1987), but the relative role of the HN component appears more dominant. Since human parainfluenza 3 virus is second only to respiratory syncytial (RS) virus as a causative agent of serious respiratory infection in infants and children, it has been considered as a target for vaccine development. In recent studies the potential use of bovine parainfluenza 3 virus for immunization against human parainfluenza 3 virus has started to be evaluated (Chanock *et al.*, 1988). Amino acid sequence data on the two viruses derived from information on the genomic nucleotide sequence show a considerable conservation. In the case of the F and HN glycoproteins, the degree of homology is 80% and 77% (Suzu *et al.*, 1987), respectively. This is in contrast to the situation in morbilliviruses, where the F component was highly conserved but the H component was divergent. Apparently the two situations must reflect different evolutionary lineages. The high degree of homology between surface glycoproteins of parainfluenza 3 virus strains of different species origin has become apparent also from studies of their antigenic properties. By use of monoclonal antibodies, the occurrence of several conserved as well as some distinguishing epitopes were demonstrated (Coelingh *et al.*, 1985; Rydbeck *et al.*, 1986). In a more detailed study that also includes analysis of the nucleotide sequence of neutralizing monoclonal antibody escape mutants of parainfluenza 3 virus (Coelingh *et al.*,1986), it was found that the humane and bovine viruses shared three epitopes in antigenic site A (recognized by neutralizing monoclonal antibodies) and two epitopes in antigenic sites D and F, (recognized by nonneutralizing monoclonal antibodies), whereas nine other epitopes in these and other sites differed between the two viruses.

Replication of bovine parainfluenza 3 virus in the respiratory tract of both cotton rats and squirrel monkeys (Coelingh et al., 1987) has induced certain resistence to replication of human parainfluenza 3 virus. The duration and magnitude of replication of prototype human and SF-4 bovine parainfluenza 3 virus strains in the upper and lower respiratory tract of squirrel monkeys was found to be similar (Coelingh et al., 1988). The animals did not develop symptoms. Protection experiments in these animals were performed by intratracheal infection with either virus strain and then challenged 4 weeks later with the human strain by the same route. Only one of six animals initially infected with the homologous human virus shed virus after challenge. In contrast all six animals with a prior infection with bovine parainfluenza 3 virus excreted virus after challenge. However, there was a marked reduction in the duration of viral shedding and the amount of virus shed compared to that in challenged nonimmunized animals. Evidence was obtained for restriction of replication of the SF-4 bovine strain in chimpanzees and rhesus monkeys. Compared with the human strain there was a 100-fold to 1000-fold reduction in the tracheal content of virus. It is likely that this reflects a property of attenuation for man, but no definite conclusion on this matter can be drawn since no illness is seen in the two monkey species studied. The degree of attenuation of bovine parainfluenza 3 virus in man and its capacity to restrict the heterologous virus replication at different times after immunization deserves further study. Reversing the approach and determining if human parainfluenza 3 virus has any capacity to protect cattle against infection with SF-4 virus may also be warranted.

Also, in the case of RS virus are there human and bovine strains that show distinct immunological cross-reactivity? Although RS viruses, like parainfluenza 3 viruses, are paramyxoviruses, there are some important unique features of its two surface glycoproteins. This difference predominantly concerns the assumed attachment protein. This protein in RS virus is denoted G for glycoprotein and carries no detectable hemagglutinating or neuraminidase activity. It is a protein with a relatively small molecular weight, 33,000 kD, and it is heavily glycosylated not only with N-linked but also, unique to this paramyxovirus, O-linked sugars (Gruber and Levine, 1985; Satake et al., 1985; Wertz et al., 1985). The RS virus attachment protein shows no homology with the corresponding protein of paramyxoviruses. The RS virus F protein shows the same basic size of its cleavage products, but only a very distant homology to the F proteins of other paramyxoviruses (Spriggs *et al.*, 1986). It is important to note that the relative immune protective role of the two glycoproteins is reversed in RS virus compared with other paramyxoviruses. Thus, as evaluated in immune protection studies employing vaccinia vector-transferred RS virus genes in cotton rats, the protection achieved by F component immunization is more pronounced than that given by G component immunization (Olmsted *et al.*, 1986; Stott *et al.*, 1986; Johnson *et al.*, 1987). To complicate the matter further, there are two subgroups of RS virus (Andersson *et al.*, 1985; Mufson *et al.*, 1985). These two subgroups of viruses, A and B, have markedly different G proteins, whereas the F proteins are more closely related. In humans it has been shown that the RS virus subgroup A gives a higher protection against a subgroup A strain infection than against a subgroup B strain infection (Mufson *et al.*, 1987). In the cotton rat model, the immune protection of the G protein is primarily against strains of the same subgroup, whereas the F protein protects against strains of both subgroups. In terms of relationships between bovine and human RS virus strains, the evolutionary difference between G proteins again is larger than between F proteins. Currently this conclusion is based on immunobiological characterization by use of monoclonal antibodies. In a recent comprehensive study (Örvell *et al.*, 1987) employing previously characterized monoclonal antibodies against a strain of subgroup A virus (Mufson *et al.*, 1985) and a new large collection of monoclonal antibodies against a subgroup B virus, it was found that none of the antibodies against the G protein reacted with bovine RS virus but that a considerable fraction of F-specific monoclonal antibodies cross-reacted. In fact all of the latter antibodies which showed neutralizing activity blocked the replication of human strains of both subgroups and bovine strains equally well. Thus, there must be dominating neutralizing epitopes shared between RS viruses in the two species. In view of this, the replicative capacity of bovine RS virus in humans might be evaluated. There already have been attempts to use human RS virus for immunization of cattle. A bovine strain of RS virus and a human strain were adapted to *in vitro* growth in bovine cell culture and then inoculated into gnotobiotic calves (Thomas *et al.*, 1984). The virus strains replicated without causing symptoms, and specific antibody responses were recorded. In further studies (Stott *et al.*, 1984), an inactivated bovine virus vaccine was compared with two candidate live vaccines. These live vaccines were a modified bovine strain and a temperature-sensitive mutant of a human strain. Only the inactivated vaccine gave complete protection, whereas the live immunogens gave an infection-permissive immunity. However, the mean peak titers and the mean duration of shedding were reduced significantly in the live vaccine candidate virus-immunized animals compared to the nonimmunized control animals.

It is possible to combine the classical Jennerian approach with the use of contemporary techniques of viral genetics. Two examples concerning viruses with segmented genomes, influenzavirus and rotavirus, will be given. For many years attempts have been made to develop live influenza A virus vaccine donor strains (Chanock and Murphy, 1980). In this context it was observed that avian influenza virus strains generally replicated poorly in the lower respiratory tract of squirrel monkeys (Murphy et al., 1982) and also in most cases showed a markedly restricted growth in primate cells in culture (Murphy et al., 1985). Departing from this observation, attempts have been made to select a certain avian virus as donor strain for use in reassortment formulations of live influenza A virus to be used in humans. To approach this problem, the relative contribution of the six genes for the internal components of avian influenza viruses to their attenuation for growth in mammalian cells has been evaluated. The individual contribution of each of the six genes for internal components (except PB2) from a selected avian virus, A/Mallard/NY/78, was determined against the background of seven human influenza A virus genes (Tian et al., 1985). This study showed complex relationships. The nucleoprotein (NP) and matrix (M) genes each played a major and independent role in host-range restriction. Also two other genes, PB1 and NS, acting in consort could cause restriction. Further similar studies were performed with another avian virus, A/Pintail/79 (Snyder et al., 1987). The reassortants were evaluated by infection experiments in monkeys. It was found that the NP gene and also certain constellations of avian and human polymerase genes each could cause attenuation. The fact that host-range restriction of avian influenza viruses is polygenic in nature offers promise for establishment of genetically stably reassortants for human use.

Virulent rotaviruses represent the single most important group of agents causing severe diarrhea in infants and young children around the world. To provide protection during the critical period of the first 2 years of life, two vaccines containing viruses of heterologous host origins have been tried. These two vaccines included animal rotaviruses, one of bovine origin (Vesikari et al., 1983) and the other of rhesus monkey origin (Kapikian et al., 1985). It was later on found that the bovine virus showed a too high a degree of attenuation and it has therefore been withdrawn from further studies. In contrast, the rhesus virus has been found to give identifiable symptoms in a certain fraction of vaccinees. These side effects currently are under consideration on the basis that they may be acceptable if an effective immunity against the more virulent human virus is obtained. Recent results from a trial in Venezuela are encouraging (Flores *et al.*, 1987). A prerequisite for these results was that the virus causing the epidemic in Venezuela was rotavirus type 3, since one of the limitations of the live rhesus rotavirus vaccine is that it only gives immunity to this type. There is a need for a multivalent rotavirus vaccine to include all four known human sero- types of the virus. To achieve this, attempts are now being made to select reassortants containing the single human rotavirus gene which codes for the protein primarily involved in immune protection (VP7) of serotypes 1, 2, and 4 against a background of simian rotavirus genes.

IV. Experimentally Produced or Selected Attenuated Virus Variants with Genomic Point Mutations, Deletions, or Insertions

In the absence of any spontaneously occurring nonpathogenic virus variants, the conventional approach to modify the virulence of a virus was to perform repeated passages *in vivo* or *in vitro* in unnatural host cells with a hope for selection of attenuated virus (*cf.* Ada, 1982; Norrby, 1983, 1987). In many cases it was found empirically that this approach yielded attractive live vaccine candidates, but frequently the act of optimizing a position between virulence that was too high and overat- tenuation of the virus was difficult. In more recent studies, this ap- proach was combined with treatment aiming at serial mutagenesis, as exemplified by a study on Rift Valley fever virus (Caplen *et al.*, 1985). However, most modern approaches to development of live vaccines have been more targeted.

Both in the case of influenza A virus and RS virus, extensive attempts have been made to produce satisfactorily attenuated and immunogenic temperature sensitive (ts) mutants. Regrettably, the mutants iden- tified were not found to be useful since they either were overattenuated or showed a genetic instability. More promising results were obtained in studies of a cold-adapted (ca) mutant of influenza A virus (Maassab and DeBorde, 1985). During selection to growth at 25°C, the virus sustained both ts and ca mutations. When the master strain ca influ- enza A/Ann Arbor/6/60 has been used as a donor for the six "internal" genes, it regularly has given reassortants with attenuated properties for susceptible human volunteers. As a means of identifying the rela- tive role of the "internal" genes from ca donor virus, each one of them was introduced against a background of the seven remaining genes from a wild-type human influenza A virus (Snyder *et al.*, 1988). The virulence of the reassortants was evaluated by infection of ferrets and hamsters. It was concluded that four genes independently could contribute to attenuation of the ca reassortant virus. One of these genes is responsible for production of M protein and the other three genes (PB2, PB1, and PA) for components of the polymerase complex. It was inferred that the PA and M genes may restrict virus replication in both the upper and lower respiratory tract of man, whereas the genes PB2 and PB1 primarily may affect attenuation for the lower respiratory tract. To understand the molecular basis for attenuation of influenza the nucleotide sequence of the six RNA segments coding for "internal" proteins was determined in the abovementioned ca virus strain and its parental wild type (Cox *et al.*, 1988). A total of 22 nucleotide changes resulting in 11 amino acid substitutions were found. This represents a 0.2% variation in nucleotide sequences for the viruses. The biologically most significant alterations were interpreted to be (1) an alanine to serine change in M2 (there were no changes in the dominant M protein deriving from the same RNA segment), (2) a leucin to proline change in PA, (3) an asparagine to serine change in PB2, and finally (4) one or more of different changes seen in PB1. In the future it may be possible to define more precisely the contribution of each of the mutations observed by sequencing revertants, by using functional assays of expressed proteins altered at only site or by using mutant rescue in expression systems having influenza genes altered in a single position.

The available genetic data relating both to ca attenuated virus and avian–human influenza A virus ressortants discussed above clearly reveal that several mutations in various genes may contribute independently to attenuation. Therefore, it should be feasible to generate genetically stable candidate vaccine strains based on the requirement for multiple reversions before virulence is restored.

Also studies with animal influenza viruses have shown that properties of virulence can be determined by several different genes. Thus, for example, the exchange of different single genes in a fowl plague influenza A virus for homologous genes of different species origin—human, equine, swine—could reduce pathogenicity of the virus (Scholtissek *et al.*, 1977). In the case of equine influenza A virus, attempts have been made to generate an attenuated virus by reassortment between a human influenza ts donor virus and a virulent equine influenza virus (Brundage-Auguish *et al.*, 1982). It should be pointed out that unlike human influenza A virus only two subtypes of equine influenza viruses have been identified, and these subtypes do not show any significant antigenic drift. This situation implies favorable conditions for establishing a long-time protection by immunization of young horses. In the above-mentioned study two ts reassortants of an equine influenza virus, subtype A1, were produced by mating a human influenza ts donor virus with an equine influenza A/Cornell/16/74 wild-type virus and by isolation of ts reassortant viruses possessing hemagglutinin and neuraminidase from the equine virus. The human ts donor virus was prepared for the purpose and had ts mutations in both one of the polymerase genes (P3) and in the nucleoprotein gene. One of the reassortant virus clones had retained six of the eight equine virus genes and was ts for the P3 gene, whereas the other reassortant had retained three genes and was ts for both P3 and NP. The growth of both clones was restricted in the lungs of hamsters, but in the nasal turbinates the growth equaled that of the virulent virus.

It would appear that the use of constructs with disrupted function of individual genes by deletion or by insertion of foreign genetic material might provide more readily for genetically stable attenuated viruses. Such deletion mutants can be constructed in DNA viruses, retroviruses, and positive-strand RNA viruses. There are several examples of attenuation of DNA viruses by this approach. Vaccinia virus is frequently used by vectorologists, and the insertion of heterologous genes most often is made into the thymidine kinase gene, which thereby loses its function. As a consequence the virulence of the virus is reduced (Buller et al., 1985; cf. chapter by Murphy and Esposito). Recently (Flexner et al., 1987; Ramshaw et al., 1987), the impact of vaccinia virus replication as determined in the sensitive host system represented by nude mice was reduced further by insertion of the gene for the T-cell interleukin 2 growth factor (IL-2) into the vector. The production of IL-2 allowed survival of these highly susceptible animals. The concept of engineering genes for factors amplifying different arms of the immune system into candidate live virus vaccines may have a broader application.

Thymidine kinase-negative (TK⁻) deletion mutants have been prepared with herpesviruses, and also in this case resulted in a reduced virulence. The herpesvirus pseudorabies virus (PRV) causes a severe disease in pigs. Attenuation of the virus was achieved by making a TK⁻ deletion mutant. This construct was the first genetically engineered modified live-virus vaccine brought from the laboratory to the marketplace. Approval for use in the United States was given in January 1986. Prior to this license it was demonstrated that the new vaccine was safer to the environment and to animals than wild virus or virus in conventional live vaccines (Kit et al., 1985). One problem in the use of this new PRV vaccine has been the lack of markers to distinguish vaccinated pigs from those infected with pathogenic field strains. U.S. federal and state regulatory agencies have considered all vaccinated pigs to be potential carriers of PRV and discouraged movements of these pigs under most circumstances. To overcome this problem a second deletion was engineered in a DNA fragment encoding the major envelope protein, gIII (Kit *et al.*, 1987), which is one of four different glycoproteins in PRV. It was subsequently found that the prototype strain chosen for preparation of the genetically engineered live vaccine also had a deletion in the glycoprotein gI gene. In spite of the occurrence of deletions in three of the vaccine virus genes, it replicated to high titers in cell cultures. Antibodies to glycoprotein gIII were not present in vaccinated pigs but could be identified in pigs infected with wild virus. This observation can be used to discriminate between a vaccine virus and wild virus infection in animals.

The findings that not only protein gIII is nonessential, but that in addition the virus can dispense with both glycoprotein gI (Mettenleiter *et al.*, 1985) and a highly sulfated glycoprotein gX (Rea *et al.*, 1985) without impairment of virus replication are both interesting and surprising. It should be noted that there are analogous nonessential glycoproteins in herpes simples virus (HSV) type 1. Glycoprotein gC, which acts as a C3b receptor, and gE, which acts as an IgG Fc receptor, can be deleted without destruction of the virus replicative capacity. These apparent pardoxical observations may be resolved by the following heuristic hypotheses. Viral thymidine kinase and glycoproteins may be of importance for persistent and/or cytolytic herpesvirus infections of macrophages and nerve cells. The glycoproteins inserted into membranes of infected cells serving potentially as decoys could cause perturbance of membrane structure and function and contribute to virus spread. If this assumption is correct, deletion of glycoproteins would lead to reduced immunopathology, hypersensitivity reactions, and immunosuppression. From the vaccine point of view it is important that the advantages gained by these losses probably will outweigh the benefit the host otherwise would derive from their role as target antigens.

Genetic engineering has also been used to obtain prototype live attenuated strains of HSV. The aim in using such a vaccine is to attenuate a virus so that it can not establish latency by itself, but it can still retain a replicative capacity to give a local immunity prohibiting infection with wild virus at the portal of entry and its subsequent colonization of ganglia. Available technology (*cf.* Roizman and Jenkins, 1985) allowing both introduction of deletions, transplantation of genetic material within a genome, and insertion of heterologous genetic material was employed for generation of these constructs (Meigner *et al.*, 1987). Two different constructs were prepared. Both had a 700-bp deletion in the coding sequences of the TK gene and in addition an approximately 13-kbp deletion encompassing genetic material between the $\alpha 27$ gene and the promoter-regulatory domain of the $\alpha 4$ gene. The latter of the two deleted sequences includes most of the internal inverted repeat sequences, and as a consequence the genome is not inverted, but instead frozen in the prototype orientation. In addition a DNA fragment derived from HSV type 2 encoding the genes specifying glycoproteins G and D was inserted into the construct at the place of the larger deletion. The only difference between the two constructs was that in one of them the TK gene was reinserted under the control of the $\alpha 4$ gene promotor. There were several rationales for the design of the two constructs, but in essence the aim was to reduce neurotropism and virulence and to provide immunity covering both types of HSV. There were no revertants of virus when the vaccine candidate strains replicated in different species. They were attenuated for rodents and owl monkeys. Somewhat unexpectedly, it was found that not only the TK^+ construct but also occasionally the TK^- construct could give a latent infection in regional sympathic ganglia. Protection against intracerebral infection of mice was observed, in particular with the TK^+ construct which allowed a better replication of virus. Protection studies were performed subsequently with genital herpes in guinea pigs, with herpetic-ocular disease in rabbits, and with generalized disease in owl monkeys (Meigner *et al.*, 1988). The two vaccine candidate constructs prevented severe or fatal disease in all three species, but had the limitation that they did not preclude replication of challenge virus. Further, only in rodent models was it possible to prevent the establishment of a latent virus infection. In contrast some owl monkeys showed recurrent symptomatic episodes caused by persistent challenge virus. It would appear that it may be difficult to generate a strain of HSV that fulfils the two requirements of giving a self-limiting, symptomless mucosal infection and concomitantly induces a long-lasting local immunity.

The fact that picornaviruses can be obtained in a complementary DNA form, which sometimes is infectious by itself as first shown with poliovirus (Racaniello and Baltimore, 1981) or after transcription into RNA, has opened up possibilities for restructuring these RNA plus-strand viruses. Both chimeric viruses (to be discussed in the next section and deletion mutants can be established. Spontaneously occurring deletion mutants have not been encountered, but multiple point mutations occur. Recently, viable deletion mutants of the Sabin strain of type 1 poliovirus were constructed (Kuge and Nomoto, 1987). Selected nucleotide sequences in the 5′ noncoding region of the genome were removed, and two different constructs were made. One of these PV1(Sab)IC-DA21 lacked the genome region of nucleotide positions 564–726, whereas the other, PV1(Sab)IC-DH, had a somewhat smaller deletion, positions 600–726. The former construct gave a reduced plaque size by comparison with the parental virus and the other construct. It is of interest to note that the additionally deleted region in strain PV1(Sab)IC-DA21 includes one part, nucleotides 564–577, which has a high uridine content in all picornaviruses studied and a region of 8 base positions (583–590) that is conserved identically in picornaviruses. Either one of these sequences may serve as a signal to enhance virus replication. The small-plaque mutant was found to have a further reduced neurovirulence compared to the parent Sabin type 1 virus. To establish if deletion of the selected area had a generalized diminishing impact on neurovirulence, the corresponding deletion was introduced into the neurovirulent Mahoney virus of type 1 polio (Nomoto *et al.*, 1988b). Again a marked reduction in neurovirulence was seen, but the residing neurovirulence of the Mahoney deletion mutant virus was in excess of that of the attenuated Sabin type 1 virus.

Unfortunately there are limitations in evaluating the use of deletion mutants in negative-strand or double-strand RNA viruses due to the absence of genetic techniques to engineer such changes. However, a spontaneously occurring viable mutant of influenza A virus, which had an in-frame 36-bp deletion about 30% into the NSI protein coding region of the eighth gene, has been identified (Buonagurio *et al.*, 1984). A reassortant virus bearing this mutant NS gene against a background of seven wild-type influenza A virus genes has been isolated (Chanock *et al.*, 1988). In this new context the mutant gene was still capable of specifying temperature specificity. Unexpectedly, it was found that infected hamsters and chimpanzees shed virus which had lost its temperature sensitivity. The revertants still possessed the truncated NS gene, but apparently compensatory alterations in the same or other genes restored temperature stability in the virus. Evidently a single deletion may not necessarily provide a stable attenuation for a candidate live virus strain. Still, segmental genomic changes should offer attractive approaches to stabilizing attenuated properties of viruses. This can be obtained by introduction of cassette genomic alterations in viruses, a technique which has yielded promising results with picornaviruses. This will be the topic of the next section of this review.

V. Attenuation by Formation of Chimeric Constructs of Different Types or Strains of Picornaviruses

Although the use of live poliovaccines has given highly successful results, the inherent problem of a low frequency of vaccine-induced or vaccine-associated cases of paralytic poliomyelitis remains with the currently used vaccine, especially with Sabin types 2 and 3 virus strains. Because of the readiness with which genomic nucleotide sequences of picornaviruses can now be derived, extensive comparisons have been made of a large number of poliovirus strains with both virulent and attenuated properties. In studies of poliovirus type 3 (Stanway *et al.*, 1984), a comparison was made of P3/Leon/37, the neurovirulent parent of the Sabin vaccine, P3/Leon/12ab, the vaccine itself, and P3/119, a virus isolate from a fatal case of vaccine-associated poliomyelitis. Attenuation of virus correlated with 10 point mutations, but only 3 of these resulted in amino acid substitutions. In the revertant neurovirulent virus, 8 out of the 10 point mutations remained, demonstrating the genealogical interlinkage between the strains (Cann *et al.*, 1984). The revertant differed from the vaccine strain by point mutations at 7 positions, with 3 resulting in amino acid substitutions. Interestingly, none of these changes represented back-mutations of the amino acid substitutions seen in the vaccine strains, and their role for reversion to neurovirulence hence appears less crucial. The only back-mutation encountered occurred in a noncoding region, position 472. This particular region, however, is highly conserved between different serotypes of poliovirus, emphasizing that it may have a critical function in the replicative cycle of the virus. Further studies have supported the observation that mutational changes at position 472 correlate to neurovirulence (Evans *et al.*, 1985). When consecutive virus isolates were made from a child who had received live polio vaccine, it was found that a mutation in position 472 had occurred already within 3 days after administration of the vaccine (Minor *et al.*, 1986). Confirmatory results were obtained in a separate study (Weeks-Levy *et al.*, 1988).

The results obtained by comparison of neurovirulent and attenuated strains of poliovirus type 1 differed markedly from those observed in the above-cited studies of poliovirus type 3 (Nomoto *et al.*, 1982). A total of 55 nucleotide substitutions scattered over the entire length of the genome were seen in a comparison of the Sabin vaccine strain P1/LSc, 2ab and its neurovirulent precursor P1/Mahoney virus strain. Twenty-one of these changes resulted in amino acid replacements. Although the predicted amino acid sequences of poliovirus types 1 and 3 show about 90% homology (Toyoda *et al.*, 1984), none of the mutations observed in the type 3 vaccine strain had an obvious counterpart in the type 1 vaccine strain. However, further studies have emphasized that some analogies can be drawn between the mechanism of attenuation in the two types.

To identify the role of different regions of poliovirus type 1 for neurovirulence, a number of recombinant viruses were constructed (Kohara *et al.*, 1985; Omata *et al.*, 1986; Nomoto *et al.*, 1988b). These *in vitro* recombinants were evaluated for their neurovirulence by intracerebral injection into *Cynomolgus* monkeys. It was found that the loci influencing attenuation of the neurovirulent phenotype were spread over wide areas of the genome, but that there were particularly strong determinants influencing neurovirulence in the 5' noncoding region. Further dissection of this region by generation of additional recombinants emphasized the occurrence of strong determinants for neurovirulence in this regon, with particular emphasis on alterations in nucleotide position 480, which has been deduced to be equivalent to position 472 in type 3.

Additional recent data emphasize the role of the 5' noncoding region for neurovirulence of polioviruses. Sequences required for the mouse neurovirulence displayed by the poliovirus type 2 Lansing strain were characterized by use of intratypic recombinants between this virus and Mahoney type 1 virus (LaMonica *et al.*, 1986). It was concluded that in the Lansing strain the capsid region was of dominating importance for neurovirulence in mice. Since most likely the capsid region determines the capacity of the Lansing virus to infect rodent cells, an obligatory dependence on these gene products is to be anticipated in any virus strain expected to display biological activities in these cells. In an attempt to develop a mouse model for neurovirulence potentially useful for control of the human vaccines, it was examined whether position 472, which contains the crucial nucleotide in determining type 3 neurovirulence in humans, also influenced neurovirulence in mice (LaMonica *et al.*, 1987). for this purpose chimeric viruses were constructed to contain the structural protein coding region which confers the mouse-adapted phenotype and the 5' noncoding region of either the type 3 vaccine virus or its neurovirulent progenitor as well as the revertant mentioned above. It was shown that a cytosine in position 472 allowed expression of the neurovirulent phenotype in mice, but that similar to the situation in humans a uracil in this position suppressed this phenotype. It is possible therefore that neurovirulence of Lansing poliovirus derivatives in mice can be exploited as a useful indicator of the genetic stability of new attenuated mutations created by site-directed mutagenesis.

As a means of improving the genetic stability of the Sabin types 2 and 3 vaccine strains, two alternative strategies offer themselves. One is to use the Sabin type 1 strain as a vector for types 2 and 3 antigenic components, viz., to make a cassette exchange of the genome section (in total or in fragmental representation) coding for structural proteins. It could be considered to produce particles with dual serotype specificity similar to the constructs of HSV discussed above. The other alternative is to perform site-directed mutagenesis in the 5′ noncoding region. The first approach has already been taken (Nomoto et al., 1988a). The appropriate chimeric constructs were made and it was confirmed that they were recognized and neutralized by antibodies against the heterologous type 2 or 3 capsid protein region in the type 1 genome. The viral constructs appeared stable during serial passages. Monkey neurovirulence tests were performed by intraspinal injection of the chimeric virus strains. The neurovirulence score was lower than with the homologous Sabin types 2 and 3 strains. It now remains to evaluate the capacity of these constructs to infect the human intestinal tract and to determine the possible changes of neurovirulence ensuing from this replication.

Chimeric viruses have also been produced to determine the genomic correlate of attenuation in another picornavirus, hepatitis A virus (Cohen et al., 1988). Difficulties have been encountered in attempts to produce a live hepatitis A virus that is sufficiently attenuated in humans and still can induce protective immunity (Provost et al., 1986). To study this problem in more detail the complete nucleotide sequence of both a wild-type virus and its derivative attenuated candidate vaccine variant were determined (Cohen et al., 1987). There were 24 nucleotide changes in the attenuated variant and 12 of these resulted in amino acid substitutions. These changes occurred along the whole genome. To evaluate their relative role in attenuation, chimeras between the two virus strains were prepared. The virus genome was divided into three regions: (1) the 5′ noncoding region, (2) the region encoding capsid proteins, and (3) the remainder of the genome. These constructs were transfected into mammalian cells and the virus produced was inoculated intravenously into marmosets. In contrast to the results obtained with poliovirus (Omata et al., 1986) which showed that the 5′ noncoding region had a dominating importance for neurovirulence, it was concluded that the virulence of hepatitis A virus depends both on the 5′ and 3′ parts of its genome. The part of the genome determining the capsid proteins may play a relatively lesser role. The generation of further chimeras of hepatitis A virus may help in identifying an appropriately attenuated virus strain. The recent identification of more effectively growing cytopathic hepatitis A virus–cell systems (Andersson, 1987; Cromeans *et al.*, 1987) may help in these endeavors.

VI. Epilogue

There are no easy victories in the field of vaccine development and application. Still the prospects are bright for successful active immunoprophylaxis of many infections because of the impressive array of genetic engineering techniques as well as immunochemical methods that have become available in the last decade. Immunoprotective epitopes can now be identified with a remarkable precision. Viral genomes can be modified extensively, allowing a controlled reduction of virus virulence. In particular, casette genetic interstrain or intertypic rearrangements offer promising approaches in the evolution of new live vaccines. Hopefully, this kind of vaccine can come into use eventually to prevent, for example, local respiratory and enteric infections, which represent the dominating disease burden in both animals and humans.

References

Ada, G. L. (1982). *Aust. J. Exp. Biol. Med.* **60**, 549–569.

Adams, J. M., Imagawa, D. T., Wright, S. W., and Tarjan, G. (1959). *Virology* **7**, 351–353.

Andersson, D. A. (1987). *J. Med. Virol.* **22**, 35–44.

Andersson, L. J., Hierholzer, J. C., Tsou, C., Hendry, R. M., Fernie, B. F., Stone, Y., and McIntosch, K. (1985). *J. Infect. Dis.* **151, 626–633**

Appel, M. J. G., Shek, W. R., Sheshberadaran, H., and Norrby, E. (1984). *Arch. Virol.* **82**, 73–82.

Barrett, T., Clarke, D. K., Evans, S. A., and Rima, B. K. (1987). *Virus Res.* **8**, 373–386.

Brundage-Auguish, L. J., Holmes, D. F., Hosier, N. T., Murphy, B. R., Massicott, J. G., Appleyard, G., and Coggins, L. (1982). *Am. J. Vet. Res.* **43**, 869–874.

Buller, R. M., Smith, G. L., Cremer, K., Notkins, A. L., and Moss, B. (1985). *Nature (London)* **317**, 813–815.

Buonagurio, D. A., Krystel, M., Palese, P., DeBorde, D. C., and Maassab, H. F. (1984). *J. Virol.* **49**, 418–425.

Cann, A. J., Stanway, G., Hughes, P. J., Minor, P. D., Evans, D. M. A., Schild, G. C., and Almond, J. W. (1984). *Nucleic Acids Res.* **12**, 7787–7792.

Caplen, H., Peters, C. J., and Bishop, D. H. L. (1985). *J. Gen. Virol.* **66**, 2271–2277.

Chanock, R. M. (1981). *J. Infect. Dis.* **143**, 364–373.

Chanock, R. M., and Murphy, B. R. (1980). *Rev. Infect. Dis.* **2**, 421–432.

Chanock, R. M., Murphy, B. R., Collins, P. L., Coelingh, K. V. W., Olmsted, R. A., Snyder, M. H., Spriggs, M. K., Prince, G. A., Moss, B., Flores, J., Gorziglia, M., and Kapikian, A. Z. (1988). *Vaccine*, **6**, 129–133.

Coelingh, K. L. W., Winter, C. C., and Murphy, B. R. (1985). *Virology* **143**, 569–582.

Coelingh, K. L. W., Winter, C. C., Murphy, B. R., Rice, J. M., Kimball, P. C., Olmstead, R. A., and Collins, P. L. (1986). *J. Virol.* **60**, 90–96.

Coelingh, K. L. W., Winter, C. C., and Murphy, B. R. (1987). *In* "Vaccines '87: Modern Approaches to New Vaccines" (R. M. Chanock, R. A. Lerner, F. Brown, and H. Ginsberg, eds.), pp. 296–301. Cold Spring Harbor Lab., Cold Spring Harbor, New York.

Coelingh, K. L. W., Battey, J., Lebacq-Verheyden, A. L., Collins, P. L., and Murphy, B. R. (1988). *In* "Vaccines '88: Modern Approaches to New Vaccines" (R. M. Chanock, R. A. Lerner, F. Brown, and H. Ginsberg, eds.), pp. 171–177. Cold Spring Harbor Lab., Cold Spring Harbor, New York.

Cohen, J. I., Rosenblum, B., Ticehurst, R. J., Daemer, R. J., Feinstone, S. M., and Purcell, R. H. (1987). *Proc. Natl. Acad. Sci. U.S.A.* **84,** 2497–2501.

Cohen, J. I., Rosenblum, B., Feinstone, S., Ticehurst, J. R., and Purcell, R. H. (1988). *In* "Vaccines '88: Modern Approaches to New Vaccines" (R. M. Chanock, R. A. Lerner, F. Brown, and H. Ginsberg, eds.), pp. 133–137. Cold Spring Harbor Lab., Cold Spring Harbor, New York.

Coulon, P., Rollin, P., Aubert, M., and Flamand, A. (1982). *J. Gen. Virol.* **61,** 97–100.

Cox, N. J., Kitame, F., and Kendal, A. P. (1988). *In* "Vaccines '88: Modern Approaches to New Vaccines" (R. M. Chanock, R. A. Lerner, F. Brown, and H. Ginsberg, eds.), pp. 139–143. Cold Spring Harbor Lab., Cold Spring Harbor, New York.

Cromeans, T., Sobsey, M. D., and Fields, H. A. (1987). *J. Med. Virol.* **22,** 45–56.

Dalziel, R., Lampert, P., Talbot, P., and Buchmeier, M. (1986). *J. Virol.* **59,** 463–471.

Evans, D. M. A., Dunn, G., Minor, P. D., Schild, G. C., Cann, A. J., Stanway, G., Almond, J. W., Currey, K., and Maizel J. V., Jr. (1985). *Nature (London)* **314,** 548–550.

Fleming, J., Trousdale, M., El-Zaatari, F., Stohlman, S., and Weiner, L. (1986). *J. Virol.* **58,** 869–875.

Flexner, C., Hügin, A., and Moss, B. (1987). *Nature (London)* **330,** 259–262.

Flores, J., Midthun, K., Hoshino, Y., Green, K., Gorziglia, M., Kapikian, A. Z., and Chanock, R. M. (1986). *J. Virol.* **60,** 972–979.

Flores, J., Perez-Schael, I., Gonzales, M., Garcia, D., Perez, M., Daond, N., Cunto, W., Chanock, R. M., and Kapikian, A. Z. (1987). *Lancet* **1,** 882–884.

Fraser, K. B., and Martin, S. J. (1978). *In* "Experimental Virology" (T. W. Tinsley and F. Brown, eds.), pp. 1–249. Academic Press, New York.

Gorziglia, M., Hoshino, Y., Buckler-White, A., Blumentals, I., Glass, R., Flores, J., Kapikian, A. Z., and Chanock, R. M. (1986). *Proc. Natl. Acad. Sci. U.S.A.* **83,** 7039–7043.

Gruber, C., and Levine, S. (1985). *J. Gen. Virol.* **64,** 417–432.

Johnson, P. R., Olmsted, R. A., Prince, G. A., Murphy, B. R., Alling, D. W., Walsh, E. E., and Collins, P. L. (1987). *J. Virol.* **61,** 3163–3166.

Kapikian, A. Z., Midthun, K., Hoshino, Y., Flores, J., Wyatt, R. G., Glass, R. J., Ashaa, J., Nakagomi, O., Nakagomi, T., and Chanock, R. M. (1985). *In* "Vaccines '85: Modern Approaches to New Vaccines" (R. A. Lerner, R. M. Chanock, and F. Brown, eds.). pp. 357–366. Cold Spring Harbor Lab., Cold Spring Harbor, New York.

Kilbourne, E. D. (1976). *J. Infect. Dis.* **134,** 395–400.

Kit, S., Kit, M., and Pirtle, E. C. (1985). *Am. J. Vet. Res.* **46,** 1359–1367.

Kit, S., Sheppard, M., Ichimura, H., and Kit, M. (1987). *Am. J. Vet. Res.* **48,** 780–793.

Kohara, M., Omata, T., Kameda, A., Semler, B. L., Itoh, H., Wimmer, E., and Nomoto, A. (1985). *J. Virol.* **53,** 786–792.

Kuge, S., and Nomoto, A. (1987). *J. Virol.* **61,** 1478–1487.

LaMonica, N., Moriam, C., and Racaniello, V. R. (1986). *J. Virol.* **57,** 515–525.

LaMonica, N., Almond, J. W., and Racaniello, V. R. (1987). *J. Virol.* **61,** 2917–2920.

Löve, A., Rydbeck, R., Kristensson, K., Örvell, C., and Norrby, E. (1985). *J. Virol.* **53,** 67–74.

Maasab, H. F., and DeBorde, D. C. (1985). *Vaccine* **3,** 355–369.

Meigner, B., Longnecker, R., and Roizman, B. (1987). *In* "Vaccines '87: Modern Approaches to New Vaccines" (R. M. Chanock, R. A. Lerner, F. Brown, and H. Ginsberg, eds.). pp. 368–373. Cold Spring Harbor Lab., Cold Spring Harbor, New York.

Meigner, B., Longnecker, R., and Roizman, B. (1988). *In* "Vaccines '88: Modern Approaches to New Vaccines" (R. M. Chanock, R. A. Lerner, F. Brown, and H. Ginsberg, eds.). pp. 193–196. Cold Spring Harbor Lab., Cold Spring Harbor, New York (in press).

Mettenleiter, T. C., Lukacs, N., and Rzika, H.-J. (1985). *J. Virol.* **56,** 307–311.

Minor, P. D., John, A., Ferguson, M., and Icenogle, J. P. (1986). *J. Gen. Virol.* **67,** 693–706.

Mufson, M. A., Örvell, C., Rafner, B., and Norrby, E. (1985). *J. Gen. Virol.* **66,** 2111–2124.

Mufson, M. A., Belshe, R. B., Örvell, C., and Norrby, E. (1987). *J. Clin. Microbiol.* **25,** 1535–1539.

Murphy, B. R., Hinshaw, V. S., Sly, D. L., London, W. T., Hosier, N. T., Wood, F. T., Webster, R. G., and Chanock, R. M. (1982). *Infect. Immun.* **37,** 1119–1126.

Murphy, B. R., Clements, M. L., Tierney, E. L., Black, R. E., Steinberg, J., and Chanock, R. M. (1985). *J. Infect. Dis.* **152,** 225–229.

Nomoto, A., Omata, T., Toyoda, H., Kuge, S., Horie, H., Kataoka, Y., Genba, Y., Nakano, Y., and Imura, N. (1982). *Proc. Natl. Acad. Sci. U.S.A.* **79,** 5793–5797.

Nomoto, A., Kohara, M., Kuge, S., Abe, S., Semder, B. L., Komatsu, T., Arita, M., and Itoh, H. (1988a). *In* "Applied Virology Research" (E. Kurstak, R. G. Marusyk, F. H. Murphy, and m. H. V. van Regenmortel, eds.), p. 43–54, Vol. 1. Plenum, New York.

Nomoto, A., Iizuka, N., Kohara, M., and Arita, M. (1988b). *Vaccine,* **6,** 134–137.

Norrby, E. (1983). *Arch. Virol.* **76,** 163–177.

Norrby, E. (1987). *Adv. Virus Res.* **32,** 1–34.

Norrby, E., Sheshberadaran, H., McCullough, K. C., Carpenter, W. C., and Örvell, C. (1985). *Intervirology* **23,** 228–232.

Olmsted, R. A., Elango, N., Prince, G. A., Murphy, B. R., Johnson, P. R., Moss, B., Chanock, R. M., and Collins, P. L. (1986). *Proc. Natl. Acad. Sci. U.S.A.* **83,** 7462–7466.

Omata, T., Kohara, M., Kuge, S., Komatzu, T., Abe, S., Semler, B., Kameda, A., Itoh, H., Arita, M., Wimmer, E., and Nomoto, A. (1986). *J. Virol.* **58,** 348–358.

Örvell, C., Norrby, E., and Mufson, M. A. (1987). *J. Gen. Virol.* **68,** 3125–3135.

Plowright, W. (1962). *Ann. N.Y. Acad. Sci.* **101,** 548–563.

Provost, P. J., Bishop, R. P., Gerety, R. J., Hilleman, M. R., McAleer, W. J., Scolnick, E. M., and Stevens, C. E. (1986). *J. Med. Virol.* **20,** 165–175.

Racaniello, V. R., and Baltimore, D. (1981). *Proc. Natl. Acad. Sci. U.S.A.* **78,** 4887–4891.

Ramshaw, J. A., Andrew, M. E., Phillips, S. M., Boyle, D. B., and Compar, B. E. H. (1987). *Nature (London)* **329,** 545–546.

Rea, T. J., Timmins, J. G., Long, G. W., and Post, L. E. (1985). *J. Virol.* **54,** 21–29.

Roizman, B., and Jenkins, F. (1985). *Science* **229,** 1208–1214.

Rydbeck, R., Örvell, C., Löve, A., and Norrby, E. (1986). *J. Gen. Virol.* **67,** 1531–1542.

Rydbeck, R., Löve, A., and Norrby, E. (1988). *J. Gen. Virol.* (in press).

Sabin, A. B. (1957). *JAMA, J. Am. Med. Assoc.* **164,** 1216–1223.

Satake, M., Coligan, J. E., Elango, N., Norrby, E., and Venkatesan, S. (1985). *Nucleic Acids Res.* **13,** 7795–7812.

Scholtissek, L., Rott, R., Orlich, M., Harms, E., and Rohde, W. (1977). *Virology* **81,** 74–80.

Sheshberadaran, H., Norrby, E., McCullough, K. C., Carpenter, W. C., and Örvell, C. (1986). *J. Gen. Virol.* **67,** 1381–1392.

Snyder, M. H., Buckler-White, A. J., London, W. T., Tierney, E. L., and Murphy, B. R. (1987). *J. Virol.* **61,** 2857–2863.

Snyder, M. H., Betts, R. F., Clements, M. L., Herrington, D., Sears, S. D., Maassab, H. F., and Murphy, B. R. (1988). *In* "Vaccines '88: Modern Approaches to New Vaccines"

(R. M. Chanock, R. A. Lerner, F. Brown, and H. Ginsberg, eds.), pp. 145–149. Cold Spring Harbor Lab., Cold Spring Harbor, New York.

Spriggs, D. R., Bronson, R. T., and Fields, B. N. (1983). *Science* **220**, 505–507.

Spriggs, M. K., Olmsted, R. A., Venkatesan, S., Coligan, J. E., and Collins, P. L. (1986). *Virology* **52**, 241–251.

Spriggs, M. K., Murphy, B. R., Prince, G. A., Olmsted, R. A., and Collins, P. (1987). *J. Virol.* **61**, 3416–3423.

Stanway, G., Hughes, P. J., Mountford, R. C., Reeve, P., Minor, P. D., Schild, G. C., and Almond, J. W. (1984). *Proc. Natl. Acad. Sci. U.S.A.* **81**, 1539–1543.

Steinhauer, D. A., and Holland, J. J. (1987). *Annu. Rev. Microbiol.* **41**, 409–433.

Stott, E. J., Thomas, L. H., Taylor, G., Collins, A. P., Jebbett, J., and Crouch, S. (1984). *J. Hyg.* **93**, 251–261.

Stott, E. J., Bell, L. A., Young, K. K., Furze, J., and Wertz, G. W. (1986). *J. Virol.* **60**, 607–613.

Suzu, S., Sakai, Y., Shioda, T., and Shibuta, H. (1987). *Nucleic Acids Res.* **15**, 2945–2958.

Takafuji, E. T., Gaydos, J. C., Allen, R. G., and Top, F. H., Jr. (1979). *J. Infect. Dis.* **140**, 48–53.

Thomas, L. H., Stott, E. J., Collins, A. P., Crouch, S., and Jebbett, J. (1984). *Arch. Virol.* **79**, 67–77.

Tian, S.-F., Buckler-White, A. J., London, W. T., Reck, L. J., Chanock, R. M., and Murphy, B. R. (1985). *J. Virol.* **53**, 771–775.

Toyoda, H., Kohara, M., Kataoka, W., Suganuma, T., Omata, T., Imura, N., and Nomoto, A. (1984). *J. Mol. Biol.* **174**, 916–925.

Vesikari, T., Isolauri, E., Delem, A., Dhondt, E., Andre, F. E., and Zissis, G. (1983). *Lancet* **1**, 807–811.

Wadell, G., Hammarskjöld, M.-L., Winberg, G., Varsanyi, T. M., and Sundell, G. (1980). *Ann. N.Y. Acad. Sci.* **354**, 16–42.

Weeks-Levy, C., Mento, S. J., Detjen, B. M., and Cano, F. R. (1988). *In* "Vaccines '88: Modern Approaches to New Vaccines" (R. M. Chanock, R. A. Lerner, F. Brown, and H. Ginsberg, eds.), pp. 223–227. Cold Spring Harbor Lab., Cold Spring Harbor, New York.

Wertz, G. W., Collins, P. L., Huang, Y., Gruber, C., Levine, S., and Ball, L. A. (1985). *Proc. Natl. Acad. Sci. U.S.A.* **82**, 4075–4079.

ADVANCES IN VETERINARY SCIENCE AND COMPARATIVE MEDICINE, VOL. 33

Live Bacterial Vaccines and Their Application as Carriers for Foreign Antigens

GORDON DOUGAN,* LAURIE SMITH,[†]
AND FRED HEFFRON[†]

* Wellcome Biotechnology Limited Beckenham, Kent, England
[†] Department of Molecular Biology, Research Institute of Scripps Clinic,
La Jolla, California

I. Introduction

This review discusses how bacterial genetics and recombinant DNA techniques are being combined to develop new attenuated bacterial vaccine strains and, in turn, how these vaccine strains are being used to

271

construct multivalent vaccines that express genes for protective antigens. We will focus on attenuated vaccines for the facultative intracellular pathogens, *Salmonella typhimurium, S. typhi,* and *Mycobacterium
tuberculosis,* because they show particular promise for the construction
of multivalent vaccines. We will also include the current status of live
vaccines for pathogenic *Brucella, Shigella,* and *Vibrio cholerae.*

In this antibiotic era why should anyone attempt to develop new
bacterial vaccines? There are several answers to that question. First,
vaccines are needed even with available antibiotics because antibiotic
treatment of many bacterial infections cannot prevent serious sequelae
(e.g., tetanus). Antibiotics are not readily available in many Third
World countries where vaccination programs have been sponsored by
the World Health Organization (WHO). Furthermore, from the patient's standpoint, vaccination is much more cost-effective and less
time-consuming than continued treatment with expensive drugs; good
vaccines can provide lifelong immunity. Additionally, the evolution of
multiply drug-resistant bacteria has reduced the effectiveness of many
antibiotics. Antibiotic-resistant strains of *Neisseria gonorrhoeae* and
Shigella spp. can be difficult to treat, and many nosocomial bacterial
infections require treatment with novel antibiotics that are very deleterious to the patient. Perhaps the most important impact living
vaccines will have in the future is as carriers for protective antigens
from other pathogens. This approach depends on construction of "ideal"
vaccine strains that not only confer solid immunity to themselves but
also to foreign antigens that they express.

What is the ideal vaccine? An effective vaccine must stimulate a
protective immune response, antibody or cell-mediated, against the
appropriate antigens at the site of infection or microbial replication. It
must protect against infection by organisms following the normal route
of infection. For example, an effective *Salmonella* vaccine must protect
against oral inoculation although it need not be given orally. Furthermore, the ideal vaccine is one that provides complete protection for the
lifetime of the animal to the largest realistic challenge dose of the most
virulent strains. There are no ideal vaccines yet, although by using
modern genetics there is now a much better understanding of what
types of *Salmonella* mutations should be considered for inclusion as
attenuated vaccines as discussed below.

Traditionally, bacterial vaccines have been either inactivated toxins
such as tetanus toxoid and diptheria toxoid or killed whole-cell vaccines
such as the pertussis vaccine. These vaccines have proved highly effective in protecting against the respective diseases. However, for many
bacterial pathogens, killed preparations, be they toxoids, lipopolysac-

charide (LPS) fractions, or bacterial cells, provide only short-term immunity and low efficacy. In general, host resistance to facultative intracellular pathogens requires a cellular immune response, and to be effective a vaccine against these pathogens must confer cellular immunity (reviewed in Collins, 1974). Facultative intracellular pathogens cause insidious diseases that are frequently not self-limiting, such as leprosy, tuberculosis, and undulant fever. Why a living vaccine works so well and elicits cellular immunity is not yet understood. High cellular immunity requires that living organisms persist in particular tissues of the host; subunit vaccines do not generally stimulate strong cellular immunity (Collins and Mackaness, 1968). The mechanisms by which persistence stimulates cellular immunity and the precise location of the persistent organisms are under investigation and discussed below.

This review will concentrate primarily on *S. typhi* and *S. typhimurium* because they have been well defined genetically and the immune response upon infection has been studied extensively. What contributes to making the best attenuated *Salmonella* vaccines is unknown but is being actively investigated in several laboratories including the authors.

II. *Salmonella* Species

There are many closely related species of *Salmonella,* all of which are capable of causing infection in humans. They can be found in all vertebrates. Turtles were sold as pets for children until it was discovered they could serve as reservoirs for *S. typhimurium. Salmonella panama* is a common intestinal bacteria of snakes. All members of this genus share at least 90% DNA homology. Recently, the Center for Disease Control (CDC) has suggested classifying most *Salmonella* as members of the *enteriditis* species, distinguishing them based on flagellar serotypes. In that classification *S. typhimurium* is a B serotype of *S. enteriditis, S. choleraesuis,* a swine pathogen, a C serotype, and *S. dublin,* a very invasive human pathogen, a D serotype. The most invasive salmonellae such as *S. paratyphi, S. dublin,* and *S. typhi* are members of the B or D serotypes. This nomenclature, however, has not been widely accepted.

Of all the *Salmonella* species, more is known about *S. typhimurium* LT2 than any other. This organism has a genome size of 4×10^6 bp and about 20% of its genes have been identified. Genes from one species of *Salmonella* can usually be moved to another species via a transducing phage such as P22. This is important in vaccine construction because an attenuating mutation that has been identified in *S. typhimurium* based on mouse studies can be moved to *S. typhi* by generalized transduction for clinical trial in humans. Excellent genetics and an inexpensive, simple animal model make *S. typhimurium* the preferred organism for study of the genetics of attenuation and for development of multivalent living vaccines.

III. Course of *Salmonella* Infection

Salmonella typhimurium is an important veterinary and human pathogen. It is the most common cause of gastroenteritis in humans in the United States. In humans, *S. typhimurium* does not invade beyond the intestinal mucosa. In horses, pigs, cattle, and mice, it can cause a disseminated infection. *Salmonella typhimurium* infection in mice is used as a genetic and immunological model for *S. typhi* infection in humans. There are substantial differences, however. *Salmonella typhi* is a more fastidious organism to culture (not to mention more dangerous to work with) that has a capsular polysaccharide, also known as the Vi antigen, and does not have the high-molecular-weight virulence plasmid present in *S. typhimurium*. Although sanitary conditions continue to improve worldwide, typhoid fever continues to be prevalent and is a major reportable cause of death globally. Less than 500 cases per year are reported in the United States because of excellent sanitation (W.H.O.W.E.R., 1986, 1987). In humans, *S. typhi* and *S. typhimurium* are foodborne diseases and are transmitted by ingestion of contaminated food products. After ingestion, *S. typhi* multiplies in the gastrointestinal tract, enters the intestinal lymphatics, and can pass into the bloodstream. After passage out of the lumen of the small intestine, it can be found in the Peyer's patches, the specialized lymphoid tissue located along the intestine. *Salmonella typhimurium,* on the other hand, is found in both the small and large intestines; mucosal invasion is confined to the gastrointestinal tract and disseminated infection is rarely observed.

The natural route of *S. typhimurium* infection in the mouse is by ingestion. During an oral infection, *S. typhimurium* passes directly through cells of the intestinal epithelium. Like the Gram-negative enteropathogens *Yersinia* spp. and *Shigella* spp., it can invade and replicate in a variety of animal cells. The elegant studies of Small *et al.* (1987), V. Miller and S. Falkow (unpublished observations), and Jones *et al.* (1981) demonstrate that *S. enteriditis* and *S. typhimurium* can invade a large variety of human and animal epithelial cells. Besides invading animal cells, the organism has been shown to pass through polarized cells such as those that line the intestine (Finley *et al.*, 1988). This ability to transcytose is probably critical to the pathogen establishing a systemic infection.

In vitro studies suggest that *S. enteriditis* and *S. typhimurium* may kill the animal cells that they invade (B. Finley and S. Falkow, unpublished observations; L. Gahring and F. Heffron, unpublished observations). The mechanism by which the killing takes place is not clear but most likely involves a cytotoxin similar to that of *Escherichia coli* LT and *V. cholerae* toxins (Chopra *et al.*, 1987). *Vibrio cholerae* toxin has been shown to inhibit macrophage chemotaxis (Aksamit *et al.*, 1985). According to one report *Salmonella* cytotoxin does not inhibit protein synthesis of Henle cells as does the toxin from *Shigella flexneri* (Hale and Formal, 1981). The cytotoxin ensures that this facultative intracellular pathogen will pass from one animal cell to another existing part of the time intracellularly and the rest of the time extracellularly. This life cycle also means that *Salmonella* will be susceptible to both bactericidal antibodies and cell-mediated immunity.

Following passage through the intestinal epithelium and the lamina propria, the bacteria can be found in the Peyer's patches. The infection spreads through the lymph system to the blood stream and the bacteria are found in the filtering organs: the liver and spleen (Collins, 1969). They replicate in these organs and are released back into the bloodstream; the mouse becomes bacterimic and soon dies. Whether or not *S. typhimurium* actually replicates within the macrophage or some other cell type within these organs has not been determined. The course of many viral infections has been studied by thin sectioning of organs or whole animals and using antibody or nucleic acid probes to identify the location of the virus within particular tissues and cells (Southern *et al.*, 1984). A similar approach for *Salmonella* would yield much new information including the precise types of cells in which the *Salmonella* replicates.

It is obvious that *S. typhimurium* encounters professional phagocytes soon after entering the host. Professional phagocytes migrate toward chemotactic factors such as bacterial initiation peptides and C5a, ensuring that they are one of the first cell types an invading microorganism will encounter (Cooper and Ziccardi, 1976). Resistance to professional phagocytes is critical to establishing an infection in the mouse whether or not it is able to replicate in the microbicidal environment of the macrophage. We have found large differences in how well *S. typhimurium* can persist in the macrophage, depending on whether it is a resident or an elicted macrophage and on the eliciting agent (N. Buchmeier, L. Gahring, and F. Heffron, unpublished observations). The strain of *S. typhimurium* that we have studied (ATCC14028) replicates in resident splenic and peritoneal macrophages from sensitive (*ity*; see below) strains of mice and in the mouse macrophage cell line J774. However, even in the most resistant macrophages there is appreciable bacterial survival (1–10%, N. Buchmeier, L. Gahring, and F. Heffron, unpublished observations). Several groups, including the authors, are attempting to identify properties of bacteria that confer bacterial resistance to antimicrobial mechanisms of the phagocyte and enable bacteria to replicate under normally hostile intracellular conditions (Fields *et al.*, 1986).

IV. Immunity to Infection

Humoral immunity is mediated by antibodies which act to opsonize bacteria and enable enhanced phagocytosis by macrophages and neutrophils or to stimulate complement deposition and lysis. Virulent strains of *Salmonella*, however, are resistant to complement-mediated lysis. Cellular immunity involves the generation of both cytotoxic T lymphocytes (CTL) directed against infected cells and specific T helper cells capable of activating CTLs and macrophages to become more microbicidal. Both cellular and humoral immunity require the participation of L3T4−, the mouse marker, or CD4−, the human marker, positive T helper cells. A few antigens, primarily those containing repetitive structures, such as LPS, elicit antibodies without T helper cell participation. Immunity against such T-cell-independent antigens is very short lived and its role in *Salmonella* immunity is unclear (see below).

The discovery that there are subclasses of T helper cells which produce various lymphokines suggests that different helper cells may interact specifically with the various cells of the immune system to modulate the type of immune response generated (Cher and Mosmann, 1987; Mosmann and Coffman, 1987). This may make current measurements of cellular immunity against bacterial pathogens more equivocal. If only certain helper T cells can activate macrophages, how can they be measured? They can be detected by assaying for production of specific lymphokines such as interleukin-2 (IL-2), IL-3, IL-4, and IFy. Normally, the total number of immune T helper cells is quantitated by determining the number of cells from regional lymph nodes or the spleen that proliferate when exposed to antigen. How much of this is due to B cells and how much to T cells can be determined with appropriate controls. T helper cells that activate macrophages are quantitated *in vivo* by assaying for lymphokine production as determined by delayed-type hypersensitivity (DTH). DTH results from release of lymphokines from T helper cells and macrophages and is measured by swelling after subcutaneous injection of an antigen, but is somewhat difficult to quantitate in the mouse.

There are several other measurements of immunity other than the proliferative response of T cells. Humoral immunity against bacteria is usually measured in an ELISA against the whole bacteria or purified components. Other assays include bactericidal assays, agglutination assays, and precipitation assays.

A. Natural Resistance to *Salmonella* Infection

Susceptibility of mice to infection by *S. typhimurium* and other facultative intracellular pathogens is polygenic just as is susceptibility in humans to *S. typhi* infection. Several loci are involved, of which three have been studied in detail (reviewed in O'Brien, 1986). The *ity* locus apparently is directly linked to the macrophage, in that macrophages from *ity* mice are less microbicidal (Lissner *et al.*, 1983). *ity* controls resistance to several intracellular pathogens besides *Salmonella* including *Leishmania donovani* and *Mycobacterium* (Taylor and O'Brien, 1982; Skamene *et al.*, 1982; Brown *et al.*, 1982). It does not correlate with resistance to *Brucella* infection, however (Ho and Cheers, 1982). The *xid* locus determines the levels of antibody response to *Salmonella* (O'Brien *et al.*, 1979, 1981) and *lps* mice contain B cells that are hyporesponsive to the mitogenic stimulus of LPS and macrophages that are not activated by LPS (Colwell *et al.*, 1986; O'Brien *et al.*, 1982).

What mouse genetic background is right to use if the goal of the research is to develop *Salmonella* vaccines that can be applied to man? Studies in human volunteers have demonstrated that some individuals are highly resistant to *S. typhi* infection, even though there is no evidence of prior exposure. Because man is a genetically complex mixture of susceptible and nonsusceptible individuals, it follows that one inbred mouse strain cannot mimic the immune response of humans to *S. typhi*. One approach to determining the correct model system is to compare the effectiveness of several vaccines in different strains of mice. Eisenstein *et al.* (1984) have carried out these studies and concluded that subunit vaccines provided no protection in sensitive strains of mice but some protection in resistant strains. However, their conclusion was that a living vaccine was far more effective in any of these mouse strain backgrounds.

B. Acquired Resistance to *Salmonella* Infection

The relative contributions of cellular and humoral immunity to resistance to *Salmonella* infection have been studied in detail. From the life cycle of *S. typhimurium* in the mouse, we might conclude that either antibodies or cellular immunity can control infection. As noted by Collins (1974), there was a raging debate more than 20 years ago about the contribution of these two arms of the immune system in controlling infection. "There has been a tendency . . . to allot a predominating role to either humoral or cellular factors, often to the virtual exclusion of the other arm of the defense system. Much of this controversy stems from the fact that the contribution made by the two defense systems can vary extensively depending upon the strain of organism, the host, and the experimental conditions selected by the individual investigator for the particular study."

Virtually all evidence favors a large contribution of cellular immunity to protection against *S. typhimurium* infection in the mouse and protection against all intracellular pathogens. All earlier adoptive transfer experiments suggested that immunity could be transferred with cells but not with serum (reviewed in F. Collins, 1974; Collins and MacKaness, 1968; F. M. Collins, 1969; Collins *et al.,* 1966; Saxén, 1984). The evidence that humoral immunity alone is sufficient to control infection comes from several experiments that demonstrate limited protection using hyperimmune serum. Using monoclonal antibodies directed against *Salmonella* LPS, Colwell *et al.* (1984), reported a slight increase in length of survival of mice injected with the monoclonal antibody. Eisenstein *et al.* (1984) used hyperimmune serum from multiply vaccinated mice and found that it conferred about a 10-fold increase in LD_{50} when resistant strains of mice subsequently were challenged with virulent organisms. These same investigators noted that with a living vaccine they obtained about 1000-fold higher levels of immunity. Our own work also shows a correlation between the most protective attenuated *Salmonella* strains (Fields *et al.,* 1986) and cellular immunity but not antibody titers against the whole organism (P. I. Fields and F. Heffron, unpublished observations). Much of the controversy about the relative contribution of cellular and humoral immunity stems from the erroneous belief that a subunit vaccine cannot provide cellular immunity. It has been known for many years that complete Freund's adjuvant is remarkable because it stimulates strong cellular immunity.

In spite of this, any subunit vaccine that protects, even if it is administered in complete Freund's adjuvant, is given as evidence for antibody protection against *Salmonella* infection without independent measurements of the level of cellular immunity. In conclusion, there is no good evidence that antibodies alone can protect against *Salmonella* infection when realistic challenge doses are given at long time periods postvaccination.

How is a *Salmonella* infection controlled in immune and in naturally resistant strains of mice? A virulent strain of *Salmonella* kills susceptible strains of mice at very low infectious doses, however, there are large differences between strains of inbred mice in their susceptibility to *Salmonella* infection. Several investigators have exploited these differences to determine where control of *Salmonella* infection can take place and, further, compared the course of infection in immune and susceptible mice. Control of a *Salmonella* infection can take place at several different points during infection and is mediated by different components of the immune system. Early in infection, control is probably due to the professional phagocyte. Nude mice (*nu*) are missing the thymus and most T-cell functions. O'Brien *et al.* (1982) have compared the course of *S. typhimurium* infection in resistant and sensitive strains of nude mice. Their results suggest that macrophages are more important for the early control of infection than are T cells because there are substantial differences between *ity* (*nu/nu*) mice and resistant (*nu/nu*) mice during the early period of infection. Thus, phagocytic cells may be primarily responsible for controlling early *Salmonella* replication. This same study demonstrated that nude *ity*[r] mice are unable to control the later stages of *Salmonella* infection, suggesting that T cells are essential, although which effector cell is required for controlling infection is not known.

Unimpaired replication of *Salmonella* takes place for up to a week in the mouse, indicating that effective cellular immunity takes this long to develop (Collins, 1969; Mackaness *et al.*, 1966). Specific immune T cells arise that are essential for stimulating T-dependent antibody production, for activating macrophages to become more microbicidal, and for generation of immune cytotoxic T lymphocytes (CTLs). Within the last few years some evidence has appeared supporting a role for CTLs in control of bacterial infections. These thymus-derived cells become activated to kill infected cells by interaction with T helper cells. They can be identified by antibodies against surface proteins that are expressed uniquely on this type of cell (such as Lyt2). Adoptive-transfer experiments suggest that CTLs may be essential for controlling infection with *Mycobacterium* (Orme and Collins, 1984; Adu *et al.*, 1983),

Brucella (Pavlov *et al.*, 1982), and *Listeria* (Cheers and Sandrin, 1983; Kaufmann *et al.*, 1985). Killing of *Listeria*-infected macrophages by CTLs has been demonstrated *in vitro* (De Libero and Kaufmann *et al.*, 1986). Similar experiments have not been reported for *Salmonella*. Activated macrophages have been strongly implicated in control of *Listeria* infection in the mouse (North, 1970, 1978), but once again less experimental evidence is available for *Salmonella*.

V. Subunit versus Living Vaccines

A. Subunit Vaccines to *Salmonella*

Current killed vaccines against *S. paratyphi* or *S. typhi* have good efficacy for periods of up to 2 years based on field trials in New Guinea and Czeckoslovakia (Ashcroft *et al.*, 1964; Tapa and Cvjetanovic, 1975). They are made by acetone-killing the organism followed by lyophilization. A successful trial in Nepal (72% efficacy) has just been reported for a vaccine made from the capsular polysaccharride of *S. typhi* (Acharya *et al.*, 1987). There is some evidence that a subunit vaccine is more effective in people who have had prior exposure to *Salmonella*, such as those in these three trials but not for travelers from industrialized nations.

An effective subunit vaccine for *S. typhimurium* appears to be a mixture of outer membrane proteins and LPS. Neither component by itself is as protective as the mixture (Kuusi *et al.*, 1981; Killion and Morrison, 1986). A ribosomal vaccine with considerable efficacy has been described (Angerman and Eisenstein, 1978; Venneman *et al.*, 1970). However, subsequent work suggests it is contaminated with both outer membrane proteins and LPS which probably accounts for its efficacy (Hoops *et al.*, 1976). A completely synthetic vaccine has been described that consists of a synthetic polysaccharide and an outer membrane protein (Svenson *et al.*, 1979). To be effective it must administered in complete Freund's adjuvant which is known to stimulate cellular immunity.

B. Efficacy of Living Attenuated Vaccines

Collins and his colleagues (1966) have provided some of the strongest evidence for the superior immunity generated by living vaccines for mouse-virulent salmonellae. In this classic paper, the authors compared protection following vaccination with strains of *Salmonella* that differed in ability to persist but were antigenically similar. Mice were challenged with a virulent strain of *S. enteriditis*. High antibody titers could be generated by vaccination with killed strains but protective immunity could not. They found that protection was correlated solely with persistence, but the difference in protective properties was not trivial. Continuous perfusion with a nonprotective strain did not generate significant cellular immunity. Angerman and Eisenstein (1978) compared the efficacy of living *Salmonella* vaccines to that of several subunit vaccines. Only a living vaccine was able to protect against the highest challenge doses, even at 3 weeks post vaccination, suggesting that the living vaccine provided better protection. Angerman and Eisenstein (1980) also correlated the duration of protection afforded with live and killed organisms. Again, they found that a living vaccine was the most efficacious. More recently, De Libero and Kauffman (1986) have shown that immunity to *Listeria* can be correlated solely with persistence of the vaccinating strain. The most recent work with *Salmonella* has verified this result but demonstrated that, while it is absolutely essential for immunity, persistence alone is insufficient as discussed below. The precise reason that living bacteria can provide such long-lasting immunity will not be clear until the pathogenesis of *Salmonella* spp. is better understood and how its survival within different tissues of the organism influences the immune response.

VI. Genetics of Attenuation of *Salmonella*

The virulence determinants of *Salmonella* are multiple and almost all have yet to be characterized. Some *Salmonella* strains produce an enterotoxin that appears to be closely related to those of *V. cholerae* and *E. coli* (Chopra *et al.*, 1987) and is implicated in virulence. The enterotoxin apparently acts like that of *V. cholerae* by causing severe fluid loss and electrolyte imbalances in the intestine (Giannella *et al.*, 1973). Other determinants, such as surface components involved in adherence or invasion through mucosal surfaces, are only now being identified (Small *et al.*, 1987; Fields *et al.*, 1986). Clinical and animal isolates of *Salmonella* vary greatly in virulence in the mouse model. Hormaeche and his collaborators (1980) have compared strains of *S. typhimurium* in sensitive mice. He found they varied greatly, presumably because of differences in genes involved in pathogenesis.

There are certainly many avirulent *Salmonella* strains available. Although individual strains, such as *S. typhimurium* LT2 variants, can be shown to be attenuated, they are not usually considered as vaccine candidates primarily because the genetic lesion is unknown. Obviously, the quality control of such a vaccine would be very difficult. How can genetics be used to construct candidate attenuated live vaccine strains? Modern genetic techniques can be used to introduce defined genetic lesions into the genomes of bacteria. This approach has led to the identification of regions in the genome that contribute to virulence in several bacterial species (Weiss *et al.*, 1983; Fields *et al.*, 1986; Smith and Linggood, 1971). Strains that carry defined mutations in virulence determinants are likely to be attenuated and can be considered as vaccine candidates.

Early studies on *Salmonella* virulence relied on less well-defined techniques for isolating mutants but concentrated on either mutations in surface components or mutations in biosynthetic pathways. Many rough variants of virulent *Salmonella* strains are less virulent than smooth parental strains (Nakano and Saito, 1969; Germanier, 1970). The smooth-to-rough phenotypic change involves loss of the ability to synthesize or assemble the O-specific side-chains of the surface LPS molecule. Different mutations give rise to different rough phenotypes. LPS is synthesized sequentially starting from a lipid (lipid A) attached to the cell surface by being imbedded in the cell membrane. In our own analysis, we found that a loss of the O-specific side-chains but maintainance of a complete core resulted in a two-log increase in LD_{50} for i.p. inoculation in BALB/c mice (*ity*) but this may depend, in part, on *Salmonella* strain background (Fields *et al.*, 1986; Fields and Heffron, unpublished observations; see Stocker and Makela, 1984, for review). A mutation in *rfaF* that affects core LPS structure increases the LD_{50} by an additional two logs (Fields *et al.*, 1986). Mutations that result in even shorter LPS structures are quite fragile, sensitive to detergents, and have lost all virulence (see Stocker and Makela, 1984; Lyman *et al.*, 1976; Germanier, 1970). Thus, LPS, on the basis of such rough mutants, has been implicated both as a virulence determinant and as a candidate protective antigen. With the exception of *galE* mutants (discussed later), rough strains have not found use as *Salmonella* vaccines, although a spontaneously rough variant of *S. dublin* has been sold for some time as a live cattle vaccine. We have isolated a number of attenuating mutations of a virulent strain of *Salmonella* (ATCC14028) that is missing the O antigen (Fields *et al.*, 1986). This rough strain has an LD_{50} in BALB/c mice that is only one to two logs higher than the smooth parent. No surface antigens, except for LPS, have been shown definitively to be virulence factors in *Salmonella*. The Vi capsule of *S. typhi* has been implicated as a virulence factor, but spontaneously Vi-negative mutants of *S. typhi* are still able to cause typhoid fever in humans (Hornick *et al.*, 1970; Woodward, 1980).

An alternative approach to attenuation is to mutate a gene or genes encoding enzymes in a biosynthetic pathway essential for survival *in vivo*. In the early 1950s, Bacon and co-workers used irradiation to isolate auxotrophic mutants of *S. typhi*. They found that mutants defective in *para*-aminobenzoic acid biosynthesis or in purine biosynthesis were less virulent in an intraperitoneal infection model of mice (Bacon *et al.*, 1950, 1951). This important observation was not followed up until Hoiseth and Stocker published a report of their work on *S. typhimurium aroA* mutants in 1981. These workers, following the ideas of Bacon and co-workers, used transposon mutagenesis to isolate deletion mutations in the *aroA* gene. *aroA* encodes the enzyme 5-enol pyruvylshikimate 3-phosphate synthase, a key enzyme in the aromatic biosynthetic pathway of bacteria. In bacteria, this pathway is the sole route of biosynthesis of several key aromatic metabolites, including *para*-aminobenzoic acids. Mammalian cells do not possess an equivalent pathway and must extract the aromatic components from their diet. Apparently there must be limiting amounts of one or more of the key aromatic metabolites *in vivo*, as *aroA* mutants of several *Salmonella* species, including *S. typhimurium*, *S. dublin*, and *S. typhi* have been shown to be attenuated in several experimental animal model systems (Killar and Eisenstein, 1985; Robertsson *et al.*, 1983; Smith *et al.*, 1984; Dougan *et al.*, 1987a). The work of Hoiseth and Stocker was also significant because they demonstrated that *Salmonella aroA* mutants could act as effective vaccines, an observation that has been confirmed by other workers. *aroA* mutants of *S. typhimurium* set up a self-limiting infection in mice which is eventually cleared. After oral infection of BALB/c mice, *S. typhimurium aroA* mutants are able to invade the gut mucosal surface and spread systemically to reach the liver and spleen (Maskell *et al.*, 1987). It takes several weeks for BALB/c mice to clear the mutant organisms from the body. The immune mechanisms by which *Salmonella aroA* vaccines induce protective immunity is not known although they are under investigation. *aroA* vaccines induce significant levels of anti-*Salmonella* antibodies in serum and at the gut mucosal surface, and cell-mediated immune responses have been demonstrated. It will be interesting to see how mutations in other *aro* genes affect *Salmonella* virulence.

Purine dependent mutants of *S. typhimurium* are also attenuated as first demonstrated by Bacon *et al.* (1950). Recent studies suggest that mutations at steps prior to the synthesis of inosine monophosphate in purine biosynthetic genes are less attenuated than after the inosine branch point. For example, *purE* mutants are much less attenuated than *purA* (O'Callaghan *et al.*, 1988). Indeed *purE* mutants of *S. typhimurium* still retain a significant degree of virulence and are not likely to be useful as vaccine candidates. *purA* mutants of *S. typhimurium* and *S. typhi* are apparently even more attenuated than *aroA* mutants (O'Callaghan *et al.*, 1988; Nnalue and Stocker, 1987; McFarland and Stocker, 1987). While *purA* mutants retain little virulence, they may not be as effective oral vaccines as *aroA* mutants. Our laboratory has compared protection of isogenic *aroA* and *purA* mutants of *S. typhimurium* in sensitive strains of mice (O'Callaghan *et al.*, 1988) and found that *aroA* gives much higher levels of protection. Interestingly, the combination of *aroA* and *purA* mutations in the same strain may further attenuate and reduce the value of the strain as an oral vaccine (O'Callaghan *et al.*, 1988). Nevertheless, *aroA* and *purA* mutants need careful evaluation as to their potential use as human typhoid vaccines.

Mutations in other genes can give rise to attenuated strains of *Salmonella*. *thyA* mutants, which are dependent on thymidine, are attenuated but to our knowledge have not been evaluated as vaccines. R. Curtiss and his collaborators (personal communication) have shown that *crp* and *cya* mutants of *S. typhimurium* are attenuated and promising vaccine candidates. A recent study by Fields *et al.* (1986) has isolated a large number of Tn*10* mutants of *S. typhimurim* which are sensitive to killing by macrophages. These mutations are being studied for potential use as live vaccines.

VII. Human Typhoid Vaccine Strains

Salmonella typhi causes typhoid fever in humans but does not cause a typhoid-like disease in any other animal. When *S. typhi* is injected i.p. in mice it undergoes only a few divisions. As a consequence it is only possible to evaluate *S. typhi* vaccines fully in humans. This has placed enormous constraints on the development of novel typhoid vaccines. A number of strains have been put forward as candidate live vaccines, but only a few have been evaluated in man. Some, but not all, were developed using information accumulated using the mouse typhoid model which employs non-*typhi* serotypes of *Salmonella*, such as *S. typhimurium* and *S. enteriditis*.

An early attempt to develop a human live oral typhoid vaccine involved using a mutant of *S. typhi* that is dependent on streptomycin for growth (Reitman, 1967). The molecular basis of this mutation was unknown but was presumed to act at the level of the ribosome. Early tests in the i.p. mouse model showed that the streptomycin-dependent mutant was less virulent than the parental strain and was able to induce significant levels of anti-O-agglutinins in the serum of infected mice. The mutation was determined to be stable enough to allow human trials to begin. Multiple doses of over 10^{10} viable streptomycin-dependent S. *typhi* were well tolerated by humans and a vaccine efficacy of between 66–78% was detected. However, the strain was found to lose viability upon lyophilization, a fact that stopped its development as a human vaccine. Efficient lyophilization is an essential step in the mass production of a live typhoid vaccine (Levine *et al.*, 1976).

The fact that rough strains of S. *typhimurium* are attenuated is decribed in the previous section. The same results hold true for S. *typhi*. In the early 1970s Germanier (1970) undertook a careful study to identify an optimal rough mutant to develop into a human typhoid vaccine. To summarize this work, he found that rough *galE* mutants of S. *typhimurium* produced the most promising vaccines, as evaluated in the mouse typhoid model. The *galE* gene encodes the enzyme uridine diphosphate (UDP)-galactose-4-epimerase, which is involved in galactose metabolism and ultimately in LPS biosynthesis because it is a constituent of the O antigen. When grown on medium lacking galactose, *galE* mutants exhibit a rough colonial morphology producing incomplete LPS. If the growth medium is supplemented with galactose, cells begin to synthesize a smooth LPS with complete O side-chain, probably utilizing galactokinase and galactose-1-phosphate-uridyl transferase. However, *galE* mutants accumulate a toxic phosphorylated derivative of galactose and autolyse. Germanier (1970) clearly showed that *galE* mutants of S. *typhimurium* were attenuated and were the most effective vaccines in mice of all the LPS biosynthesis mutations he examined. One problem with *galE* mutants is that secondary mutations affecting galactose sensitivity of the cell and expression of *galE* genes rapidly accumulate. Recombinant DNA techniques were used recently to introduce a defined deletion into the *galE* gene of a virulent S. *typhimurium* strain. The *galE* deletion mutant was found to be attenuated and to be an effective vaccine in mice (Hone *et al.*, 1987).

In 1975 Germanier and Furer reported the construction of Ty21a as a live typhoid vaccine. This strain is a *galE* mutant of S. *typhi* Ty2 generated by mutagenizing with nitrosoguanidine, a potent chemical mutagen. It was isolated by treating with at least two rounds of nitrosoguanidine to obtain a stable, attenuated *galE* mutant as judged by infection of S. *typhi* in mice. The levels of other galactose metabolizing enzymes were found to be reduced in Ty21a. The nature of the genetic lesions in Ty21a induced by mutagenesis are still unknown, but the strain is likely to contain multiple mutations by analogy with other strains constructed with this mutagen. Furthermore, Ty21a appears to differ significantly from Ty2 (Silva *et al.*, 1987). Certainly, Ty21a has lost the ability to produce Vi capsular antigen. Other workers have claimed that they can isolate spontaneous galE-positive revertants of the strain (Silva-Salinas et al., 1985). Despite the uncertainty of the genetic lesions in Ty21a, there is no disputing the fact that the strain is attenuated and it has now been carefully evaluated in humans.

Initially Ty21a was tested in human volunteers for safety and immunogenicity. Doses of over 10^{10} organisms were found to be well tolerated. Subsequently the volunteers were challenged with virulent S. typhi either with or without prior vaccination with Ty21a. The vaccine showed an efficacy of 87%, clearly providing protection against typhoid (Gilman et al., 1977). Encouraged by this data, field trials of Ty21a were carried out in Egypt and Chile. The Egyptian trial involved 32,000 children who received three doses of the vaccine in liquid form following treatment with bicarbonate. An efficacy of 96% was reported in this trial. The Chilean trial was set up in an area with a much higher endemic rate of typhoid. Unfortunately, several changes were made to the vaccine formulation during this trial and only recently has data become generally available. Despite a poor performance with some vaccination regimens, a Ty21a vaccine delivered in enteric-coated capsules gave an efficacy of 67% over three years (Wahdan et al., 1980, 1982; Levine et al., 1982). This reflects favorably with the data obtained with whole cell vaccine. One of the problems with the trial in Chile is that the strain lost viability on lyophilization. This problem appears to have been overcome and Ty21a is now licensed as a vaccine for typhoid in a number of countries including the United States. Nevertheless, because of the above-mentioned problems with Ty21a and because more recent data have identified highly protective attenuating mutations in S. typhimurium, a search is still on for a better typhoid vaccine. Mäkelä and Stocker (1984) constructed a S. typhi aroA purA mutant which was tested in humans and found to be well tolerated. Evidence for cell-mediated immune responses were detected although seroconversion to S. typhi antigens was poor (Levine et al., 1987b). Our own results with the same double mutant in S. typhimurium suggests that this combination may have been a poor choice (see above). The double mutant persists surprisingly well but provides very low levels of protection for reasons that are not clear (O'Callaghan et al., 1988). The single aroA mutation may be a better choice because it is attenuated sufficiently to be used in a vaccine, and results in mice suggest that it is among the most protective mutants tested (D. Maskell and G. Dougan, unpublished observations). A derivative of Ty2 containing this mutation has been constructed and is being evaluated in humans (Dougan et al., 1987b).

VIII. The Use of *Salmonella* as a Carrier of Foreign Antigens

The immune response to an antigen depends on how it is presented to the immune system and is the subject of much ongoing research. Some protein antigens can be extremely poor immunogens unless administered with adjuvant. Haptens are completely nonimmunogenic unless coupled to a carrier. By expressing foreign antigens in live attenuated *Salmonella* vaccines, the vaccine appears to serve as an adjuvant stimulating a greater B- and T-cell response than if the antigen were administered alone (see below). This is important not only because *Salmonella* vaccines can be given orally and are easy to produce, but also because potentially protective antigens have been identified for many parasites, pathogenic viruses, and bacteria. Pure antigen can be made by recombinant DNA technology for assessment as protective subunit vaccines. Very few adjuvants are available for use in humans and parenteral delivery of purified proteins or carbohydrates often fails to stimulate a good level of serum antibody and almost always fails to stimulate secretory immune responses at mucosal surfaces or an effective cell-mediated response. In contrast, certain live vaccines such as *Vaccinia*, BCG, and *Salmonella* can be potent stimulators of the immune system. *Vaccinia* has already been developed as a carrier for cloned foreign antigens. It has several features that might limit its usefulness as a multivalent vaccine delivery system. First, the current information suggests that the virus vaccine is not that effective as a carrier system. Second, single-dose oral vaccines would be more acceptable globally and the *Vaccinia* vaccine must be injected. Last, there are size constraints implicit in the overall size of the virus, limiting the number of antigenic determinants that realistically can be introduced into the system. Oral *Salmonella* vaccines are of particular interest because, when taken orally, they can stimulate mucosal, humoral, and cell-mediated responses in the host. Because of the close relationship between *Salmonella* and *E. coli*, the same techniques that have been developed for expression and overproduction in *E. coli* are at least partly applicable to *Salmonella*.

The strategy for constructing a new vaccine strain might be as follows. DNA from the pathogen in question (or mRNA if the pathogen is a eukaryote) is isolated and used to construct either a λgt11 or other expression library. These libraries are screened for protective antigens using identified immune sera. The coding sequence(s) for the antigens are identified by transposon insertional inactivation, direct sequencing, or any of several other techniques and the identified gene is subcloned into a plasmid expression vector. This can be as simple as cloning the gene downstream from the weak tetracycline promoter in pBR322, as was done in constructing a vaccine against the B subunit of the *E. coli* enterotoxin. These plasmids are then transformed into *Salmonella*. The most convenient way to do this is by transformation of a restriction-minus host, just as is done in *E. coli*. Most (and probably every) plasmid that can replicate in *E. coli* can also replicate in *Salmonella*. However, the problem has been that many plasmids are not stable once the vaccine strain is injected into the test animal. Also, this method would certainly not be approved for the construction of human vaccines because of antibiotic resistance encoded on the plasmid. Eventually, methods must be developed to introduce the gene(s) into the *Salmonella* chromosome in such a way that the strain is nonreverting for virulence, expresses the cloned antigen stably, and expresses no antibiotic resistance following the strain construction.

In theory, it should be possible to express protective antigens from any pathogen in *Salmonella* vaccine strains and thus deliver heterologous antigens to the immune system (Dougan *et al.,* 1987a). In practice, there are many variables that need to be examined to make the method of general utility. These include:

1. What controls stability of the vector from which the antigen is expressed?
2. How is the amount of antigen expressed related to stability, attenuation of the strain, and immune response?
3. How is the immune response to a given antigen related to cell location within the bacteria, fusion to other proteins, and location of an epitope within a single protein?
4. How does the immune response to a given expressed antigen vary with attenuating strain and route of infection?
5. Can an immune response to only one antigen in a particular pathogen provide protection to subsequent infection?

There are many unknowns but considerable progress has been made in constructing multivalent vaccines.

Formal and colleagues (1981) were the first to use *Salmonella* as a multivalent vaccine by introducing *Shigella sonnei* antigens into Ty21a. The shigellae are highly pathogenic enteric pathogens that produce potent cytotoxins and are differentiated from the salmonellae by their lack of motility. They cause bacillary dysentery and are of importance worldwide. The shigellae rapidly invade a variety of animal cells and just as quickly kill them, causing massive destruction of the superficial layer of the colonic epithelium. Lesions caused by *Shigella* spp. generally are confined to the terminal ileum and colon and are characteristically covered by pseudomembranes consisting of PMNs, cell debris, and bacteria in fibrin. Fatality rates often reach more than 20% during outbreaks and multiply drug-resistant bacteria commonly are isolated. In 1986, 17,138 cases of shigellosis were diagnosed in the United States alone and although this is one of the lowest rates in the world it points to the importance of developing a good vaccine.

Killed vaccines have shown no efficacy and there is no evidence for long-term immunity following a shigellosis infection. However, an attenuated strain produced good immunity both in animals and in a field trial (Mel *et al.*, 1965). Immunity is group specific and therefore immunity to the LPS moiety appears to be critical for protection. To construct the vaccine, a virulence plasmid of *Shigella sonnei* that encodes production of the Form I antigen was transferred to Ty21a (Kopecko *et al.*, 1980). Cells harboring the plasmid expressed *Shigella* Form I antigen at their surface as well as O9 and O12 somatic antigens of *S. typhi*. Mice vaccinated with the hybrid strain, named 5076-1C, raised antibodies to both *Shigella* and *Salmonella* antigens. 5076-1C was shown to be safe following oral administration to humans, although seroconversion to *Shigella* antigen was not detected (Tramont *et al.*, 1984) and thus the hybrid most likely has limited efficacy. More recently a hybrid Ty21a strain was developed that contains sequences which encode the group-specific *Shigella* LPS antigens (Baron *et al.*, 1987). This strain protects against *Shigella*, based on results from a field trial, but no longer provides protection against *Salmonella*. A combined dysentery and typhoid vaccine would be of great potential use. Baron *et al.* (1987) suggested using a mixture of Ty21a and Ty21a expressing *Shigella* type-specific antigens to make the vaccine multivalent.

Vaccination with *Shigella–Salmonella* hybrids demonstrated that a *Salmonella* derivative that expresses *Shigella* group-specific antigen could result in antibody response against the group-specific antigen. Expression of *E. coli* β-galactosidase in *Salmonella*, a cytoplasmic protein, results in a cellular response against β-galactosidase as well as a humoral response. This result shows that a cellular response can be induced against heterologous antigens and also shows that an antigen need not be expressed on the bacterial cell surface to generate a strong response (Brown *et al.*, 1987). In this respect the immune response to bacteria may be similar to the immune response to influenze virus. Townsend *et al.* (1986) have shown that the greatest T-cell response is directed against internal components and not viral surface components. In view of the results with β-galactosidase, these authors and several others have started construction of multivalent vaccines against many other pathogens.

Vibrio cholerae and enterotoxigenic strains of *E. coli* secrete an immunologically related enterotoxin which is a major virulence factor and a potentially protective antigen. The toxins are composed of two functional subunits—an A subunit with enzymatic and toxic activity and an immunodominant B subunit which on its own is nontoxic but serves to deliver subunit A to the eukaryotic cell membrane. Plasmids that direct the expression of the B-subunit toxoid have been introduced into *Salmonella* vaccine strains, including Ty21a (Clements and El-Morshidy, 1984), *S. enteritidis aroA* (Clements *et al.*, 1986), and *S. typhimurium aroA* (Maskell *et al.*, 1986a,b, 1987). Immunization of mice with these strains expressing the B subunit results in production of toxin-neutralizing antibodies in serum and at the gut mucosal surface, including antibodies of the IgA isotype. The mice are also protected against subsequent virulent *Salmonella* challenge, suggesting that expression of B subunit was not affecting the protective immune response to *Salmonella* challenge, suggesting that expression of B subunit was not affecting the protective immune response to *Salmonella* itself (Maskell *et al.*, 1987). Evidence suggests that, in the case of cholera, anti-toxin immunity may not be sufficient to give full protection against disease and that *Vibrio* somatic antigens may also be required. Recently, the LPS determinant of *V. cholerae* has been cloned and expressed in Ty21a, another step toward a combined cholera and typhoid vaccine (Guidolin and Manning, 1987).

The K88 adhesive antigen determinant of porcine enterotoxigenic *E. coli,* which is a proteinacious surface fimbriae involved in attachment to gut mucosal surfaces, has also been expressed from recombinant plasmids in *S. typhimurium galE* strains (Stevenson and Manning, 1985) and *aroA* (Dougan *et al.*, 1986) vaccine strains. Such strains appear to assemble the K88 antigen on their cell surfaces, and mice vaccinated with *Salmonella* strains expressing K88 produce anti-K88 antibodies.

All of the above examples of heterologous antigens expressed in *Salmonella* vaccine strains come from related enteric bacterial pathogens. How far has work progressed with antigens from other organisms? It is theoretically feasible to express protective antigens from any pathogen in *Salmonella*. However, to incorporate such antigens into viable vaccines may be much more difficult for several reasons. Foreign proteins normally are expressed in *E. coli* using regulated promoter systems. Controlled induction of promoters using organisms growing *in vivo* would be difficult and several constitutive expression systems will have to be developed. Overexpression of proteins to produce more antigen may seem advantagous at first but can lead to instability of a plasmid particularly *in vivo* (G. Dougan and D. Maskell, unpublished observations). Another problem is that many recombinant antigens may accumulate in the cytoplasm of the cell and surface expression may be required for optimal recognition of antigens by the immune system. Protection studies that correlate the amount of protection with expression of a given antigen in particular cellular locations in the bacteria, amount of antigen expressed, whether it is or is not fused to particular immunogenic *Salmonella* proteins, route of immunization, and many other variables will have to be carried out in the next few years.

IX. Vaccines against Other Pathogens

A. CURRENT *Brucella* VACCINES

The brucellae are also Gram-negative facultative intracellular pathogens. Three species, which all utilize the four carbon alcohol erythritol preferentially over glucose, cause the majority of disease: *B. abortus, B. suis,* and *B. melitensis*. The diseases caused by these broad host-range microorganisms are more insidious than typhoid fever, producing a number of nonspecific symptoms in humans that can make diagnosis difficult. As is the case with other intracellular pathogens, cell-mediated immunity is thought to play a larger role than humoral immunity and the balance between the immune response and the pathogen can be tipped to give persistent infection that can reoccur many years after an infection apparently has been resolved.

Diseases caused by the brucellae generally follow similar courses. Brucellosis is a zoonosis in industrialized countries; infection results from exposure to infected animals or dairy products. The organisms enter through the oral mucosa, nasopharynx, conjunctivae, or genitalia, although they have the capacity to penetrate unbroken skin (Cotton and Buck, 1932). Bacteremia ensues, followed by localization in regional lymph nodes, the reticuloendothelial tissues, reproductive tissues, bones, and joints. In ungulates, they often cause lesions of the female reproductive tract leading to fetal death and abortion. Lesions can also occur in the male reproductive tract, resulting in sterility. In humans, the disease manifests itself as a chronic debilitating disease characterized by intermittent chills and fever, joint and muscle pain, and generalized malaise and is difficult to diagnose. Sequelae are often extremely serious, sometimes resulting in death because of the difficulty in diagnosis. Control of infection is costly and almost unattainable at present in Third World countries where the disease is endemic.

There is, at present, no accepted human vaccine against any of the brucellae. Vaccination of the primary hosts (cattle, hogs, sheep, goats) would prevent transmission to humans.

Brucella melitensis is the causative agent of Malta fever and is prevalent in goats and sheep. It has broad host-range specificity. A bacterin, killed adjuvant 53H38 (Bosseray, 1978), and a live avirulent vaccine (Rev. 1 mutant vaccine) have been used to vaccinate sheep (Alton and Elberg, 1967) and goats (Elberg and Faunce, 1957; Alton, 1970). There is no report of the nature of the attenuating mutation or the efficacy of the live vaccine.

There are several vaccines against *B. abortus,* the cause of infectious bovine abortions. Although bacterins and killed vaccines have been tested, they have proven to be largely ineffective in providing long-lasting immunity and subsequent control of the disease (Bosseray, 1978). Several (PI, 4A fraction, Fraction 5, peptidoglycan) have been suggested for use as vaccines in humans at risk (Plommet *et al.,* 1987). However, none of these subunit vaccines has been demonstrated to stimulate long-lasting immunity. As with the *Salmonella,* it is likely that transient persistence is required to stimulate long-lasting immunity to infection. Several live, attenuated vaccines have been developed: McEwen 45/20, *B. abortus* "Russian strain" (a strain used in Eastern bloc countries about which there is little information) and Strain 19.

The McEwen 45/20 strain (McEwen and Priestly, 1938) is a rough strain of *B. abortus* that regained pathogenicity after serial passage through guinea pigs and was apparently quite immunogenic. It was discontinued as a vaccine because Strain 19 was more efficacious. It is, however, sometimes used as a killed adjuvant vaccine, but two doses are required for induction of resistance and localized tissue reactions are common (Alton, 1978). Annual boosters are also required to maintain optimal resistance but this is not cost effective. In Eastern bloc countries, the *B. abortus* "Russian strain" has been used extensively for vaccination against both *B. abortus* and *B. melitensis.* The nature of the attenuating mutation is not described. However, it has been used as a human vaccine and reportedly has some efficacy since, when last reported (Zdrodowski *et al.,* 1957), it had helped to decrease morbidity 3- to 11-fold in regions of the Soviet Union where *B. melitenesis* is endemic. This is the only case where a *B. abortus* vaccine has been shown to be effective against *B. melitensis* and no further reports have followed.

The predominant vaccine, however, remains Strain 19. First described by Buck (1930), it is a live, smooth, stable strain discovered to have little virulence in cattle or guinea pigs. The major difference between this strain and a virulent isolate, other than reduced severity of infection, is growth inhibition, rather than stimulation, by erythritol. It is lacking a single enzyme, D-erythulose 1-phosphate dehydrogenase, in the catabolic pathway; however, whether or not this is the attenuating mutation is unknown. Strain 19, is about 70% effective in cattle, and is most likely less virulent in ungulates because the organism cannot localize to the erythritol-rich placenta. Strain 19 does not provide cross-protection against other brucellae. This vaccine has several drawbacks. First, it retains considerable virulence for humans. Second, it causes persistent infection in a small population of vaccinated calves. Last, some animals retain persistently high antibody titers post-vaccination. This is the most important drawback because of its economic impact; cattle that show high brucellae titers must be destroyed. Naturally, farmers are reluctant to vaccinate their herds because of this drawback and brucellosis persists in the United States. Identification of a protective antigen and inclusion in a multivalent veterinary vaccine would substantially reduce the economic impact of these pathogens on the cattle and swine industry.

B. CURRENT *Vibrio cholerae* VACCINES

Vibrio cholerae, another foodborne pathogen, also causes severe diarrhea. Infection is localized in the intestine, and an enterotoxin that acts on the luminal surface of the small bowel and mucosal cells activates cell membrane adenyl cyclase resulting in increased levels of cAMP. There have been seven pandemics since 1817 but the incidence of disease in the United States has dropped due to better sanitation. However, it is still of major importance worldwide.

Convalescence from cholera confers immunity from further disease. Despite this fact, no good vaccine has been developed. *Vibrio cholerae* encodes a toxin related to that found in *E. coli* (Clements and Finkelstein, 1978). Texas star is a mutated derivative of the Ogawa cholera strain isolated by Finkelstein and his collaborators (Honda and Finkelstein, 1979). In adult volunteers it provided substantial protection but resulted in diarrhea (Levine *et al.*, 1984). A derivative that has been completely deleted for the toxin still gave diarrhea to volunteers (Kaper *et al.*, 1984). A possible explanation is that cholera encodes a second toxin more closely related to Shiga toxin. An effective vaccine may require a strain that is deleted for both toxin genes but that can still persist.

C. CURRENT *Mycobacterium* VACCINES

The pathogenic *Mycobacterium* are agonizingly slow-growing, facultative, intracellular pathogens. The two most notable human pathogens are *M. leprae* and *M. tuberculosis,* the causative agents of leprosy and tuberculosis. Tuberculosis is primarily a disease of man which is transferred person to person by the droplet nuclei route. It begins as a disease of the lower respiratory tract and lungs but can disseminate from its primary pulmonary focus. The incidence of new infections in the United States has remained relatively constant with the annual incidence somewhere in the range of 12 cases per 100,000 population over the last 10 years (Centers for Disease Control, 1987). In spite of the fact that both pathogens can be treated, they cause about 20 million infections a year worldwide with a mortality that exceeds 3 million deaths (Joint International Union Against Tuberculosis and WHO Study Group). High cellular immunity to the disease is necessary for protective immunity. Much progress has been made in the last 5 years in understanding the immune response to *Mycobacterium* infections and to the development of new *Mycobacterium* vaccines to reduce the worldwide significance of these diseases.

The mycobacteria are particularly well evolved to survive in phagocytic cells. Immunity to *M. tuberculosis* is believed to involve cell-mediated immune responses (Collins, 1984). Like *S. typhi, M. tuberculosis* exists *in vivo* as an intracellular parasite and can survive for long periods of time establishing persistent infections. They inhibit phagolysosome fusion apparently via release of sulfatides (Goren *et al.,* 1976) and they are very resistant to superoxides because a phenolic glycolipid surface component is a free radical scavenger (Brennan and B. Bloom, personal communication; S. Klebenoff, personal communication). Mycobacterial proteins against which cellular and humoral responses are generated have been studied in detail (see Mustafa *et al.,* 1986, for most recent work). Several of the major cellular antigens appear to be stress-induced proteins (R. Young, personal communication).

BCG *(Bacillus Calmette-Guerin)* has been used as an attenuated vaccine against *M. tuberculosis* infections for many years. BCG is an avirulent derivative of *M. bovis* and is the most widely given human living vaccine. A lifelong positive skin test results from single immunization within the first few weeks of life. It was developed in the early 1900s by passaging a strain of *M. bovis in vitro* for about 10 years until it lost virulence. This original strain was then distributed to several centers around the world for vaccine production. Unfortunately, the original BCG isolated by Calmette and Guérin has been lost and the subcultured variants undoubtably underwent genetic drift to generate strains that differed in immunological properties. Efficacy studies as a vaccine against TB have given puzzling results perhaps because of this genetic drift or for other reasons (Collins, 1974). The vaccine is highly effective in England but shows limited efficacy in adults in southern India (Hart and Sutherland, 1977; Tub. Prev. Trial Madras). One explanation for this puzzling result is that the efficacy of the vaccine strain may depend on the prior exposure of the individual. If an individual is exposed to another *Mycobacterium,* they may develop immunty that prevents the vaccine strain from persisting long enough to provide cellular immunity. Thus, the relationship with age and location is linked to exposure to other *Mycobacterium* spp. (B. Bloom, personal communication).

X. BCG as a Carrier of Heterologous Antigens

Whether or not BCG is effective as a vaccine against tuberculosis, it shows terrific promise as an immunological vehicle to vaccinate against foreign antigens both in subunit vaccines and by expression of foreign antigens in the living bacteria. BCG has been administered to about a billion people within the first months of life with remarkably few side-effects (Lotte *et al.,* 1984). Its adjuvant qualities have been well documented. Killed BCG included in Freund's adjuvant stimulates cellular immunity against other included antigens. The most exciting demonstration of its adjuvant qualities is that it can be given live with other killed microorganisms, such as *M. leprae,* stimulating high cellular immunity against the killed bacteria. The most striking demonstration of this is that the immunological anergy present in lepromatous leprosy can be overcome. Individuals with this disease normally have a very poor prognosis but when given this combination vaccine, many have recovered.

The first hurdle in developing BCG for expression of foreign antigens is to develop a method of introducing cloned antigens into living BCG. A two-step procedure has been developed (Jacobs *et al.,* 1987). The cosmid vector pHC79 was used to clone large random fragments of a double-stranded DNA bacteriophage from *M. smegmatis* (TM4) in *E. coli.* DNA from these TM4 cosmid recombinants was used to transfect *M. smegmatis* to regenerate viable phage, called phasmids by the authors because they were composites of functional plasmid and phage DNA. The phasmid DNA propagated as phage in *M. smegmatis* was used successfully to infect several strains of BCG. Obviously many other hurdles will have to be overcome before this system is practical, including identification of suitable cloning sites in the hybrid vector, expression of foreign antigens, and stable expression of new genes in BCG.

XI. Conclusions

Recombinant DNA techniques, transposon mutagenesis, and other modern methods are only now having an impact on the development of new bacterial vaccines. The primary reason vaccine development has lagged behind advances in bacterial antibiotic therapy is the small investment made by the National Institute of Health and pharmaceutical companies, the latter because of low profit margins for vaccines and high costs of liability insurance. In spite of this, we feel that the types of attenuating mutations that make ideal bacterial vaccines will be discovered in the next few years. Furthermore, from the standpoint of multivalent protection against other pathogens, there is now evidence that the immune response to *Salmonella* may be changed by the attenuating mutation (O'Callaghan *et al.,* 1988). Thus, vaccine strains may be engineered to provide the optimum immunity to a particular pathogen by changing how and in what organ a bacteria persists. The likely consequence of these new developments is that within the next 10 years several *Salmonella* strains, as well as strains of *Mycobacterium,* will be developed as carriers for antigens from many different pathogens. These vaccine strains will be optimized to provide the type of immunity appropriate to the disease. Strains will be developed that provide high IgA response as carriers for inactivated enterotoxins such as those found in *V. cholerae, Shigella* spp., and enterotoxigenic *E. coli.* Multivalent *Salmonella* and *Mycobacterium* vaccines that include protective antigens from *Brucella, Listeria, Legionella,* and *Franciscella* will be constructed because these pathogens require a high cellular response for protection. Efficient human and veterinary vaccination with easily prepared and administered vaccine strains could then ensue, resulting in decreased incidences of these insidious diseases worldwide.

REFERENCES

Acharya, I. L., Lowe, C. U., Thapa, R., Gurubacharya, V. L., Shrestha, M. B., Bact, D., Cadoz, M., Schulz, D., Armand, J., Bryla, D., Trollfors, B., Cramton, T., Schneerson, R., and Robbins, J. B. (1987). *N. Engl. J. Med.* **317,** 1101–1104.
Adu, H. O., Curtis, J., and Turk, J. L. (1983). *Cell. Immunol.* **78,** 249–256.
Aksamit, R. R., Backlund, P. S., and Cantoni, G. L. (1985). *Proc. Natl. Acad. Sci. U. S. A.* **82,** 7475–7479.

Alton, G. G. (1970). *Res. Vet. Sci.* **11,** 54–59.

Alton, G. G. (1978). *Aust. Vet. J.* **54,** 551.

Alton, G. G., and Elberg, S. S. (1967). *Vet. Bull.* **37,** 793–800.

Angerman, C. R., and Eisenstein, T. K. (1978). *Infect. Immun.* **19,** 575–582.

Angerman, C. R., and Eisenstein, T. K. (1980). *Infect. Immun.* **27,** 435–443.

Ashcroft, M. T., Ritchie, J. M., and Nicholson, C. C. (1964). *Am. J. Hyg.* **79,** 196–206.

Bacon, G. A., Burrows, T. W., and Yates, M. (1950). *Br. J. Exp. Pathol.* **31,** 714–724.

Bacon, G. A., Burrows, T. W., and Yates, M. (1951). *Br. J. Exp. Pathol.* **32,** 85–96.

Baron, L. S., Kopecko, D. J., Formal, S. B., Seid, R., Guerry, P., and Powell, C. (1987). *Infect. Immun.* **55,** 2797–2801.

Bosseray, N. (1978). *Br. J. Exp. Pathol.* **59,** 354–365.

Brown, A., Hormaeche, C. E., Demarco de Hormaeche, R., Winther, M. D., Dougan, G., Maskell, D. J., and Stocker, B. A. D. (1987). *J. Infect. Dis.* **155,** 86–92.

Brown, I. N., Glynn, A. A., and Plant, J. (1982). *Immunology* **47,** 149–156.

Buck, J. M. (1930). *J. Agric. Res. (Washington, D.C.)* **41,** 667–689.

Centers for Disease Control (1987). *Morbid. Mortal. Wkly. Rep.* **35,** 585–593

Cheers, C., and Sandrin, M. S. (1983). *Cell. Immunol.* **78,** 199–205.

Cher, D. J., and Mosmann, T. R. (1987). *J. Immunol.* **138,** 3688–3694.

Chopra, A. K., Houston, C. W., Peterson, J. W., Prasad, R., and Mekalanos, J. J. (1987). *J. Bacteriol.* **169,** 5095–5100.

Clements, J. D., and El-Morshidy, S. (1984). *Infect. Immun.* **46,** 564–569.

Clements, J. D., and Finkelstein, R. A. (1978). *Infect. Immun.* **21,** 1036–1039.

Clements, J. D., Lyon, F. L., Lowe, K. L., Farrand, A. L., and el-Morshidy, S. (1986). *Infect. Immun.* **53,** 685–693.

Collins, F. (1974). *Bacteriol. Rev.* **38,** 371–402.

Collins, F. (1984). *In* "Bacterial Vaccines" (R. Germanier, ed.), p. 373. Academic Press, New York.

Collins, F. M. (1969). *J. Bacteriol.* **97,** 676–683.

Collins, F. M., and Mackaness, G. B. (1968). *J. Immunol.* **101,** 830–845.

Collins, F. M., Mackaness, G. B., and Blanden, R. V. (1966). *J. Exp. Med.* **124,** 601–619.

Colwell, D. E., Michalek, S. M., Briles, D. E., Jirillo, E., and McGhee, J. R. (1984). *J. Immunol.* **133,** 950–957.

Colwell, D. E., Michalek, S. M., and McGhee, J. R. (1986). *Curr. Top. Microbiol. Immunol.* **124,** 121–147.

Cooper, N. R., and Ziccardi, R. J. (1976). *Miami Winter Symp.* **11,** 167.

Cotton, W. E., and Buck, J. M. (1932). *J. Am. Vet. Med. Assoc.* **33,** 342–355.

De Libero, G., and Kaufmann, H. E. (1986). *J. Immunol.* **137,** 2688–2694.

Dougan, G., Sellwood, R., Maskell, D., Sweeney, K., Beesley, J., and Hormaeche, C. (1986). *Infect. Immun.* **52,** 344–347.

Dougan, G., Hormaeche, C. E., and Maskell, D. J. (1987a). *Parasite Immunol.* **9,** 151–160.

Dougan, G., Maskell, D., Pickard, D., and Hormaeche, C. (1987b). *Mol. Gen. Genet.* **207,** 402–405.

Eisenstein, T. K., and Sultzer, B. M. (1983). *Adv. Exp. Med. Biol.* **162.**

Eisenstein, T. K., Killar, L. M., and Sultzer, B. M. (1984). *J. Infect. Dis.* **150,** 425–435.

Elberg, S. S., and Faunce, K., Jr. (1957). *J. Bacteriol.* **73,** 211–217.

Fields, P. I., Swanson, R. V., Haidaris, C. G., and Heffron, F. L. (1986). *Proc. Natl. Acad. Sci. U.S.A.* **83,** 5189–5193.

Finley, B. B., Gumbiner, B., and Falkow, S. (1988). Submitted for publication.

Formal, S. B., Baron, L. S., Kopecko, D. J., Washington, O., Powell, C., and Life, C. A. (1981). *Infect. Immun.* **34,** 746–751.

Germanier, R. (1970). *Infect. Immun.* **2**, 309–315.

Germanier, R., and Furer, E. (1975). *J. Infect. Dis.* **131**, 553–558.

Giannella, R. A., Formal, S. B., Dammin, G. J., and Collins, H. (1973). *J. Clin. Invest.* **52**, 441–453.

Gilman, R. H., Hornick, R. B., Woodward, W. E., DuPont, H. L., Snyder, M. J., Levine, M. M., and Libonati, J. P. (1977). J. Infect. Dis. 136, 717–723.

Goren, M. N., D'Arey Hart, P., Young, M. R., and Armstrong, J. R. (1976). *Proc. Natl. Acad. Sci. U.S.A.* **73**, 2510–2514.

Guidolin, A., and Manning, P. A. (1987). *Microbiol. Rev.* **51**, 285–299.

Hale, T. L., and Formal, S. B. (1981). *Infect Immun.* **32**, 137–144.

Hale, T. L., and Formal, S. B. (1986). *Microb. Pathog.* **1**, 511–518.

Hart, P. D., and Sutherland, I. (1977). *Br. Med. J.* **2**, 293–295.

Hirschel, B., Wuthrich, R., Somaini, B., and Steffen, R. (1985). *Eur. J. Clin. Microbiol.* **4**, 295–298.

Ho, M., and Cheers, C. (1982). *J. Infect. Dis.* **146**, 381–387.

Hoiseth, S. K., and Stocker, B. A. D. (1981). *Nature (London)* **291**, 238–239.

Honda, T., and Finkelstein, R. A. (1979). *Proc. Natl. Acad. Sci. U.S.A.* **76**, 2052–2056.

Hone, D., Morona, R., Attridge, S., and Hackett, J. (1987). *J. Infect. Dis.* **156**, 167–174.

Hoops, P., Prather, N. E., Berry, L. J., and Ravel, J. M. (1976). *Infect. Immun.* **13**, 1184–1192.

Hormaeche, C. E. (1979a). *Immunology* **37**, 311–318.

Hormaeche, C. E. (1979b). *Immunology* **37**, 319–327.

Hormaeche, C. E., Fahrenkrog, M. C., Pettifor, R. A., and Brock, J. (1980). *Immunology* **43**, 547–553.

Hornick, R. B., Greisman, S. E., Woodward, T. E., DuPont, H. L., Dawkins, A. T., and Snyder, M. J. (1970). *N. Engl. J. Med.* **283**, 686–691, 739–746.

Jacobs, W. R., Tuckman, M., and Bloom, B. R. (1987). *Nature (London)* **327**, 532.

Jones, G. W., Richardons, L. A., and Uhlman, D. (1981). *J. Gen. Microbiol.* **127**, 351–360.

Kaper, T. B., Lockman, H., Baldini, M. M., and Levine, M. (1984). *Nature (London)* **308**, 655–658.

Kaufmann, S. H., Hug, E., Vath, U., and Muller, I. (1985). *Infect. Immun.* **48**, 263–266.

Killar, L. M., and Eisenstein, T. K. (1984). *J. Immunol.* **133**, 1190–1196.

Killar, L. M., and Eisenstein, T. K. (1985). *Infect. Immun.* **47**, 605–612.

Killar, L. M., and Eisenstein, T. K. (1986). *Infect. Immun.* **52**, 504–508.

Killion, J. W., and Morrison, D. C. (1986). *Infect. Immun.* **54**, 1–8.

Kopecko, D. J., Washington, O., and Formal, S. B. (1980). *Infect. Immunol.* **29**, 207–214.

Kopecko, D. J., Baron, L. S., and Buysse, J. (1985a). *Curr. Top. Microbiol. Immunol.* **118**, 71–95.

Kopecko, D. J., Washington, D., and Formal, S. B. (1985b). *Infect. Immun.* **29**, 207–211.

Kuusi, N., Nurminen, M., Saxén, H., and Makela, P. H. (1981). *Infect. Immun.* **34**, 328–332.

Levine, M. M., DuPont, H. L., Hornick, R. B., Snyder, M. J., Woodward, W., Gilman, R. H., and Libonati, J. P. (1976). *J. Infect. Dis.* **133**, 424–429.

Levine, M. M., Black, R. E., Clements, M. L., Cisneros, L., Saah, A., Nalin, D. R., Gill, D. M., Craig, J. P., Young, C. R., and Ristaino, P. (1982). J. Infect. Dis. 145, 296–299.

Levine, M. M., Black, R. E., Clements, M. L., Lanata, C., Sears, S. *et al.* (1984). *Infect. Immun.* **43**, 515–522.

Levine, M. M., Ferreccio, C., Black, R. E., Germanier, R., and Chilean Typhoid Committee (1987a). *Lancet* **1**, 1049–1052.

Levine, M. M., Herrington, D., Murphy, J. R., Morris, J. G., Losonsky, G., Tall, B., Lindberg, A. A., Svenson, S., Bagar, S., Edwards, M. F., and Stocker, B. (1987b). *J. Clin. Invest.* **79**, 888–902.

Lissner, C. R., Swanson, R. N., and O'Brien, A. D. (1983). *J. Immunol.* **131**, 3006–3013.

Lotte, A. *et al.* (1984). *Adv. Tuber. Res.* **32**, 107–193.

Lyman, M. B., Steward, J. P., and Roantree, R. J. (1976). *Infect. Immun.* **13**, 1539–1542.

Mackaness, G. B., Blanden, R. V., and Collins, F. M. (1966). *J. Exp. Med.* **124**, 573–583.

Mäkelä, P. H., and Stocker, B. A. D. (1984). "Genetics of Lipopolysaccharide. Handbook of Endotoxin, Vol. 1: Chemistry of Endotoxin."

McEwen, A. D., and Priestly, F. W. (1938). *Vet. Rec.* **50**, 1097–1105.

McFarland, W. C., and Stocker, B. A. D. (1987). *Microb. Pathog.* (in press).

Maskell, D., Liew, F. Y., Sweeny, K., Dougan, G., and Hormaeche, C. (1986a). *In* "Vaccines '86" (F. Brown, R. M. Chanock, and R. A. Lerner, eds.), pp. 213–217. Cold Spring Harbor Lab., Cold Spring Harbor, New York.

Maskell, D., Liew, F. Y., Sweeney, K., Dougan, G., and Hormaeche, C. (1986b). *In* "Vaccines '86" (F. Brown, R. M. Chanock, and R. A. Lerner, eds.), pp. 213–217. Cold Spring Harbor Lab., Cold Spring Harbor, New York.

Maskell, D. J., Sweeney, K. J., O'Callaghan, D., Hormaeche, C. E., Liew, F. Y., and Dougan, G. (1987). *Microb. Pathog.* **2**, 211–220.

Mekalanos, J. J., Swarts, D. J., Pearson, G. D. N., Harford, N., Groyne, F., and De Wilde, M. (1983). *Nature (London)* **306**, 551–556.

Mel, D. M., Terzin, A. L., and Vüksić, L. (1965). *Bull. W.H.O.* **32**, 647–655.

Mosmann, T. R., and Coffman, R. L. (1987). *Immunol. Today* 223–227.

Mustafa, A. S., Gill, H. K., Nerland, A., Britton, W. J., Mehra, V., Bloom, B. R., Young, R. A., and Godal, T. (1986). *Nature (London)* **319**, 63–66.

Nakano, N., and Saito, K. (1969). *Nature (London)* **222**, 1085–1086.

Nnalue, N. A., and Stocker, B. A. D. (1987). *Infect. Immun.* **55**, 955–962.

North, R. J. (1970). *J. Exp. Med.* **132**, 521–534.

North, R. J. (1978). *J. Immunol.* **121**, 806–809.

O'Brien, A. D. (1986). *Curr. Top. Microbiol. Immunol.* **124**, 37–48.

O'Brien, A. D., and Metcalf, E. S. (1982). *J. Immunol.* **129**, 1349–1351.

O'Brien, A. D., Scher, I., Campbell, G. H., MacDermott, R. P., and Formal, S. B. (1979). *J. Immunol.* **123**, 720–724.

O'Brien, A. D., Scher, I., and Metcalf, E. S. (1981). *J. Immunol.* **126**, 1368–1372.

O'Brien, A. D., Metcalf, E. S., and Rosenstreich, D. L. (1982). *Cell Immunol.* **67**, 325–333.

O'Callaghan, D., Maskell, D., Liew, F. Y., Easman, C. S. F., and Dougan, G. (1988). *Infect. Immun.* (submitted for publication).

Orme, I. M., and Collins, F. M. (1984). *Cell. Immunol.* **84**, 113–120.

Panicali, D., Davis, S. W., Weinberg, R. L., and Paoletti, E. (1983). *Proc. Natl. Acad. Sci. U.S.A.* **80**, 5364–5369.

Pavlov, H., Hogarth, M., McKenzie, I. F. C., and Cheers, C. (1982). *Cell. Immunol.* **71**, 127–138.

Plommet, M., Serre, A., and Fensterbank, R. (1987). *Ann. Microbiol. (Paris)* **138**, 69–144.

Reitman, M. (1967). *J. Infect. Dis.* **117**, 101–108.

Robertsson, J. A., Lindberg, A. A., Hoiseth, S. K., and Stocker, B. A. D. (1983). *Infect. Immun.* **41**, 742–750.

Saxén, H. (1984). *J. Gen. Microbiol.* **130**, 2277–2283.

Shinnick, T. M., Sweetser, D. S., Thole, J., van Embden, J., and Young, R. A. (1987). *Infect. Immun.* **55**, 1932–1935.

Silva, B. A., Gonzalez, C., Mora, G. C., and Cabellao, F. (1987). *J. Infect. Dis.* **155,** 1077–1078.

Silva-Salinas, B. A., Rodriguez-Aguayo, L., Maldonado-Ballesteros, A., Valenzuela-Montero, M. E., and Sesane-Montecinos, M. (1985). *Bol. Med. Hosp. Infant. Mex. (Span. Ed.)* **42,** 234–239.

Skamene, E. P., Gros, A., Forget, P. A. L., Kongshavn, C., and Taylor, B. A. (1982). *Nature (London)* **297,** 506–509.

Small, P. L. C., Isberg, R. R., and Falkow, S. (1987). *Infect. Immun.* **55,** 1674–1679.

Smith, B. P., Reina-Guerra, M., Hoiseth, S. K., Stocker, B. A. D., Habasha, F., Johnson, E., and Merritt, F. (1984). *Am. J. Vet. Res.* **45,** 59–66.

Smith, H. W., and Linggood, M. A. (1971). *J. Med. Microbiol.* **4,** 467–485.

Southern, P. J., Blount, P., and Oldstone, M. B. A. (1984). *Nature (London)* **312,** 555–558.

Stevenson, G., and Manning, P. A. (1985). *FEMS Microbiol. Lett.* **28,** 317–321.

Svenson, S. B., Nurminen, M., and Lindberg, A. A. (1979). *Infect. Immun.* **25,** 863–872.

Tapa, S., and Cvjetanovic, B. (1975). *Bull. W.H.O.* **52,** 75–80.

Taylor, B. A., and O'Brien, A. D. (1982). *Immunology* **36,** 1257–1260.

Townsend, A. R. M., Rothbard, J., Gotch, F. M., Bahadur, G., Wraith, D., and McMichael, A. J. (1986). *Cell* **44,** 959–968.

Tramont, E. C., Chung, R., Gernan, S., Keren, D., Kapfer, C., and Formal, S. B. (1984). *J. Infect. Dis.* **149,** 133–140.

Venneman, M. R., Bigley, N. J., and Berry, L. J. (1970). *Infect. Immun.* **1,** 574–582.

Wahdan, M. H., Seri, C., Germanier, R., Lackany, A., Carisier, Y., Guerin, N., Salam, S., Geoffrey, P., Saadekn El Tantawi, A., and Guesry, P. (1980). *Bull. W.H.O.* **58,** 469–474.

Wahdan, M. H., Seri, C., Cerisier, Y., Salam, S., and Germanier, R. (1982). *J. Infect. Dis.* **145,** 292–295.

Weiss, A. A., Hewlett, E. L., Myers, G. A., and Falkow, S. (1983). *Infect. Immun.* **42,** 33–41.

Woodward, W. E. (1980). *Trans. R. Soc. Trop. Med. Hyg.* **74,** 553–556.

World Health Organization (1986). *Wkly. Epidemiol. Rec.* **61,** 197–198.

World Health Organization (1987). *Wkly. Epidemiol. Rec.* **62,** 141–142.

Zdrodowski, P., Vershilova, P., and Kotlarova, H. (1957). *J. Infect. Dis.* **101,** 1–7.

Immunomodifiers in Vaccines

AMNON ALTMAN[1] AND FRANK J. DIXON

*Department of Immunology, Research Institute of Scripps Clinic,
La Jolla, California*

I. Introduction

Despite rapid progress in all branches of science and technology, infectious diseases still afflict hundreds of millions of persons throughout the world, mostly in developing countries, resulting in physical

[1] A. A. is a Scholar of the Leukemia Society of America, Inc.

disabilities and death. Even for diseases such as hepatitis B, although a vaccine has been developed, it is not available to the majority of the estimated 200 million individuals infected with this virus due to economic and other reasons (Moss *et al.*, 1984). For many other diseases, such as malaria, no appropriate vaccines exist. Furthermore, there are considerable deficiencies in existing vaccines, including unwanted side effects and difficulties in production, storage, and delivery systems. This scenario and the recent emergence of the acquired immunodeficiency syndrome (AIDS) have highlighted the need for innovative strategies in the production of a new generation of vaccines against infectious diseases.

An ideal vaccine should elicit strong and long-lasting protective immunity with few injections, evoke minimal side effects, be readily available, inexpensive, stable, and easily administered. One traditional problem in vaccine development has, until recently, been the difficulty of producing sufficiently large and pure preparations of antigenic material from various pathogens. However, owing to recent developments in molecular biology, chemistry, and immunology, this problem has been solved to a large extent, and economical and efficient methods are now available to produce antigenic material in large quantities (see Section II). At the same time, it has become clear that such antigens, while providing specific and appropriate epitopes that can serve as targets for recognition by the immune system, usually are not, in themselves, sufficiently immunogenic, due either to their small size or to the lack of intrinsic immunostimulatory properties. Therefore, appropriate means are necessary to augment the immunogenicity of these antigen preparations.

The purpose of this review article is to focus on the components of a successful vaccine other than the antigen itself, namely, the vehicle used for antigen delivery, immunostimulatory substances designed to enhance its immunogenicity and, in the case of small antigens such as synthetic peptides, appropriate carrier molecules that may be required for an optimal immune response. These components are included in the vaccine preparation to enhance the immune response to the antigen in a way that is beneficial to the host, and fall, therefore, under the definition of immunomodifiers. In this respect, we will describe recent developments in these areas as well as our own experience with a model immune response to a synthetic peptide antigen. Several reviews in this field have been published (Allison, 1979; Waksman, 1979; Edelman, 1980; Warren *et al.*, 1986).

Other considerations important in the design of successful vaccines are the desired balance between, and relative importance of, humoral *versus* cell-mediated immunity, the presence of epitopes capable of stimulating an effective T helper cell response, elimination of epitopes that induce immune suppression, the relationship between immuno-dominant and protective epitopes, and the need for specialized humoral responses such as IgA antibodies in immune defense mechanisms of the gut mucosa.

II. New Strategies for Preparation of Vaccine Antigens

The new experimental approaches for preparing vaccine antigens in large quantities are described in detail in other chapters of this volume. However, in the interest of completeness of this presentation, we would like to describe briefly the main features of these approaches. New strategies for preparation of antigenic material fall into two main categories: (1) those that rely on nonreplicating vaccines, and (2) those that use live vaccines. The three main experimental approaches for generating nonreplicating vaccines are:

1. Expression in prokaryotic or eukaryotic cells. This approach is a direct derivative of recent advances in molecular biology that have allowed expression of genes encoding various proteins in bacterial, yeast, and mammalian cells using appropriate expression vectors. The transfected genes are usually expressed at a high level, but the biological activity of the expressed products is usually low, with the exception of hepatitis B surface antigen (HBsAg), which self-assembles in the expressing host into immunogenic 22-nm particles similar to those isolated from plasma of infected individuals (Valenzuela *et al.*, 1982). The expressed antigens can be purified by conventional biochemical methods combined, where available, with affinity purification using appropriate monoclonal antibodies.

2. Synthetic peptides. This approach is based on the demonstration that chemically synthesized linear peptides derived from the primary sequences of numerous proteins can elicit antibodies reactive with the native protein (reviewed by Lerner, 1982; Sutcliffe *et al.*, 1983). A number of predictive methods have been employed to identify potential antigenic determinants on protein sequences, and antibodies prepared against several virally derived synthetic peptides have been shown to neutralize the corresponding viruses *in vitro* and, in some isntances, to confer protection against infectious virus *in vivo*.

3. Anti-idiotypic vaccines. The idiotype of an antibody molecule is located on, or close to, its antigen-binding site. Thus, antibodies

generated against an idiotypic site are expected, in at least some cases, to mimic the configuration of the antigen that induced the original antibody response (Nisonoff and Lamoyi, 1981). This was, in fact, found to be the case in several experimental systems. Immunization with anti-idiotypic antibodies directed against virus-specific antibodies was found to stimulate neutralizing antibody formation against the relevant virus. Although anti-idiotypic vaccines are not in themselves potent enough to stimulate a protective immune response, they can prime hosts for such a response following challenge with a subimmunogenic dose of the corresponding pathogen (Kennedy et al., 1985).

For the production of live vaccines, two major strategies have been used:

4. Attenuation by gene reassortment or deletion. These approaches are based on genetic recombination between related viruses that differ in some properties, as in the case of influenza A (Chanock and Murphy, 1980), or experimentally induced deletion of genes that are not essential for replication, an approach actively pursued with herpes simplex virus (Post and Roizman, 1981). The result is an attenuated genetic variant that can replicate and thus provide a constant source of antigen for immune stimulation without inducing disease.

5. Use of attenuated virus vectors for carrying foreign genes. This strategy depends on the insertion of genes encoding protective microbial antigens into a virus that is attenuated for humans, an approach that is being intensively pursued using vaccinia virus as the attenuated vector (Panicali and Paoletti, 1982; Mackett et al., 1982). A large part of the vaccinia virus genome can be replaced by foreign genes without affecting its ability to grow. This virus has a long history of safe use in humans, and antigens expressed by a replicating vaccinia virus have the advantage of appearing on the cell surface in the context of host major histocompatibility complex (MHC) antigens, thus being capable of stimulating appropriate cell-mediated immunity. Immunization with recombinant vaccinia virus carrying genes of malaria sporozoite, influenza, herpes simplex, hepatitis B, and several other viruses was found to stimulate production of neutralizing antibodies and confer protection against these pathogens (Paoletti et al., 1984; Smith et al., 1984).

III. Components of an Effective Vaccine

Until very recently, most vaccines consisted of either attenuated live pathogens or killed whole organisms that present to the immune system a large complex of multiple antigenic determinants, combining to confer upon such immunogens intrinsic immunostimulatory properties. Newly available subunit vaccines of single antigens produced by recombinant DNA technology or small, hapten-like synthetic peptides generally represent products of low immunogenicity. Thus, since the synthetic antigens of the future are likely to be relatively weak immunogens, they will require appropriate manipulations to enhance their immunogenic properties.

Effective vaccine formulations in the form of complete Freund's adjuvant (CFA) have, in fact, been known for a long time. The key characteristic of CFA is the emulsification of the aqueous antigen solution in mineral oil to ensure the formation of a slow-release antigen depot at the site of injection, and killed mycobacteria as nonspecific immunostimulators (IS; Freund *et al.*, 1937; Freund, 1956). An emulsifier, Arlacel A, is used to form a stable water-in-oil (w/o) emulsion. The powerful immunostimulatory effect of CFA has not been surpassed by any other adjuvant. However, neither CFA nor incomplete Freund's adjuvant (IFA, which lacks mycobacteria) has been licensed for use in this country in human or veterinary vaccines because of the adverse reactions they may produce, i.e., local granulomas, pain, fever, and possibly malignancies. Thus, a major goal in the area of vaccine development is the production of vaccine formulations that will have the desirable effects, and lack the deleterious side effects, of CFA
.   As mentioned earlier, the essential components of a vaccine, in addition to the specific antigen itself, are the vehicle and the IS and, in the case of small hapten-like antigens, also the carrier. The remainder of this presentation will cover these three components. This division is arbitrary to some extent since, in many instances, it is difficult to draw the line between the activity of a given substance as a vehicle or an IS. For example, substances herein refered to as vehicles (such as w/o emulsions) have intrinsic immunostimulatory properties, and certain IS have been coupled to small antigens and, hence, used as carriers. However, this division is convenient and simplifies the presentation. The use of the term "adjuvant" will be avoided as much as possible, since it can be confusing. If this term is used to define, in a general way, agents that increase antigen-specific immune responses, then both true immunostimulators as well as some vehicles (e.g., w/o emulsions) can be considered as adjuvants.

IV. The Experimental System

During the past 5 years, we conducted a series of studies designed to define effective vaccine formulations in terms of carriers, vehicles, and

IS. The model antigen selected for these studies is peptide 72 (p72), a chemically synthesized 28 amino acid peptide corresponding to residues 110–137 of the surface glycoprotein of the hepatitis B virus, subtype *ad*. The majority of amino acid changes among hepatitis B subtypes occur within this hydrophilic region, which specifies the major *d/y* subtype system (Gerin *et al.*, 1983). Antibodies prepared against a highly similar synthetic peptide corresponding to residues 110–137 of HBsAg, subtype *ay*, were shown to bind to the native HBsAg, and chimpanzees immunized with this synthetic peptide (conjugated to keyhole limpet hemocyanin) were partially protected against subsequent challenge with infectious virus (Gerin *et al.*, 1983).

The general design of the experiments consisted of injecting various formulations of p72 (with respect to carriers, vehicles, and IS) at several sites by the subcutaneous or intramuscular routes into (BALB/c × A/J)F_1 hybrid mice or outbred rabbits, respectively. One group in each experiment was injected with a p72-tetanus toxoid (TT) conjugate incorporated in IFA. This group served as a positive control and a reference, since high titer and long-lasting anti-p72 responses were usually achieved under these conditions. Animals were bled at regular intervals beginning at 2 weeks post priming. Antibody titers against p72 or the carrier protein were determined by a standard enzyme-linked immunosorbent assay (ELISA). Titers were calculated as the reciprocal serum dilution that produced half of the maximal optical density value in a given ELISA (averaged for 5 animals per group), and the use of a high-titered anti-p72 reference serum allowed comparison of titers in sequential bleeds during the course of an experiment. If reasonably high antibody titers were not detected following priming with a certain vaccine formulation, the animals were boosted with the vaccine later, usually 3–6 months after the first injection. In many experiments, testing of the animals continued for 1–2 years to examine the persistence of the antibody response. In addition, most experiments were accompanied by a histologic evaluation of the injection site to determine the cellular infiltrates that may be indicative of the types of ongoing inflammatory tissue reactions.

V. Carriers

The introduction of defined haptenic groups onto immunogenic carriers by Landsteiner has provided a powerful tool for the analysis of specific interactions between antigens and cells of the immune system. For many years, it has been known that immunization with a hapten elicits antibody responses only when the hapten is coupled to a carrier substance that is itself immunogenic; nonimmunogenic substances serve only poorly, or not at all, as carriers for haptens (Benacerraf *et al.*, 1963). The first direct evidence for cooperative participation of two immunocytes with distinct determinant specificities in the antibody response to hapten–carrier conjugates was obtained by Mitchison (1969). It was later demonstrated that this cooperation occurs between carrier-specific T helper (Th) cells and hapten-specific, antibody-producing B cells. Thus, the inability of free haptens, including most small synthetic peptide antigens, to stimulate an antibody response results from their lack of determinants capable of stimulating T-cell help. Therefore, if the use of synthetic peptides as efficient vaccines is to be realized, in most cases they will have to be introduced to their hosts in the form of conjugates with appropriate T-cell-stimulating carriers. The importance of conjugating antigenic peptides to carriers is demonstrated in Fig. 1. Thus, glutaraldehyde-polymerized peptide or a mixture of monomeric or polymerized peptide plus carrier is not

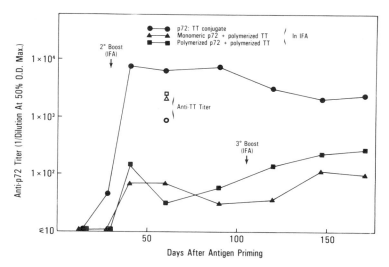

FIG. 1.   Coupling of p72 to a protein carrier is required for the induction of optimal antipeptide responses. Mice were primed with 40 μg of p72:TT conjugate, or with combinations (20 μg each) of monomeric p72 plus glutaraldehyde cross-linked TT, or cross-linked p72 plus TT, all given in IFA. A booster injection of the same antigen preparations in IFA was given on day 29 (secondary boost), and an additional injection given to two of the groups on day 105 (tertiary boost). Antibody titers against TT on day 60 are shown by the open symbols for each of the three groups.

sufficient for stimulating a strong antibody response. Such a response
is seen only when the peptide and carrier are covalently linked.

A. CARRIER-INDEPENDENT ANTIBODY RESPONSES

As mentioned previously, most short synthetic peptides must be
coupled to immunogenic carriers to elicit peptide-specific antibodies.
However, in some studies, synthetic peptides were found to be immunogenic in their free form, and yet also stimulated T-cell-dependent
IgG antibody responses and immunologic memory (Neurath et al.,
1984). These results suggested that such peptides must contain distinct T- and B-cell epitopes, both of which are necessary for an optimal
antibody response. This point was addressed directly in recent studies
(Milich et al., 1986; Good et al., 1987). A 26-amino-acid synthetic
peptide derived from the pre-S(2) region of the HBsAg was found to
contain distinct T- and B-cell recognition sites in its amino- and
carboxy-terminal regions, respectively. This synthetic peptide was
highly immunogenic in responder mouse strains in its free form.
Moreover, the synthetic T-cell site provided T-cell help for an antibody
response against the synthetic B-cell epitope, which was cross-reative
with the native pre-S(2) antigen (Milich et al., 1986). Using an
algorithm designed to predict Th sites on proteins, Good et al. (1987)
identified a T-cell site on the circumsporozoite protein of Plasmodium
falciparum. When a synthetic peptide corresponding to this site was
covalently linked to a synthetic peptide representing the major B-cell
epitope on the molecule, an immunogen capable of eliciting a high-
titer antibody response was obtained. This peptide primed Th cells for
a secondary response to the intact malarial antigen (Good et al., 1987).
Thus, combination of T- and B-cell epitopes in a synthetic peptide,
either by selecting sequences that naturally contain such epitopes in
proximity, or by artifically coupling B- and T-cell epitopes that lie
apart in the natural sequence, may be a useful approach to bypass the
requirement for coupling an antigenic peptide to a large carrier.

Dreesman et al. (1982) reported that cyclization of an HBsAg-
derived synthetic peptide by oxidation-mediated formation of a disulfide bond between two cysteine residues present in this peptide
conferred upon this free synthetic antigen immunogenic properties so
that antibodies raised against it cross-reacted with the native HBsAg.
The assumption was that peptide cyclization locked in a secondary
structure that mimicked an immunodominant epitope of the natural
antigen. On the basis of the studies cited above, it is likely that
cyclization of the peptide generated a T-cell epitope that provided help

for an antibody response. Alternative approaches to bypass the requirement for a large carrier protein are to polymerize the synthetic peptide (Jolivet *et al.*, 1983; however, this method was unsuccessful with p72, as shown in Fig. 1), or to create a large polyvalent synthetic vaccine by coupling peptides from several pathogens (Jolivet *et al.*, 1987).

B. PROTEIN CARRIERS

Diphteria toxoid (DT), and, particularly TT, commonly have been used as protein carriers for synthetic peptide antigens, based on their safe record as human vaccines. Moreover, because most humans are immune to DT and TT, the response to a synthetic peptide conjugated to such carriers should be improved by the preexisting immune response to the carrier. This assumption is based on the classical carrier effect in which the secondary antibody response to challenge with a hatpen-carrier conjugate is optimal if the same hapten–carrier combination was used for priming (Ovary and Benacerraf, 1963). Similarly, under appropriate conditions, animals preimmunized with a free carrier manifest enhanced anti-hapten antibody responses following primary immunization with the hapten coupled to the same carrier (Katz *et al.*, 1970). This effect reflects numerical expansion of carrier-specific Th cells during priming; the expanded population can then provide augmented help for the anti-hapten (peptide) antibody response when that hapten is seen in the context of the original carrier.

These concepts have, however, been challenged recently by studies on a new immunoregulatory mechanism, termed epitope suppression. Herzenberg *et al.* (1980) demonstrated that preimmunization of mice with a given carrier suppressed a primary immune response to a new hapten presented on the same carrier without affecting the antibody response to the carrier itself or the development of B-cell memory against the hapten. Schutze *et al.* (1985) reported that the antibody response to a synthetic peptide conjugated to TT could be suppressed by preexisting TT-specific immunity, although this suppression was overcome by including killed *Bordetella pertussis* microbes or muramyl dipeptides (MDP) with the first carrier immunization (Vogel *et al.*, 1987). Thus, it may be that complex immunoregulatory interactions and the status of the immune system during carrier challenge (i.e., whether help or suppression dominate) determine the final outcome, that is, whether the carrier effect will be stimulatory or suppressive. Another potential problem associated with the use of a carrier to which an individual had previously been immunized is that the preexisting antibodies form immune complexes with the carrier–peptide conjugate, resulting in rapid clearance of the conjugate. Such problems cast doubt about the routine or repeated use of DT or TT as carriers for synthetic peptide vaccines and necessitate evaluation of other proteins as potential carriers.

We have evaluated two inexpensive and readily available plant proteins, i.e., pumpkin seed globulin and hemp seed protein (edestin) as carriers for p72 in rabbits or mice. These two proteins were compared to TT, the conventional carrier used in our studies. The results demonstrated that the two plant proteins, particularly pumpkin seed globulin, were effective carriers for an anti-p72 antibody response (Fig. 2). Thus, a choice of protein carriers is available for coupling to synthetic peptide antigens and, among the three vaccine components that are the subject of this review, the carrier problem appears to be the easiest one to solve.

C. Synthetic Amino Acid Polymers

Synthetic copolymers of selected amino acids have been used as carriers. The use of such polymers bypassed the problems associated with natural protein carriers to which individuals have been preim-

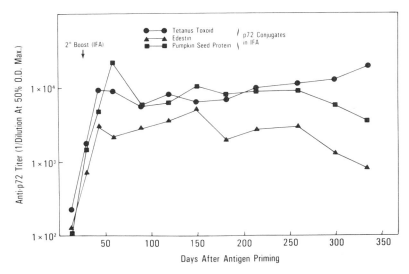

FIG. 2. Comparison of three carrier proteins in rabbit anti-p72 antibody responses. Rabbits were injected with 400 μg of p72-protein carrier conjugates (at a 1 : 1 ratio) in IFA and boosted with the same antigen preparation on day 29.

munized, e.g., DT and TT. Such polymers can be designed at will according to specific needs and synthesized with built-in immuno-stimulatory properties. The feasibility of this approach was demon-strated when synthetic peptides derived from bacteriophage MS-2, or DT were conjugated to a multichain copolymer of DL-alanine and L-lysine (Langbeheim *et al.*, 1976; Audibert *et al.*, 1982). Immunization of animals with such conjugates incorporated in CFA stimulated formation of antibodies reactive against the natural proteins. These antibodies neutralized the virus or protected against the dermonecro-tic effect of DT. Efficient responses were obtained even in an aqueous vehicle, provided the immunostimulator MDP was added to the vaccine or, even better, chemically coupled to the peptide–synthetic polymer conjugate (Audibert *et al.*, 1982).

D. Specific Antibodies and MHC Molecules as Targeted Carriers

A protective antibody response to a pathogen requires collaboration between defined cell types of the immune system. The minimal list of participants in the response includes the antibody-forming B cell, the Th cell, and the antigen-processing cell, usually a macrophage. If antigens could be targeted specifically to one or more of these cellular components, then this approach could potentially result in a more effective antibody response. This possibility was addressed in a recent study that borrowed from an experimental approach currently being tested widely in the field of cancer treatment, i.e., targeting cytotoxic drugs to tumor cells by means of conjugated monoclonal antibodies specific for such tumor cells. Based on recent findings that B cells can function as antigen-presenting cells (Chesnut and Grey, 1981), Kawa-mura and Berzofsky (1986) attempted specific targeting of a protein antigen (ferritin) to B cells by coupling the antigen to anti-murine IgM or IgG antibodies. Such conjugates were tested for their ability to stimulate the proliferation of a ferritin-specific T-cell line *in vitro* (using irradiated spleen cells as a source of antigen-presenting B cells), and to elicit an anti-ferritin antibody response *in vivo* when incorpo-rated in IFA. The ferritin–anti-Ig conjugates were compared to free ferritin as an immunogen. The results clearly demonstrated that the anti-Ig-conjugated ferritin was much more immunogenic than the free ferritin, both *in vitro* and *in vivo*.

Using a similar rationale, Carayanniotis and Barber (1987) at-tempted to target antigen specifically to the antigen-presenting cells by attaching the antigen (avidin) to anti-MHC class II monoclonal antibodies (via biotin molecules conjugated to the antibodies). They reported that such conjugates elicited an anti-avidin antibody response in the absence of an added adjuvant, whereas equivalent amounts of avidin mixed with the nonbiotinylated form of the same antibodies failed to elicit a response. A targeting effect occurred at low levels of the injected conjugate, because only mice bearing the appropriate class II MHC antigens responded. Antibodies to class I MHC antigens similarly enhanced the immunogenicity of avidin when conjugated to it. This study suggests that by employing appropriate methods to target antigens to the relevant cells of the immune system, one may avoid the use of adjuvants such as water-in-mineral oil emulsions, which cannot be used in human or veterinary vaccines. In future work, it will be important to determine which cell-surface molecules represent target structures capable of mediating this enhancement of immunogenicity, and then define the role of Th cells in this effect. In addition to B cells and macrophages, some T-cell-specific markers could also serve as potential structures for such targeting effects.

A somewhat less specific approach to target an antigen to the immune system has been that of attaching a hapten (dinitrophenyl, DNP) to class I MHC molecules (Sanderson, 1984). The rationale behind this approach is that allogeneic MHC antigens (the so-called strong transplantation antigens) are potent immunogens and stimulate a large fraction of T cells. Thus, the strong cell-mediated immunity against MHC alloantigens should be expected to provide potent help for an antibody response to an antigen linked to such MHC molecules. In support of this concept was the demonstration that attaching DNP to a purified human class I MHC (HLA) antigen, but not to an ovalbumin carrier, stimulated an efficient anti-DNP antibody response in monkeys (Sanderson, 1984). The practicality of this approach is questionable, however, since (1) MHC molecules are considered to be much more immunogenic in their native, i.e., cell-bound, form that in solution and (2) preparation of purified MHC antigens in the large quantities necessary for a mass vaccination may present significant technical problems.

E. NONPROTEIN CARRIERS

Because of the potential problems associated with the use of immunogenic carriers, especially in hosts with preexisting immunity to the carrier (see Section V,B), it might be advantageous to use carriers that are, in themselves, nonimmunogenic. Thus, Hopp (1984), demonstrated that conjugation of a synthetic hepatitis B virus peptide at its amino terminus to two molecules of palmitic acid via the α and ϵ amino groups of a lysine spacer resulted in an immunogen that stimulated antibody responses against HBsAg, but not against the palmitic acid carrier. The antibody titers obtained with this conjugate were considerably higher than when the same peptide was conjugated to a keyhole limpet hemocyanin carrier. Since these conjugates were incorporated into CFA, which is unacceptable in humans, it remains to be determined whether palmitic acid can serve as an efficient carrier for a peptide antigen formulated in other vehicles that may be acceptable for human, or at least veterinary, use.

VI. Vehicles

For an antigen to function as an efficient vaccine, it must stimulate a persistent, long-term immune response. In diseases of relatively long incubation periods, such as poliomyelitis, the stimulation of immunologic memory may be sufficient for induction of long-term immunity since an anamnestic antibody response can reach high levels within approximately 3 days after infection. However, in diseases with a short incubation period, e.g., influenza, long-term persistence of sufficiently high and protective antibody titers in the circulation is critical. One way to maintain high antibody responses for long periods after vaccination is to create an antigen depot at the injection site. The persistence of the antigen in such a depot and its slow rate of release ensure continuous stimulation of the immune system. This effect is achieved by incorporating the antigen in an appropriate vehicle. In the absence of such a vehicle, that is, when antigen is injected in an aqueous solution, the immune response is transient and consists primarily of IgM antibodies. As mentioned earlier, the distinction between vehicles and IS is not always clear-cut; in the context of this presentation, we refer to those materials included in a vaccine to slow the release of antigen (and added IS) as vehicles.

A. ALUMINUM SALTS

Aluminum compounds are the most widely used vehicles in vaccines licensed for veterinary or human use since the discovery that a suspension of alum-precipitated DT is more immunogenic than the same toxoid in an aqueous solution (Glenny et al., 1926). Although they occasionally induce sterile abscesses, aluminum salts have an excellent record of safety. These compounds consist of insoluble salts of aluminum hydroxide or aluminum phosphate. The hydrated form of the aluminum gel adsorbs protein due mainly to the electropositive net charge of the alum compounds below pH 9. Thus, the lower the pI of the antigen, the more efficient its adsorption, which may explain why antibody responses to some antigens are not enhanced by incorporation in alum vehicles. Presumably, such antigens are not adsorbed efficiently onto the alum. The stable adsorption of antigen to the alum compound creates an antigen depot, thus slowing the release of the antigen and extending the antibody response.

In addition to this effect, alum compounds probably act as true IS by virtue of their chemotactic properties. They stimulate a local production of granulomas consisting largely of macrophages. The inflammation-inducing properties of alum salts contribute to their immunostimulatory activity by attracting various cell types that may secrete biologically active cytokines.

Characteristically, the antibody response to a single injection of an alum-containing vaccine is brief, probably due to the relatively rapid clearance of antigen from the injection site and the lack of stimulation of cell-mediated immunity (Edelman, 1980; Bomford, 1980b). This problem may be partially overcome by repeated injections of the antigen, which is undesirable from a practical standpoint, as exemplified by the experiment summarized in Fig. 3. Following vaccination of mice with a p72:TT conjugate in alum gel, the primary antibody response against the synthetic peptide is lower by about one order of magnitude than that against the same antigen formulated in IFA. Second, the antibody response to the IFA-formulated vaccine can persist for up to 12 months, but the antibody titers against the alum-containing vaccine start to decline about 6 weeks after priming. Finally, the antibody response to the alum vaccine can be augmented to levels similar to those elicited with the IFA vaccine by boosting the mice with same vaccine preparation. However, this boosted response is also usually short-term and declines within 1–3 months, suggesting that alum vehicles may not be effective inducers of immunologic memory. Another problem with aluminum compounds is the difficulty of their manufacture under physicochemically reproducible conditions. As a result, variations in the stability of antigen adsorption and overall immunogenicity may exist between different batches of the same vaccine.

Although alum compounds may not be the ideal vehicles for primary immunization, they serve as efficient vehicles for booster injections provided an optimal immunization is obtained with the first vaccination. In such a case, the titer and duration of the secondary response

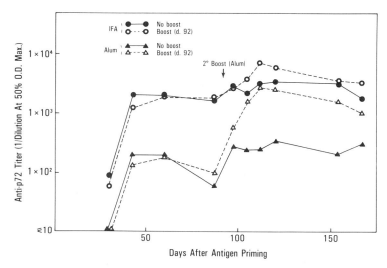

FIG. 3. Comparison of IFA and alum vehicles and the effect of antigen boost on murine anti-p72 antibody responses. Mice (ten per group) were primed with 40 μg of p72:TT in IFA or alum. Each group was divided into two subgroups, which were either unboosted or boosted with p72:TT in alum on day 92.

induced by a booster injection given in either alum or IFA are similar. This situation is illustrated in Table I.

In summary, aluminum salts may be a sufficient vehicle for strong immunogens, or when used as vehicles for booster injections, yet they may be inadequate in other situations. Thus, there is a clear need for

TABLE I

SECONDARY ANTI-p72 ANTIBODY RESPONSES IN MICE BOOSTED WITH p72:TT IN DIFFERENT VEHICLES[a]

	Secondary anti-p72 titers				
Boost	Day 14	Day 28	Day 40	Day 61	Day 180
None	320	220	410	330	300
p72:TT in alum	19,230	16,360	22,660	17,900	3,010
p72:TT in IFA	20,570	26,120	20,220	34,180	8,520

[a] CAF$_1$ mice were primed with 40 μg of p72:TT + TDM + MPL (100 μg each) in 2% squalene-in-water. Peak primary antibody response on day 60 was 1,410. Fourteen months after priming, when the anti-p72 antibody titer declined to less than 300, the mice were divided into three groups that were not boosted or boosted with p72:TT in alum or in IFA.

more effective vehicles, particularly in situations where cell-mediated immunity is important for a protective response.

B. WATER-IN-OIL (w/o) EMULSIONS

The development of w/o emulsions as vaccines emerged from early studies on tuberculosis in which both the antibody and the delayed type hypersensitivity (DTH) responses to killed mycobacteria were clearly enhanced when the organisms were incorporated in mineral oil emulsions (Freund *et al.*, 1937). Freund's adjuvant, which eventually evolved from these studies, consists of an aqueous solution of antigen emulsified at a 1 : 1 ratio in mineral oil, typically Drakeol 6-VR, by using an appropriate emulsifier. This mineral oil is a highly complex mixture of linear, cyclic, and branched-chain hydrocarbons and aromatics. Arlacel A, which is defined as mannide monooleate but also contains poorly defined fat and carbohydrate compounds, is commonly used as an emulsifier at a ratio of 1 : 9 parts Arlacel A to mineral oil, respectively. Addition of killed mycobacteria to this IFA emulsion converts it to CFA. Although IFA is an efficient vehicle for antibody responses, it does not stimulate a significant DTH response indicative of cell-mediated immunity (Edelman, 1980; Bomford, 1980b; Warren *et al.*, 1986).

As in the case of alum compounds, w/o emulsions mediate their immunopotentiating effects via two major mechanisms. First, the antigen is trapped within the water droplet phase of the lipid emulsion, creating a depot that releases antigen at a much slower rate than the alum compounds. This probably accounts for the fact that, with w/o emulsions, one injection is often sufficient to stimulate a high-titer, persistent antibody response. Second, the oil emulsion stimulates a local inflammatory reaction that consists of oil-ingesting macrophages, lymphocytes, and plasma cells, and persists for at least several months. This local reaction probably involves the production of active mediators that potentiate different arms of the immune response.

The powerful immunostimulatory effects of w/o emulsions, in particular CFA, have not been surpassed by any other vehicle–IS combination, and they still serve as the vaccine formulation of choice for laboratory experiments in animals. However, the use of w/o emulsions has been associated with a number of deleterious side effects that have excluded their routine use in veterinary and human vaccines, including local abscesses and granulomas, pain, fever, and possible carcinogenic effects (Edelman, 1980). Some of the toxic effects have been attributed to the presence in the mineral oil of linear short-chain hydrocarbons that act as lipid solvents and, therfore, cause damage to mammalian cell membranes. Mineral oils have also been known to induce plasmacytomas in BALB/c and NZB mice when administered intraperitoneally (Potter and Boyce, 1962). The emulsifier Arlacel A was found to be carcinogenic in males of one mouse strain, and to act as a tumor promoter in other strains (Murray *et al.*, 1972). IFA vehicles have been made more practical, however, by the use of highly refined mineral oils and Arlacel A that are free of toxic substances, and by injecting the vaccines intramuscularly rather than subcutaneously (Salk *et al.*, 1952, 1953). Many trials, involving a total of more than one million human subjects, have demonstrated the immunogenicity, safety, and efficacy of IFA combined with influenza and poliomyelitis vaccines (Edelman, 1980; Prigal, 1972). The only undesirable side effect of the mineral oil-containing w/o emulsions in humans was the infrequent occurrence of local nodules. Evaluators of long-term, follow-up studies of 18,000 army personnel immunized with an influenza vaccine in IFA concluded that no increases in malignant, allergic, or collagen diseases occurred (Beebe *et al.*, 1972).

The side effects associated with the use of mineral oils and Arlacel A, and the fact that mineral oils are not biodegradable, prompted an intense search for alternative and more acceptable oil vehicles. This effort has proceeded in three major directions, namely, the use of biodegradable oils, reduction of the oil content in the emulsion, and replacement of Arlacel A with safer emulsifiers.

C. BIODEGRADABLE OIL VEHICLES

Several formulations of w/o emulsions containing metabolizable oils instead of mineral oil have been developed. One of these is Adjuvant 65, a preparation of peanut oil, aluminum monostearate stabilizer, and Arlacel A emulsifier. This formulation contains only components that can be metabolized or are secreted by the body (Woodhour *et al.*, 1964). This vehicle was found to be safe and relatively potent in humans when combined with influenza vaccines (Hilleman *et al.*, 1972), although others found it to be less effective than IFA (Stuart-Harris, 1969).

Other encouraging modifications of oil emulsions have been reported, although they have not been extensively tested, including a preparation of highly refined peanut oil emulsified in aqueous vaccines using glycerol and lecithin as emulsifiers. This formulation potentiated antibody responses and protective immunity in several experimental models with marginally immunogenic doses of nonreplicating viral antigens (Reynolds *et al.*, 1980a). The oil components are metabolizable or normal constituents of the host, and are more readily emulsified than other w/o emulsions.

Whitehouse *et al.* (1974) demonstrated that squalene, a natural unsaturated oil that is an intermediate in the biosynthesis of cholesterol, as well as its hydrogenated form, squalane, functioned as potent vehicles for inducing allergic encephalitis in rats when emulsified with an aqueous solution of homogenized guinea pig spinal cord as the antigen. The immunostimulatory activity of these vehicles was high even in the absence of added mycobacteria, i.e., as biodegradable analogs of IFA. Squalane was more effective than squalene, probably due to its lower biodegradability and resultant slower rate of antigen release. Similarly, squalane was found to be as effective as mineral oil in providing a vehicle for immunization against a protein antigen (ovalbumin) in terms of antibody titers. Neither oil stimulated a DTH response to the antigen, requiring the addition of IS to the vaccines (Whitehouse *et al.*, 1974). Emulsions of squalane or squalene were also effective substitutes for mineral oil in an experimental model of tumor eradication by intralesional injection of bacterial products (Yarkoni and Rapp, 1979).

We evaluated the activity of squalane or squalene and compared them to mineral oil as vehicles for mmunization with p72 : TT. These studies also included a comparison of Arlacel A and Montanide 888 as emulsifiers. Montanide 888 is an oil of the mannide oleate family. When used at 5% vol/vol as an emulsifier, the w/o emulsions obtained are considerably less viscous than those prepared with Arlacel A; they are reported to be stable for more than 6 months at 4°C, and sterilizable by filtration.

Montanide 888 was found to be an appropriate emulsifier for mineral oil emulsions. In general, antibody responses were elicited earlier with Montanide-emulsified, than in Arlacel A-emulsified, vaccines and, in some instances, reached higher levels, although they tended to persist for a somewhat shorter time. This effect may be due to the lower stability and viscosity of the Montanide emulsions. The particular oil-emulsifier combination also affected the magnitude of antibody responses to p72. The main conclusions from these studies can be summarized as follows:

1. When Montanide 888 is used as an emulsifier, mineral oil is a more effective vehicle than squalene or squalane during the primary response. However, when Arlacel A is used as the emulsifying agent, the primary anti-p72 antibody responses elicited in mice by mineral oil or biodegradable oil-formulated vaccines are similar (Fig. 4). Squalane

or squalene were inferior vehicles in rabbits compared to mineral oil, even when Arlacel A was used as the emulsifier (not shown). As shown in more detail later (Section VII,A,3) squalane or squalene are effective vehicles when supplemented with defined bacterial IS (Fig. 4).

2. Although mineral oil is a more efficient vehicle than squalane or squalene (with Montanide 888 as the emulsifier) in terms of the primary antibody responses, no significant differences in secondary responses among these three oil vehicles were seen in mice following an antigen boost given in an alum vehicle 6 months after priming

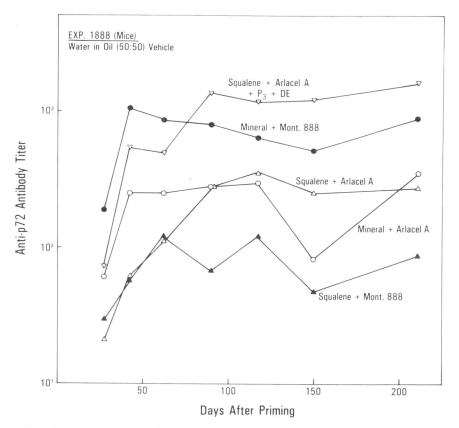

FIG. 4. Comparison of oil vehicles (mineral oil versus squalene) and emulsifiers (Arlacel A versus Montanide 888) in murine anti-p72 antibody responses. In one of the groups, the vaccine was supplemented with 100 μg each of P_3 (TDM, see Section VII,A,1,b) plus DE (MPL, see Section VII,A,2).

(Fig. 5). The persistence of the secondary antibody responses was similar among the three groups for at least 9 months after the boost. Following the initial decline in antibody titer after the boost, as seen in Fig. 5, the titers remained fairly constant and were, 9 months after the boost, 1,660, 2,620, and 1,360 in groups primed with antigen in mineral oil, squalane, or squalene, respectively. In contrast, recall responses in rabbits were markedly lower in groups primed with squalane- or squalene-formulated vaccines than in a group primed with a mineral oil-containing vaccine (not shown). Thus, the efficacy of s1qualane or squalene as vehicles clearly varied between the two species tested, and was far better in mice. The cause could be more rapid metabolism and clearance of the biodegradable oils in the rabbits. Since Montanide 888 served as an emulsifier in these experiments, and since Arlacel A is clearly a better emulsifier than Montanide 888 for squalane and squalene, it remains to be seen whether these two biodegradable oils will be more effective in rabbits (or other species) when formulated with an optimal emusifying agent (e.g., Arlacel A).

In summary, biodegradable oils such as squalane and squalene are potential candidates for effective vaccine vehicles that might be

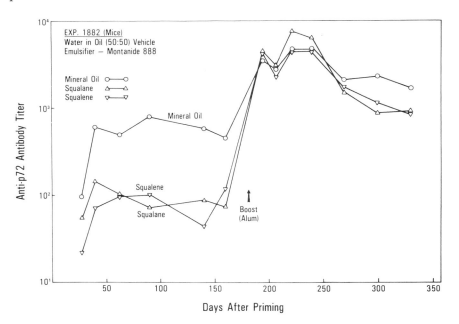

FIG. 5. Comparison of three oils as vehicles for primary and secondary anti-p72 responses. All mice were boosted with p72:TT in alum on day 180.

acceptable in humans. However, more detailed studies are necessary to evaluate their potential.

D. Oil-in-Water Emulsions

In an attempt to reduce the amount of oil in the emulsion, Ribi and his colleagues developed an oil-in-water (o/w) emulsion that contained only 1–2% oil (Meyer *et al.*, 1974) and, in addition, substituted metabolizable oils (squalane or squalene) for the mineral oil used conventionally in IFA-emulsified vaccines (Yarkoni and Rapp, 1979). In preparing these vaccines, antigen is first incorporated into a minimal volume of oil by grinding or blending, and these antigen-containing oil droplets were then emulsified in saline plus 0.2% Tween 80 (Ribi *et al.*, 1975). These formulations are considerably less viscous than IFA emulsions and can be readily sterilized by filtration. However, these o/w emulsions function as effective immuogenic vaccines only when supplemented with defined bacterial IS. Unlike the w/o emulsions (such as IFA), they elicit very weak antibody responses in the absence of the added stimulators even when mineral oil is used. They will, therefore, be reviewed in more detail later (see Section VII,A,3).

E. Biodegradable Microcapsules

The process of microencapsulation has found many applications in agriculture and medicine. Microcapsules manufactured by several established procedures serve as microreservoirs in situations where controlled or sustained release of their contents is desired. Thus, their potential as vehicles for vaccine preparations is obvious, since they have the properties necessary to ensure sustained antigen release. One of the newer promising types of microcapsule is that made of biodegradable polymers. Preferably, the biodegradable polymers are natural substances, thus reducing potential toxicity. Among the various types of biodegradable microcapsules, those manufactured from copolymers of lactic and glycolic acids have attracted special attention (Gresser and Sanderson, 1984). They are characterized by a homogeneous distribution of the encapsulated material(s) in the polymeric matrix. Release from such microcapsules is dependent on polymer degradation and diffusion through the matrix. The rate of release from these microcapsules is determined mainly by the polymer composition (e.g., ratio of lactic to glycolic acids) and drug content or loading. The components of this polymer are natural, safe, and nontoxic materials that have been used to manufacture surgical sutures.

We have examined microcapsules manufactured by Southern Research Institute (Birmingham, AL) made of poly(DL-lactate-co-glycolide) as a vehicle for the delivery of synthetic peptide vaccines. These microcapsules were designed as a free-flowing powder of spherical particles less than 100 μm in diameter that can be injected with a coventional syringe and hypodermic needle. Free p72 or a p72:TT conjugate with or without various IS were incorporated into the microcapsules. These preparations were designed to release their contents at a controlled rate over a period of 1–12 months.

Our studies demonstrated that, first, p72:TT incorporated in microcapsules retained its antigenicity, since incorporation of the p72:TT-containing microcapsules in IFA elicited high primary antibody responses in rabbits. Second, microencapsulated p72:TT elicited very weak primary antibody responses in vehicles other than IFA, such as alum or 2% carboxymethylcellulose. This is probably due to the fact that the microcapsules are made of an inert material that fails to stimulate a beneficial local inflammatory reaction. Third, some preparations of microencapsulated p72:TT apparently stimulated memory B cells, since several groups boosted with p72:TT in alum several months after priming with antigen-containing microcapsules produced early, high-titered anti-p72 antibodies characteristic of an anamnestic response. However, an adequate secondary response to microencapsulated p72:TT required a 10-fold higher primary antigen dose compared to free p72:TT in IFA. Finally, p72:TT in microcapsules can boost efficient secondary responses in animals primed with p72:TT in optimal vehicle–IS combinations. As can be seen in Fig. 6, mice primed with p72:TT in alum in the presence of two defined bacterial IS, P_3 (or TDM) and DE (or MPL) (see Section VII,A,3) mount moderate p72-specific antibody responses. An antigen boost given in alum about 4 months after priming results in a high-titered ($>1 \times 10^4$) antibody response, but a similar effect can be obtained by boosting the mice with p72:TT-containing microcapsules.

Overall, these findings suggest that, although microencapsulated antigen may not serve as an effective primary vaccine even when supplemented with active IS, it might function well as a vaccine for booster injections. This, plus the controlled release of antigen from the microcapsules, which can be extended for up to 12 months, raises an interesting possibility: It might be possible to obtain a long-term protective antibody response by combining in one single injection an optimally immunogenic vaccine (e.g., antigen in a biodegradable oil

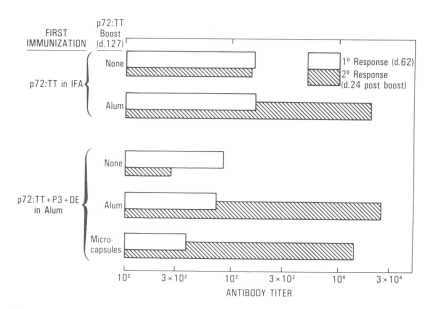

FIG. 6. Boosting of secondary anti-p72 antibody responses by microencapsulated antigen. Mice were primed with 40 μg of p72:TT in IFA or with the same antigen supplemented with P₃ plus DE (100 μg each) in alum. Some of the groups were not boosted, and others were boosted with p72:TT in alum or in biodegradable p72:TT microcapsules on day 127. Peak primary antibody responses on day 62 after priming are represented by the open bars and responses measured 24 days after the booster injection are represented by the striped bars.

emulsion containing appropriate IS) with antigen-containing micro-capsules. The former might stimulate an effective primary response as well as memory B cells, while the latter could provide an antigen depot for continually boosting a high-titered secondary response. If this is indeed the case, then antigen-containing microcapsules could find wide application in vaccines by replacing the need for booster injections.

F. LIPOSOMES

Liposomes, which are artificial spheres of phospholipid bilayers separated by aqueous compartments, can act as vehicles for the delivery of water- or lipid-soluble molecules. Incorporation within liposomes protects such molecules from degradation. Liposomes can be made from safe, natural phospholipids, and their composition and properties can be varied at will. They have been safely administered parenterally to patients as drug carriers. Other properties that are advantageous for considering liposomes as a vaccine vehicle include their mobilization into draining lymph nodes at the site of injection, and their interaction with antigen-presenting macrophages that ingest them (reviewed by Allison and Gregoriadis, 1976).

Allison and Gregoriadis (1974) were the first to report that a protein antigen, DT, entrapped within liposomes stimulated higher antibody responses than in its free form. This finding has been extended to many other systems. The immunogenic potency of liposomes can be increased further by the inclusion of immunostimulators such as bacterial lipopolysaccharide, lipid A, or MDP (Jolivet *et al.*, 1981; Alving and Richardson, 1984; Desiderio and Campbell, 1985). Liposomes injected intradermally or intramuscularly form a depot that releases the antigen slowly over a period of days to weeks (Kramp *et al.*, 1982). This is one mechanism responsible for their ability to enhance immunologic responses. Other mechanisms of action probably exist as well because, unlike vaccines injected in alum salts or oil emulsions, which also form a local antigen depot, antigens entrapped in liposomes stimulate cellular immunity in addition to antibody responses (Sanchez *et al.*, 1980). The reason for this is unclear, but may be related to the preferential uptake of liposomes by macrophages and the resulting antigen presentation in a hydrophobic microenvironment that may be particularly effective for stimulation of T cells. It is known, for example, that protein antigens coupled to lipid moieties induce increased DTH responses in proportion to their hydrophobicity (Coon and Hunter, 1975). Although further studies are needed to confirm the efficacy and stability of liposomes, they are a potentially promising delivery system for vaccines.

VII. Immunostimulators (IS)

The concept of immunoadjuvants, which are substances that can augment specific antibody responses when combined with the antigen, was introduced by Ramon (1926), who first demonstrated that antibody levels against DT or TT could be increased by addition of various substances such as lecithin or saponin. Numerous substances have since been reported to have immunostimulatory activity. Originally, many IS were crude preparations or whole microbes in which the active principle was not clearly defined. Moreover, the mechanism of action of most of these IS has never been fully elucidated. The realization that future vaccines will consist of poorly immunogenic antigens requiring immunopotentiation, and that various crude IS preparations induce deleterious side effects, led to an intensified effort to isolate and identify chemically defined, nontoxic IS.

Rather than catalog the immense number of substances with IS activity, we will focus our discussion on those with which we have had considerable experience as well as those for which extensive information exists regarding their chemical nature and/or mechanism of action.

A. MICROBIAL IS AND SYNTHETIC DERIVATIVES

1. Microbacterial Products

The use of mycobacteria as IS dates back to the original development of mycobacteria-containing oil emulsions, i.e., CFA (Freund et al., 1937; Freund, 1956). This is one of the most potent vaccine formulations, known to stimulate both humoral and cell-mediated immunity, but it is too toxic for use outside the laboratory. Since the discovery of CFA, a progressive series of studies have been undertaken in several laboratories to purify and define the active mycobacterial principle(s).

The insoluble material obtained by centrifugation of disrupted mycobacteria consists primarily of bacterial cell walls that retain the IS properties of the whole microbe. Proteolytic removal of proteins from cell walls and extraction with organic solvents results in an insoluble polymeric complex consisting of mycolic acid linked to an arabinogalactan, which is in turn attached to a mucopeptide (Ribi et al., 1975). This rigid complex, termed "cell wall skeleton," contains the IS, MDP (see Section VII,A,1,a) as a sturctural subunit, and has reduced antitumor, antimicrobial, and IS activities compared with the cell wall preparation. Full biologic activity is restored when cell wall skeleton is combined with trehalose dimycolate (TDM; see Section VII,A,1,b) or with an active derivative of bacterial lipopolysaccharide (LPS; see Section VII,A,2). The lipid fraction of mycobacteria contains TDM as the active moiety (Ribi et al., 1975).

  a. MDP and Derivatives   (reviewed by Adam et al., 1981; Kotani et al., 1986; Bahr and Chédid, 1986; Warren et al., 1986). The synthetic MDP, N-acetylmuramyl-L-alanine-D-isoglutamine, represents the minimal structure analogous to bacterial peptidoglycan, which retains IS activity and can substitute for the whole mycobacteria used in CFA (Adam et al., 1974; Ellouz et al., 1974; Kotani et al., 1975). It is probably the most extensively characterized microbial IS. MDP and its derivatives have numerous activities in the immune and central nervous system that include, in addition to their ability to stimulate

humoral and cell-mediated immunity, augmentation of nonspecific
host resistance mechanisms to tumor and infection, polyclonal B cell
activation and mitogenesis, and pyrogenicity. Unlike the mycobacteria
or peptidoglycan from which it is derived, MDP is not itself immunogenic (Audibert *et al.*, 1976), and does not stimulate a tuberculin
reaction (Audibert *et al.*, 1978). Several hundred analogs of MDP have
been synthesized in studies designed to elucidate the structure–
function relationship of this molecule, and to dissociate the clinically
undesirable effects of MDP from its beneficial activity. This effort has
allowed the selection of compounds that retain the IS activity but are
nontoxic and nonpyrogenic (Chédid *et al.*, 1976; Azuma *et al.*, 1976;
Adam *et al.*, 1981; Kotani *et al.*, 1986). Also, indomethacin inhibits the
pyrogenicity of MDP without affecting its IS property (Masek, 1986).
MDP can replace the mycobacteria in CFA to induce both humoral and
cell-mediated immunity (Ellouz *et al.*, 1974). Depending on the mode of
MDP administration, it can preferentially stimulate the production of
distinct immunoglobulin classes or subclasses (Leclerc *et al.*, 1978;
Kishimoto *et al.*, 1979).

MDP and related compounds have been shown to stimulate specific
antibody production to a wide range of bacterial, viral, protozoan, and
protein antigens as well as to numerous synthetic peptides derived
from them (reviewed by Audibert *et al.*, 1985). They retain this effect
when administered with antigen in saline rather than in an oil
emulsion (Audibert *et al.*, 1976), even by the oral route (Chédid *et al.*,
1976). Under these conditions, however, they do not significantly
augment cell-mediated immunity, indicated by a DTH reaction (Bomford, 1980b). MDP and its active derivatives do, however, stimulate
potent cell-mediated immunity when incorporated into oil emulsions
(Carelli *et al.*, 1981; Bomford, 1980b) or liposomes (Masek *et al.*, 1978),
or even in an aqueous solution if made lipophilic by appropriate
chemical modifications (Parant *et al.*, 1980). Examples of the stimulation of cell-mediated immunity by MDP in oil are the anti-tumor
effects and the induction of experimental autoimmunity (reviewed by
Warren *et al.*, 1986).

The IS activity of MDP can be augmented by direct conjugation to
protein antigens, or by attachment of synthetic peptide antigens by
means of synthetic carriers, e.g., copolymers of DL-alanine and L-lysine
(Mozes *et al.*, 1980; Arnon *et al.*, 1980; Audibert *et al.*, 1982; Carelli *et
al.*, 1982). The result is a totally synthetic vaccine in which antigen,
carrier, and IS are synthesized chemically.

MDP possesses several properties that make it an attractive IS in
veterinary and human vaccines, including the detailed information

available on structure–function relationship, lack of intrinsic immunogenicity, the availability of immunologically-active, nonpyrogenic derivatives and the ability of MDP to stimulate potent cell-mediated immunity when appropriately modified or incorporated into biodegradable vehicles such as liposomes and metabolizable oils. Unfortunately, MDP can, under some conditions, suppress the immune response (Leclerc et al., 1979, 1982; Fergusson et al., 1983); moreover, factors such as the nature and concentration of the antigen, the procedure for coupling MDP to the antigen, and the degree of substitution, can modify the IS activity of MDP. Thus, it is questionable whether a universal "recipe" for using MDP as an IS in vaccines will emerge. We have conducted several experiments in which MDP was mixed at several doses (1–100 μg) with, or chemically coupled to, p72 : TT, but have not stimulated the anti-p72 antibody response. Nevertheless, MDP may serve as an important IS in future vaccines once its safety and parameters for effective use have been determined.

b. *Trehalose Dimycolate (TDM)*. A lipid component of mycobacteria termed cord factor, defined on the basis of its exclusive occurrence in virulent strains of mycobacteria and its delayed toxic effect in mice, was originally isolated by Noll and Bloch (1955) and Noll et al. (1956) and defined as trehalose-6,6'-dimycolate. Improved fractionation procedures led to the isolation of an active P_3 fraction from cord factor. The active principle of cord factor was defined on the basis of its ability to cooperate with cell wall skeleton, a cell wall-derived peptidoglycolipid, in inducing regression of established tumors in guinea pigs (Azuma et al., 1974). Since the active moiety of P_3 is trehalose dimycolate, the purified, biologically active material has been termed TDM. Unlike MDP, which is derived from the cell wall peptidoglycan, a ubiquitous component of many bacterial species, TDM is unique to virulent strains of mycobacteria. The toxicity of TDM depends on the mycobacterial strain of origin. For example, the TDM used in our experiments (see Section VII,A,3) obtained from RIBI Immunochem Research, Inc. (Hamilton, MT) is derived from *Mycobacterium phleii* and is nontoxic (J. Cantrell, personal communication).

TDM is nonimmunogenic and has little biological activity itself in terms of granuloma induction, antitumor, and IS effects. However, when TDM is combined in oil–water emulsions together with other bacterial products such as the cell wall skeleton cited above, LPS, or MDP, it exerts potent biological effects, including augmentation of antigen-specific humoral and cell-mediated immunity, induction of tumor regression, and resistance to bacterial infection (Azuma et al., 1974; Ribi et al., 1975, 1982). It is thought that, when incorporated in

50% w/o or 1% o/w emulsions, TDM becomes attached to the oil droplets via its lipophilic (mycolic acid) residues and to the antigen in a vaccine preparation via its polar (trehalose) end. The subsequent presentation of the antigen in a lipophilic microenvironment augments its immunogenicity, particularly for Th cells and, therefore, results in a strengthened immune response. Studies that examined the IS effect of TDM combined with other bacterial products on the antibody response to p72 will be summarized later (see Section VII,A,3).

2. Lipopolysaccharides (LPS)

LPS obtained from the cell walls of Gram-negative bacteria possesses a broad spectrum of biological activities. It is a potent B-cell mitogen (Andersson *et al.*, 1972; Gery *et al.*, 1972) and an IS of antibody formation (Johnson *et al.*, 1956), and is highly immunogenic by itself (Landy and Baker, 1966; Rudbach, 1971). LPS is a macromolecule composed of three principal regions. The *O*-polysaccharide, which carries the main serologic specificity of bacteria, is covalently linked to the core polysaccharide common to groups of Gram-negative bacteria; the latter is, in turn, covalently linked to lipid A via a trisaccharide of 2-keto-3-deoxyoctanoic acid (KDO). Lipid A is the biologically active moiety of LPS (Andersson *et al.*, 1973; Chiller *et al.*, 1973).

The principal drawback for the clinical use of LPS is the toxicity attributed to its lipid A portion. This toxic effect is elicited with minute quantities of lipid A or LPS, which are best known for causing pyrogenicity and changes in blood clotting and blood pressure that can lead to shock and death (Tanamoto *et al.*, 1984). Efforts have been made to separate the clinically beneficial effects of LPS, e.g., stimulation of leukopoiesis and immune responses, protection against lethal irradiation and induction of antitumor and bacterial resistance, from its toxicity. Two approaches that have met with considerable success are alkylation, which decreased toxicity by 100,000-fold (Chédid *et al.*, 1975), and removal of a phosphate group from the reducing end of lipid A, which converted the toxic diphosphoryl lipid A into nontoxic monophosphoryl lipid A (MPL; referred to as DE, or detoxified endotoxin, in Figs. 4, 6–9; Ribi *et al.*, 1984). MPL fully retains the other biological activities of lipid A, including mitogenicity for B cells. The latter procedure reduced the toxicity of lipid A by a factor of 2,000–10,000 in dogs and rabbits, two species similar to humans in their endotoxin susceptibility.

Synthetic or natural lipid A maintain their IS activity when incorporated into liposomes (Yasuda *et al.*, 1982; Alving and Richardson, 1984) and also increase cell-mediated immunity to an antigen mixed with LPS. As noted above, MPL cooperates with TDM to potentiate immune and other beneficial host responses; some experiments documenting this effect are reported in Section VII,A,3. The dissociation of LPS toxic effects from those effects that may be clinically desirable provides hope that nontoxic LPS derivatives may eventually find use in vaccines and some clinical applications.

A lipoprotein that is unrelated to LPS but also from membranes of *E. coli* and some other enteral bacteria, similarly acts as a B-cell mitogen and IS in several species. This lipoprotein has been characterized, and the moiety responsible for B-cell activation was defined as a group of three fatty acids bound to glyceryl cysteine attached to an oligopeptide (Resch and Bessler, 1981). A corresponding synthetic lipopeptide, tripalmitoyl pentapeptide, was constructed and found to be a potent B-cell mitogen (Bessler *et al.*, 1985). Moreover, tripalmitoyl pentapeptide, in its free or antigen-conjugated forms, enhanced murine antibody responses of the IgM and IgG classes to sheep red blood cells and to protein antigens both *in vitro* and *in vivo* (Lex *et al.*, 1986). The lack of apparent toxicity of this compound, its ease of synthesis, and its activity on human cells (unlike lipid A) make this molecule a potential alternative to LPS derivatives as an IS in vaccine preparations. However, as with other IS that are polyclonal B-cell activators, the potential risk of inducing autoimmunity must be considered, and more pharmacologic studies are necessary to evaluate the safety and efficacy of this synthetic lipopeptide.

3. Influence of MPL Combined with Mycobacterial Products on Antibody Responses to p72

The remarkable synergism in biological activity between MPL and mycobacterial products, and the apparent lack of toxicity of these materials, stimulated particular interest in this IS combination. The mixture of MPL and cell wall skeleton, in fact, underwent clinical trials in humans with advanced melanoma (by intralesional injection) and was found to induce regression of tumor nodules (Vosika *et al.*, 1979).

We extensively evaluated the effect of a combination of TDM plus MPL (referred to as P_3 plus DE, respectively, in Figs. 4, 6–9) on primary and secondary anti-p72 antibody responses in mice and rabbits primed with p72:TT plus these two IS. The oils used were either mineral or biodegradable (squalane and squalene). Since previous studies indicated that administration of p72:TT in alum as a

330 AMNON ALTMAN AND FRANK J. DIXON

booster injection stimulated efficient secondary antibody responses (see Section VI,A), groups primed with different vaccine formulations were boosted uniformly with p72:TT in alum.

TDM + MPL were added to p72:TT vaccines formulated in several vehicles, i.e., w/o (50:50) or o/w (1–2%) emulsions, and aluminum hydroxide gel, and tested for stimulation of anti-p72 antibody responses. The effect of these IS on primary antibody responses (i.e., after a single injection) was variable and was determined by the type of vehicle used for priming. For example, if an optimal vehicle, such as a water-in-mineral oil emulsion (essentially IFA) was used for priming, the addition of TDM plus MPL did not significantly augment the primary antibody response. If, on the other hand, the vehicle used for priming was less than optimal, e.g., water-in-biodegradable oil emulsions (using Montanide 888 as an emulsifier), or 2% o/w emulsions (with any of the three oils studied), MPL plus TDM had a marked immunostimulatory effect (Fig. 7). This effect was more pronounced in the 2% o/w emulsions that are relatively poor vehicles (peak antibody titers of less than 1×10^2 in the absence of IS; see bottom of Fig. 7). The

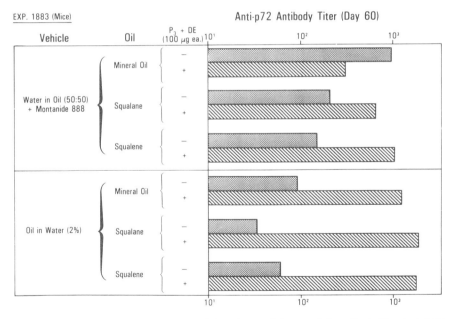

FIG. 7. Comparison of 50% w/o and 2% o/w emulsions and the effect of bacterial IS on murine anti-p72 antibody responses. Antibody titers shown were determined 60 days after priming.

addition of the microbial IS augmented the primary antibody response by at least one order of magnitude. Moreover, the responses obtained with the IS-containing metabolizable oils, squalane or squalene (either as w/o or 2% o/w emulsions) were similar to, or even better than, those elicited by a water-in-mineral oil (IFA) emulsion (Fig. 7).

More importantly, the effect of adding the bacterial IS combination of TDM plus MPL to the primary vaccine was remarkably potent when secondary responses were examined following a booster injection of p72:TT in alum (without further addition of TDM + MPL). Thus, as shown in Fig. 8, the secondary antibody responses of mice primed with p72:TT plus bacterial IS in alum increased significantly ($>3 \times 10^4$) after the boost. In contrast, the group primed with the same vaccine without the IS combination produced much lower titers after a booster injection. In this experiment, antibody titers were compared to those elicited by an IFA vaccine without a booster injection.

An experiment using 2% squalene-in-water emulsion instead of alum as a vehicle gave similar results (Fig. 9). Thus, addition of TDM plus MPL to the primary vaccine resulted in a secondary antibody

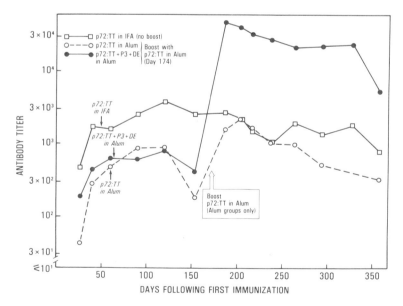

FIG. 8. The immunostimulatory effect of bacterial IS (P_3 and DE) on anti-p72 antibody responses of mice primed with an alum-formulated vaccine. The two groups primed with antigen in alum (with or without bacterial IS) were boosted on day 174 with p72:TT in alum.

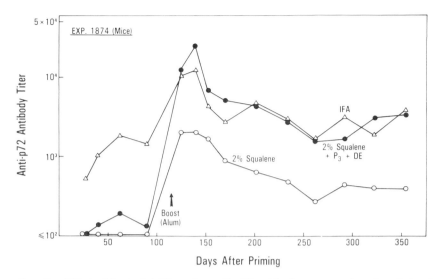

FIG. 9. Effect of bacterial IS on the anti-p72 antibody response in mice. Animals were primed with p72 : TT in IFA or in 2% squalene-in-water emulsion with or without P_3 + DE (100 μg each). The three groups were boosted on day 112 with antigen in alum.

response similar to that elicited by priming with an IFA-formulated vaccine in terms of magnitude and persistence. Typically, the secondary antibody responses peak rapidly and start to decline, but then stabilize and remain at fairly high levels for at least 6–8 months (Fig. 9). In contrast to mice, rabbits had a less remarkable reaction to the immunostimulatory property of the TDM + MPL combination, particularly in secondary antibody responses. It remains to be seen whether addition of the same IS to the booster injection will increase their effectiveness in rabbits.

These results imply that vaccine formulations potentially acceptable for human use, i.e., emulsions (w/o or o/w) of biodegradable oils, or perhaps even alum gels, supplemented with defined bacterial products, might be an adequate and efficient replacement for IFA. Their ability to stimulate B-cell memory, as evidenced by the potent secondary antibody responses, is of particular importance in this respect.

4. Other Bacteria

Various bacteria, in addition to those described in previous sections, were found to potentiate immune responses upon mixing with antigens. Two of the more prominent examples are *Bordetella pertussis* and *Corynebacterium parvum*.

Corynebacterium parvum augmented antibody responses to sheep red blood cells in mice (Bomford, 1980a) and also stimulated cell-mediated immunity to admixed antigens (Bomford, 1980b). *Bordetella pertussis* was studied more extensively, and found to possess several immunomodulatory components that act together to enhance the immune response (reviewed by Warren *et al.*, 1986). The principal IS components are LPS (described earlier) and pertussis toxin (PT). Recently, purified preparations of PT were used to study its immuno-modulatory effects in the absence of LPS contamination. The results established PT as a T-cell mitogen that augments immune responses, particularly cell-mediated responses, partly through its ability to alter recirculation of T cells. *Bordetella pertussis* or the purified PT preferentially enhances antibody response of the IgE class, and, as noted earlier, also overcomes the phenomenon of epitope suppression observed when a hapten-carrier conjugate is injected into animals with preexisting immunity to the same carrier (see Section V,B). Since sufficient information concerning the safety, efficacy, and nature of the active components in these bacteria is missing, it is unlikely that these microbes or their derivatives will be used in veterinary or human vaccines in the near future.

5. Glucan

Glucan is a β-1,3-polyglucose isolated from the cell wall of the yeast *Saccharomyces cerevisiae* in a particulate or soluble form. Its intravenous administration into several animal species stimulates a marked increase in the phagocytic and proliferative activity of the reticuloendothelial system. The proliferation of macrophages is accompanied by reversible hepatosplenomegaly and granuloma formation (only in response to particulate glucan). Glucan, which localizes exclusively in macrophages and activates them, was found in numerous studies to induce antitumor effects and resistance to microbial pathogens, and to stimulate antibody responses to a host of antigens, including to microbial vaccines (Reynolds *et al.*, 1980b; reviewed by DiLuzio, 1983). Since particulate glucan may be toxic, it remains to be seen whether soluble glucan preparations will be equally effective as IS in vaccines. We found that addition of glucan to p72:TT vaccines formulated in an alum vehicle (but not in IFA) resulted in a 3- to 4-fold enhancement of the primary antibody response to p72 and, furthermore, that the secondary response elicited by a p72:TT (*without* glucan) in alum, was also significantly higher in mice that were primed with antigen plus glucan.

B. Nonmicrobial IS

An extremely large number of nonmicrobial substances with different degrees of purity were reported to act as IS in various experimental systems. These include, among others, salts, sugars, surface active compounds, polyribonucleotides, and some biologically derived immunomodulators, i.e., lymphokines and monokines.

The saponins are a group of glycosidic compounds of plant origin that have been used widely as IS in veterinary vaccines against foot-and-mouth disease and found to be active in other systems (Bomford, 19080a). This amphipathic surface active substance is not considered adequate, however, for human vaccines because of its hemolytic and irritant properties. In attempts to eliminate the toxicity of crude saponin preparations, Dalsgaard (1974) isolated an active extract from the bark of the tree *Quillaja saponaria* Molina, referred to as Quil A, which had significantly reduced toxicity. The reported immunostimulatory activity of saponin may explain the increased immunogenicity of antigen formulated in an immunostimulating coplex termed Iscom (Morein *et al.*, 1984). This complex is formed by mixing the antigen (virus glycoprotein) with a solution of Quil A in the presence of a detergent, Triton X-100, resulting in the formation of micelles with a distinct morphology. It has been suggested that Quil A has regions accessible to hydrophobic interaction with the cell membrane proteins in this complex, enhancing the effectiveness of antigen presentation (Morein *et al.*, 1984). We tested a commercial preparation of Quil A (Superfos A/S, Denmark) with p72 : TT vaccines formulated in alum or in a w/o emulsion, but have not observed any enhancing effect of this purified saponin preparation on the antibody response.

Selenium and vitamin E have also been reported to enhance antibody responses. In our hands, a commercial preparation of these two substances in oil (Seletoc) augmented the anti-p72 antibody response 8- to 10-fold when added to an IFA- but not to an alum-formulated vaccine.

Goodman and Weigle (1981) have described a new class of B-cell activators, the C8-substituted guanine ribonucleosides, that traverse the cell membrane, bypassing conventional triggering mechanisms to activate B cells at an intracellular site. These compounds act as potent polyclonal B-cell mitogens *in vitro* and as IS capable of augmenting specific antibody responses *in vitro* and *in vivo* (Weinstein *et al.*, 1975; Goodman and Weigle, 1983a,b). We tested one of these compounds, 7-methyl-8-oxoguanosine, in our experimental system. This compound was active in IFA-formulated, but not in alum-formulated, vaccines of p72 : TT, and considerably augmented the anti-p72 antibody responses at doses of 1 or 10 mg per mouse. The immunopotentiating effect was most pronounced when a suboptimal antigen dose (4 instead of 40 μg p72 : TT) was injected into the mice. In another experiment, 50 mg of this compound augmented the primary antibody response of rabbits to p72 (given in a water-in-squalene emulsion) by 3- to 5-fold. These effects were not consistent, however, and additional studies may be necessary to establish optimal doses and vaccine formulations for the effective use of these defined compounds.

Finally, we examined a surface active quaternary amine salt, dimethyldioctadecylammonium bromide as an IS. Addition of this salt to an alum-formulated vaccine of p72 : TT, at 2 μmoles per mouse, augmented by about eightfold the peak primary antibody response measured on day 60 after immunization and, in addition, led to enhanced secondary responses following a booster injection of p72 : TT in alum (without the salt).

Nonionic block polymer surfactants, termed pluronic polyols and composed of polymers of hydrophilic polyoxyethylene and lipophilic polyoxypropylene, were found to serve as potent IS when formulated in 2.5% o/w emulsions (Hunter et al., 1981). The immunostimulatory activity of these polymers correlated with their hydrophile/lipophile ratio such that more lipophilic polymers, which promoted the retention of antigen molecules by oil droplets in the emulsion, were more active. This action may be common to other surfactants described earlier in this article, or reported by others to have immunostimulatory activity.

Biologically derived, i.e., natural, substances of mammalian origin have also been tested for their activity as IS. Such substances offer the advantage of being naturally involved in immune response regulation, and thus have less likelihood of eliciting adverse reactions. These include fragments of the Fc portion of immunoglobulin (Morgan and Weigle, 1981), a tetrapeptide derived from a conserved region of a leukophilic IgG fraction termed "tuftsin" (Florentin et al., 1978; Fridkin and Gottlieb, 1981), specific antibodies to admixed antigens (Harte et al., 1983; Celis and Change, 1984), and, finally, physiologic regulators of the immune response in the form of lymphocyte-derived lymphokines and macrophage-derived monokines. These biological response modifiers have been reviewed extensively elsewhere (Feldmann, 1985; Merluzzi and Last-Barney, 1985; Dinarello, 1985). In general, these natural immunoregulatory molecules, many of which have by now been molecularly cloned and characterized, have a very short biological half-life. As a result, it will be necessary to formulate slow-release depots of these cytokines together with the antigen to prolong their retention and activity.

C. Mechanisms of Action of IS

As noted earlier, an extremely large and diverse collection of substances is known to act as IS, and multiple independent mechanisms may be responsible for their biological activities. The complexity of the immune system, which involves finely tuned interactions among cells and soluble mediators with diverse effector and regulatory functions, further obscures conclusions about the mechanisms of action by the IS. Nevertheless, attempts have been made to formulate some unifying hypotheses in this area.

One important mechanism of action that may be common to many of the IS studied is the activation of macrophages. These cells and their products play a central role in regulation of immune responses (reviewed by Unanue, 1984). Macrophages provide at least two different obligatory signals for the immune response. First, they display on their surfaces Ia antigens specified by the MHC of the species (the so-called class II MHC antigens), which are critical for the antigen presentation function of macrophages. Thus, after processing an antigen, macrophages present it to T cells (which are required as helpers in the antibody response) in association with Ia determinants on their surface (Sette *et al.*, 1987). The second signal is the macrophage-soluble product, interleukin 1 (IL-1), a well-characterized polypeptide that exerts a spectrum of biological effects through interaction with various immune and nonimmune cells (Dinarello, 1985). IL-1 was actually found to stimulate antigen-specific antibody responses *in vivo* (Staruch and Wood, 1983).

Thus, it is highly likely that many of the IS exert their immunostimulatory influence by activating macrophages to secrete active mediators, predominantly IL-1, and to increase their surface Ia antigen expression. Indeed, MDP, LPS, and other microbial and nonmicrobial IS have been shown to activate macrophages. However, stimulation of IL-1 production and induction of increased Ia expression may be independent events since, for example, MDP can stimulate IL-1 production by macrophages (Oppenheim *et al.*, 1980; Bahr *et al.*, 1987) without affecting their Ia expression (Behbehani *et al.*, 1985). Furthermore, increased Ia expression by macrophages may not be a direct effect of the IS. Rather, they may initiate and amplify cellular interactions resulting in activation of T and/or B cells, which then go on to produce and secrete lymphokines. These lymphokines, in turn, may induce an increase in Ia expression (as well as other parameters of activation) in macrophages. One defined T-cell-derived lymphokine, interferon-γ, is known to act as a macrophage-activating factor (Schreiber *et al.*, 1983; Pace *et al.*, 1983). Macrophage activation *in vitro* has been found to correlate with, and is essential for, induction of protective immunity against *Schistosoma* (Lewis *et al.*, 1987), and it has been proposed that macrophage activation, particularly IL-1 induction, might serve as a convenient and reliable assay to screen various substances as potential IS (Bahr *et al.*, 1987). Although macrophage activation may not be the universal mechanism of action by all IS, it is certainly common to many of them.

Another important mechanism of action of many IS may be based on their physicochemical properties as amphipathic, surface active substances. Many IS are surfactants that act to lower the tension between two immiscible phases such as oil and water. They have discrete hydrophilic and hydrophobic regions, and preferentially localize on hydrophobic surfaces in contact with aqueous media. In this manner, these amphipathic compounds may anchor antigens to the hydrophobic microenvironment of oil droplets or cell membranes. As a result, antigen is concentrated locally and can, in association with the oil droplets, activate inflammatory mechanisms and cells of the immune system and be presented more efficiently to macrophages or T cells. The IS activity of pluronic polyols (see Section VII,B) has been established as not simply a function of their surface-active properties but, rather, critically dependent on their hydrophile/lipophile balance, which can be determined by physicochemical methods (Hunter *et al.*, 1981). As noted earlier, modifications of MDP that result in more lipophilic derivatives improve its IS activity, particularly with respect to stimulation of cell-mediated DTH responses (Parant *et al.*, 1980). It has also been claimed that Th cells recognize primarily amphipathic regions as dominant epitopes on protein antigens (DeLisi and Berzofsky, 1985).

This mechanism of action may be shared by several of the IS reviewed here, e.g., TDM, the lipid A moiety of LPS, liposomes, saponin, Iscoms, and the cationic surfactant, dimethyldioctadecylammonium bromide. As noted earlier, TDM probably anchors itself to the oil droplets via its hydrophobic region and concentrates antigen on the surface of the oil droplet via its hydrophilic portion (see Section VII,A,1,b).

Some of the IS may utilize yet another mechanism to enhance immune responses by directly activating either Th cells to release immunomodulatory lymphokines, or the B-cell precursors of antibody-forming cells. IS such as LPS or C8-substituted guanine ribonucleosides are direct polyclonal activators of B cells and may, therefore, cooperate with antigen and T-cell-derived mediators to promote B-cell differentiation and proliferation. This action may not necessarily be regarded as beneficial to the host since polyclonal B cell activation can lead to hyperglobulinemia and production of autoantibodies, resulting in pathologic manifestations such as immune complex diseases and autoimmunity.

VIII. Concluding Remarks

The process of developing efficient and safe vaccine formulations is long and laborious, involving titration of each component and its combinations, toxicity studies, and the process of regulatory controls. In the past, the development of new vaccines has been largely empirical. Today, however, we are better equipped to approach the problem of vaccine development. Technological advances in biochemistry and molecular biology have facilitated the preparation of protein antigens from various pathogens in a pure form and large quantities. Moreover, our understanding of the way the immune system works, particularly the rules governing the recognition of antigenic epitopes by T and B lymphocytes, has improved to a large extent. Finally, more efficient methods to isolate and characterize defined molecules with immunomodulatory activity are now available, and thus, vaccine development can proceed more expediently.

Yet it is quite possible that a universal vaccine formulation, in terms of optimal combinations of vehicles and IS, will not be available in the near future. Examination of the vast literature in this area reveals that for almost every vehicle and/or IS found to be effective with a given antigen and a certain vaccination schedule, a contrasting report documents the lack of activity of the same immunomodifier(s) with another antigen or under slightly different conditions. Perhaps this is to be expected because of the immense complexity of cellular and humoral interactions in the immune system, and the multiple mechanisms involved in IS action.

Detailed structure–function studies accompanied by rational modifications of biologically active substances constitute a powerful approach for developing defined molecules that retain the desirable properties of an IS, i.e., increased protection and immunity against a pathogen, but are devoid of toxic effects. In this respect, it is often emphasized that the inflammatory properties of many IS or vehicles make them unacceptable in human, or even veterinary, vaccines. However, it is important to remember that a certain level of an inflammatory response is an integral part of an effective and long-lasting immunity. The cellular constituents of the local inflammatory reaction are active participants in the immune response, either as antigen-presenting cells or as producers of immunopotentiating soluble mediators. Therefore, one important task would be to define substances and conditions that stimulate a controlled and beneficial inflamamtory process with minimal toxicity. Biodegradable oils formulated as o/w emulsions containing very little oil (and not requiring emulsifiers such as Arlacel A), detoxified derivatives of LPS, and/or liposomes come to mind in this respect. Natural immunomodulatory molecules, i.e., lymphokines and monokines, are another good example provided they can be delivered in an appropriate slow-release depot. Finally, the demonstrated efficacy of IS (e.g., MDP) covalently linked to an antigen is encouraging, because this method may allow targeting of the desired IS molecules to clones of antigen-specific B (or T) cells without inducing the undesirable polyclonal activation of the immune system.

ACKNOWLEDGMENT

This is Publication No. 5034IMM from the Immunology Department, Research Institute of Scripps Clinic, 10666 North Torrey Pines, La Jolla, CA, 92037. The work reported herein was supported, in part, by National Institutes of Health grants AI-07007, AG-01743, CA-27489, CA-35299, AR-35411, and a grant from Johnson and Johnson.

We are grateful to M. K. Occhipinti and P. Minick for expert editorial assistance.

REFERENCES

Adam, A., Ciorbaru, R., Ellouz, F., Petit, J.-F., and Lederer, E. (1974). *Biochem. Biophys. Res. Commun.* **56**, 561–567.

Adam, A., Petit, J.-F., Lefrancier, P., and Lederer, E. (1981). *Mol. Cell. Biochem.* **41**, 27–47.

Allison, A. C. (1979). *J. Reticuloendothel. Soc.* **26**, 619–630.

Allison, A. C., and Gregoriadis, G. (1974). *Nature (London)* **252**, 252.

Allison, A. C., and Gregoriadis, G. (1976). *Recent Results Cancer Res.* **56**, 58–64.

Alving, C. R., and Richardson, E. C. (1984). *Rev. Infect. Dis.* **6**, 493–506.

Andersson, J., Möller, G., and Sjöberg, O. (1972). *Cell Immunol.* **4**, 381–393.

Andersson, J., Melchers, F., Galanos, C., and Luderitz, O. J. (1973). *J. Exp. Med.* **137**, 943–953.

Arnon, R., Sela, M., Parant, M., and Chedad, L. (1980). *Proc. Natl. Acad. Sci. U.S.A.* **77**, 6769–6772.

Audibert, F., Chédid, L., Lefrancier, P. and Choay, J. (1976). *Cell. Immunol.* **21,** 243–249.
Audibert, F., Heymer, B., Gros, C., Schleifer, K. H., Seidl, P. H., and Chédid, L. (1978). *J. Immunol.* **121,** 1219–1222.
Audibert, F., Jolivet, M., Chédid, L., Arnon, R., and Sela, M. (1982). *Proc. Natl. Acad. Sci. U.S.A.* **79,** 5042–5046.
Audibert, F., Leclerc, C., and Chédid, L. (1986). *In* "Biological Response Modifiers" (P. F. Torrence, ed.), pp. 307–327. Academic Press, Orlando, Florida.
Azuma, I., Ribi, E., Meyer, T. J., and Zbar, B. (1974). *J. Natl. Cancer Inst. (U.S.)* **52,** 95–100.
Azuma, I., Sugimura, K., Taniyama, T., Yamawaki, M., Yamamura, Y., Kusumoto, S., Okada, S., and Shiba, T. (1976). *Infect. Immun.* **14,** 18–27.
Bahr, G. M., and Chédid, L. (1986). *Fed. Proc., Fed. Am. Soc. Exp. Biol.* **45,** 2534–2540.
Bahr, G. M., Chédid, L. A., and Behbehani, K. (1987). *Cell. Immunol.* **107,** 443–454.
Beebe, G. W., Simon, A. H., and Vivona, S. (1972). *Am. J. Epidemiol.* **95,** 337–344.
Behbehani, K., Beller, D. I., and Unanue, E. R. (1985). *J. Immunol.* **134,** 2047–2049.
Benacerraf, B., Ojeda, A., and Maurer, P. H. (1963). *J. Exp. Med.* **118,** 945–952.
Bessler, W. G., Cox, M., Lex, A., Suhr, B., Wiessmuller, K. H., and Jung, G. (1985). *J. Immunol.* **135,** 1900–1905.
Bomford, R. (1980a). *Clin. Exp. Immunol.* **39,** 426–434.
Bomford, R. (1980b). *Clin. Exp. Immunol.* **39,** 435–441.
Carayanniotis, G., and Barber, B. H. (1987). *Nature (London)* **327,** 59–61.
Carelli, C., Audibert, F., and Chédid, L. (1981). *Infect. Immun.* **33,** 312–314.
Carelli, C., Audibert, F., Gaillard, J., and Chédid, L. (1982). *Proc. Natl. Acad. Sci. U.S.A.* **79,** 5392–5395.
Celis, E., and Chang, T. W. (1984). *Science* **224,** 297–299.
Chanock, R. M., and Murphy, B. R. (1980). *Rev. Infect. Dis.* **2,** 421–428.
Chédid, L., Audibert, F., Bona, C., Damais, C., Parant, F., and Parant, M. (1975). *Infect. Immun.* **12,** 714–721.
Chédid, L., Audibert, F., Lefrancier, P., Choay, J., and Lederer, E. (1976). *Proc. Natl. Acadi. Sci. U.S.A.* **73,** 2472–2475.
Chesnut, R. W., and Grey, H. M. (1981). *J. Immunol.* **126,** 1075–1079.
Chiller, J. M., Skidmore, B. J., Morrison, D. C., and Weigle, W. O. (1973). *Proc. Natl. Acad. Sci. U.S.A.* **70,** 2129–2133.
Coon, J., and Hunter, R. (1975). *J. Immunol.* **114,** 1518–1522.
Dalsgaard, K. (1974). *Arch. Gesamte Virusforsch.* **44,** 243–254.
DeLisi, C., and Berzofsky, J. A. (1985). *Proc. Natl. Acad. Sci. U.S.A.* **80,** 3782–3786.
Desiderio, J. V., and Campbell, S. G. (1985). *Infect. Immun.* **48,** 658–663.
DiLuzio, N. R. (1983). *Trends Pharmacol. Sci.* **4,** 344–347.
Dinarello, C. A. (1985). *J. Clin. Immunol.* **5,** 287–297.
Dreesman, G. R., Sanches, Y., Ionescu-Matiu, I., Sparrow, J. T., Six, H. R., Peterson, D. L., Hollinger, F. B., and Melnick, J. L. (1982). *Nature (London)* **295,** 158–160.
Edelman, R. (1980). *Rev. Infect. Dis.* **2,** 370–383.
Ellouz, F., Adam, A., Ciorbaru, R., and Lederer, E. (1974). *Biochem. Biophys. Res. Commun.* **59,** 1317–1325.
Feldmann, M. (1985). *Nature (London)* **313,** 351–352.
Fergusson, T. A., Krieger, M. J., Pesce, A., and Michael, J. G. (1983). *Infect. Immun.* **39,** 800–806.
Florentin, I., Bruley-Rosse, M., Kiger, N., Imbach, J. L., Winternitz, F., and Mathé, G. (1978). *Cancer Immunol. Immunother.* **5,** 211–216.

Freund, J. (1956). *Adv. Tuberc. Res.* **7**, 130–148.
Freund, J., Casals, J., and Hosmer, E. P. (1937). *Proc. Soc. Exp. Biol. Med.* **37**, 509–513.
Fridkin, M., and Gottlieb, P. (1981). *Mol. Cell. Biochem.* **41**, 73–97.
Gerin, J. L., Alexander, H., Wai-Kuo Shih, J., Purcell, R. H., Dapolito, G., Engle, R., Green, N., Sutcliffe, J. G., Shinnick, T. M., and Lerner, R. A. (1983). *Proc. Natl. Acad. Sci. U.S.A.* **80**, 2365–2369.
Gery, I., Kruger, K., and Spiesel, S. Z. (1972). *J. Immunol.* **108**, 1088–1091.
Glenny, A. T., Pope, C. G., Waddington, H., and Wallace, U. (1926). *J. Pathol. Bacteriol.* **29**, 38–39.
Good, M. F., Maloy, W. L., Lunde, M. N., Margalit, H., Cornette, J. L., Smith, G. L., Moss, B., Miller, L. H., and Berzofsky, J. A. (1987). *Science* **235**, 1059–1062.
Goodman, M. G., and Weigle, W. O. (1981). *Proc. Natl. Acad. Sci. U.S.A.* **79**, 4933–4937.
Goodman, M. G., and Weigle, W. O. (1983a). *J. Immunol.* **130**, 2580–2585.
Goodman, M. G., and Weigle, W. O. (1983b). *Proc. Natl. Acad. Sci. U.S.A.* **80**, 3452–3456.
Gresser, J. D., and Sanderson, J. E. (1984). *In* "Biopolymeric Controlled Release Systems" (D. L. Wise, ed.), pp. 127–138. CRC Press, Boca Raton, Florida.
Harte, P. G., Cooke, A., and Playfair, J. H. L. (1983). *Nature (London)* **302**, 256–258.
Herzenberg, L. A., Tokuhisa, T., and Herzenberg, L. A. (1980). *Nature (London)* **285**, 664–667.
Hilleman, M. R., Woodhour, A. F., Friedman, A., and Phelps, A. H. (1972). *Ann. Allergy* **30**, 477–483.
Hopp, T. P. (1984). *Mol. Immunol.* **21**, 13–16.
Hunter, R., Strickland, F., and Kezdy, F. (1981). *J. Immunol.* **127**, 1244–1250.
Johnson, A. G., Gaines, S., and Landy, M. (1956). *J. Exp. Med.* **103**, 225–246.
Jolivet, M., Sache, E., and Audibert, F. (1981). *Immunol. Commun.* **10**, 511–522.
Jolivet, M., Audibert, F., Beachey, E. H., Tartar, A., Gras-Masse, H., and Chédid, L. (1983). *Biochem. Biophys. Res. Commun.* **117**, 359–366.
Jolivet, M., Audibert, F. M., Gras-Masse, H., Tartar, A. L., Schlesinger, D. H., Wirtz, R., and Chédid, L. A. (1987). *Infect. Immun.* **55**, 1498–1502.
Katz, D. H., Paul, W. E., Goidl, E. A., and Benacerraf, B. (1970). *J. Exp. Med.* **132**, 261–282.
Kawamura, H., and Berzofsky, J. A. (1986). *J. Immunol.* **136**, 58–65.
Kennedy, R. C., Dreesman, G. R., and Kohler, H. (1985). *BioTechniques* **3**, 404–409.
Kishimoto, T., Hirai, Y., Nakanishi, K., Azuma, I., Nagamatsu, A., and Yamamura, Y. (1979). *J. Immunol.* **123**, 2709–2715.
Kotani, S., Watanabe, Y., Kinoshita, F., Shimono, T., Morisaki, I., Shiba, T., Kusumoto, S., Tarumi, Y., and Ikenaka, K. (1975). *Biken J.* **18**, 105–112.
Kotani, S., Tsujimoto, M., Koga, T., Nagao, S., Tanaka, A., and Kawata, S. (1986). *Fed. Proc., Fed. Am. Soc. Exp. Biol.* **45**, 2534–2540.
Kramp, W. J., Six, H. R., and Kasel, J. A. (1982). *Proc. Soc. Exp. Biol. Med.* **169**, 135–139.
Landy, M., and Baker, P. J. (1966). *J. Immunol.* **97**, 670–679.
Langbeheim, H., Arnon, R., and Sela, M. (1976). *Proc. Natl. Acad. Sci. U.S.A.* **73**, 4636–4640.
Leclerc, C., Audibert, F., and Chédid, L. (1978). *Immunology* **35**, 963–970.
Leclerc, C., Juy, D., Bourgeois, E., and Chédid, L. (1979). *Cell. Immunol.* **45**, 199–206.
Leclerc, C., Bourgeois, E., and Chédid, L. (1982). *Eur. J. Immunol.* **12**, 249–252.
Lerner, R. A. (1982). *Nature (London)* **299**, 592–596.
Lewis, F. A., Winestock, J., and James, S. L. (1987). *Infect. Immun.* **55**, 1339–1345.

Lex, A., Wiesmuller, K. H., Jung, G., and Bessler, W. G. (1986). J. Immunol. 137, 2676–2681.

Mackett, M., Smith, G. L., and Moss, B. (1982). Proc. Natl. Acad. Sci. U.S.A. 79, 7415–7419.

Masek, K. (1986). Fed. Proc., Fed. Am. Soc. Exp. Biol. 45, 2549–2551.

Masek, K., Zaoral, M., Jezek, J., Zuchmeir, L., and Straka, R. (1978). Experientia 34, 1363–1364.

Merluzzi, U. J., and Last-Barne, K. (1985). Int. J. Immunopharmacol. 7, 31–39.

Meyer, T. J., Ribi, E. E., Azuma, I., and Zbar, B. (1974). J. Natl. Cancer Inst. (U.S.) 52, 103–111.

Milich, D. R., McLachlan, A., Chisari, F. V., and Thornton, G. B. (1986). J. Exp. Med. 164, 532–547.

Mitchison, N. A. (1969). In "Immunological Tolerance" (M. Landy and W. Braun, eds.), pp. 149–158. Academic Press, New York.

Morein, B., Sundquist, B., Hoglund, S., Dalsgaard, K., and Osterhaus, A. (1984). Nature (London) 308, 457–460.

Morgan, E. L., and Weigle, W. O. (1981). J. Exp. Med. 154, 778–790.

Moss, B., Smith, G. L., Gerin, J. L., and Purcell, R. H. (1984). Nature (London) 311, 67–69.

Mozes, E., Sela, M., and Chédid, L. (1980). Proc. Natl. Acad. Sci. U.S.A. 79, 4933–4937.

Murray, R., Cohen, P., and Hardegree, M. D. (1972). Ann. Allergy 30, 146–151.

Neurath, A. R., Kent, S. B. H., and Strick, N. (1984). Science 224, 392–395.

Nisonoff, A., and Lamoyi, E. (1981). Clin. Immunol. Immunopathol. 21, 397–406.

Noll, H., and Bloch, H. (1955). J. Biol. Chem. 214, 251–265.

Noll, H., Bloch, H., Asselineau, J., Bromakolyarowitz, A. N., and Lederer, E. (1956). Biochim. Biophys. Acta 20, 299–309.

Oppenheim, J. J., Togawa, A., Chédid, L., and Mizel, S. (1980). Cell. Immunol. 50, 71–81.

Ovary, Z., and Benacerraf, B. (1963). Proc. Soc. Exp. Biol. Med. 114, 72–76.

Pace, J. L., Russell, S. W., Schreiber, R. D., Altman, A., and Katz, D. H. (1983). Proc. Natl. Acad. Sci. U.S.A. 80, 3782–3786.

Panicali, D., and Paoletti, E. (1982). Proc. Natl. Acad. Sci. U.S.A. 79, 4927–4931.

Paoletti, E., Lipinskas, B. R., Samsonoff, C., Mercer, S., and Panicali, D. (1984). Proc. Natl. Acad. Sci. U.S.A. 81, 193–197.

Parant, M., Audibert, F., Chédid, L., Level, M., Lefrancier, P., Choay, J., and Lederer, E. (1980). Infect. Immun. 27, 826–831.

Post, L. E., and Roizman, B. (1981). Cell (Cambridge, Mass.) 25, 227–232.

Potter, M., and Boyce, C. R. (1962). Nature (London) 193, 1086–1087.

Prigal, S. J. (1972). Ann. Allergy 30, 529–535.

Ramon, G. (1926). Ann. Inst. Pasteur, Paris 40, 1–10.

Resch, K., and Bessler, W. (1981). Eur. J. Biochem. 115, 247–252.

Reynolds, J. A., Harrington, D. G., Crabbs, C. L., Peters, C. J., and DiLuzio, N. R. (1980a). Infect. Immun. 28, 937–943.

Reynolds, J. A., Kastello, M. G., Harrington, D. G., Crabbs, C. L., Peters, C. J., Jemski, J. V., Scott, G. H., and DiLuzio, N. R. (1980b). Infect. Immun. 30, 51–57.

Ribi, E., Meyer, T. J., Azuma, I., Parker, R., and Brehmer, W. (1975). Cell. Immunol. 16, 1–10.

Ribi, E., Granger, D. L., Milner, K. C., Yamamoto, K., Strain, S. M., Parker, R., Smith, R. W., Brehmer, W., and Azuma, I. (1982). Immunology 46, 297–305.

Ribi, E., Cantrell, J. L., Takayama, K., Qureshi, N., Peterson, J., and Ribi, H. O. (1984). Rev. Infect. Dis. 6, 567–584.

Rudbach, J. A. (1971). *J. Immunol.* **106**, 993–1001.

Salk, J. E., Bailey, M. L., and Leurent, A. M. (1952). *Am. J. Hyg.* **55**, 439–456.

Salk, J. E., Contakos, M., Laruent, A. M., Sorensen, M., Rapalski, A. J., Simmons, I. H., and Sandberg, H. (1953). *JAMA, J. Am. Med. Assoc.* **151**, 1169–1175.

Sanchex, Y., Ionescu-Matiu, I., Dreesman, G. R., Kramp, W., Six, H. R., Hollinger, F. B., and Melnick, J. L. (1980). *Infect. Immun.* **30**, 728–733.

Sanderson, A. R. (1984). *In* "Vaccines '84: Modern Approaches to Vaccines" (R. M. Chanock and R. A. Lerner, eds.), pp. 379–383. Cold Spring Harbor Lab., Cold Spring Harbor, New York.

Schreiber, R. D., Pace, J. L., Russell, S. W., Altman, A., and Katz, D. H. (1983). *J. Immunol.* **131**, 826–832.

Schutze, M.-P., Leclerc, C., Jolivet, M., Audibert, F., and Chédid, L. (1985). *J. Immunol.* **135**, 2319–2322.

Sette, A., Buus, S., Colon, S., Smith, J. A., Miles, C., and Grey, H. M. (1987). *Nature (London)* **328**, 395–399.

Smith, G. L., Godson, G. N., Nussenzweig, V., Nussenzweig, R. S., Barnwell, J., and Moss, B. (1984). *Science* **224**, 397–399.

Staruch, M. J., and Wood, D. D. (1983). *J. Immunol.* **130**, 2191–2194.

Stuart-Harris, C. H. (1969). *Bull. W.H.O.* **41**, 617–621.

Sutcliffe, J. G., Shinnick, T. M., Green, N., and Lerner, R. A. (1983). *Science* **219**, 660–666.

Tanamoto, K., Zahringer, U., McKenzie, G. R., Galanos, C., Rietschel, E., Luderitz, O., Kusumoto, S., and Shiba, T. (1984). *Infect. Immun.* **44**, 421–426.

Unanue, E. R. (1984). *Annu. Rev. Immunol.* **2**, 395–428.

Valenzuela, P., Medina, A., Rutter, W. J., Ammerer, G., and Hall, B. D. (1982). *Nature (London)* **298**, 347–350.

Vogel, F. R., Leclerc, C., Schutze, M.-P., Jolivet, M., Audibert, F., Klein, T. W., and Chédid, L. (1987). *Cell. Immunol.* **107**, 40–51.

Vosika, G. J., Schmidtke, J. R., Goldman, A., Ribi, E., Parker, R., and Gray, G. R. (1979). *Cancer (Philadelphia)* **44**, 495–503.

Waksman, G. H. (1979). *Springer Semin. Immunopathol.* **2**, 5–33.

Warren, H. S., Vogel, F. R., and Chédid, L. A. (1986). *Annu. Rev. Immunol.* **4**, 369–388.

Weinstein, Y., Segal, S., and Melmon, K. L. (1975). *J. Immunol.* **115**, 112–117.

Whitehouse, M. W., Orr, K. J., Beck, F. W. J., and Pearson, C. M. (1974). *Immunology* **27**, 311–330.

Woodhour, A. F., Metzgar, D. P., Stim, T. B., Tutell, A. A., and Hilleman, M. R. (1964). *Proc. Soc. Exp. Biol. Med.* **116**, 516–523.

Yarkoni, E., and Rapp, H. J. (1979). *Cancer Res.* **39**, 1518–1520.

Yasuda, T., Kanegasaki, S., Tsumita, T., Takakuma, T., Homma, J. Y., Inage, M., Kusumoto, S., and Shiba, T. (1982). *Eur. J. Biochem.* **124**, 405–407.

Vaccines for Parasitic Infections

ANTHONY F. BARBET

Department of Infectious Diseases, College of Veterinary Medicine, University of Florida, Gainesville, Florida

I. Introduction

A. HISTORICAL PERSPECTIVE

Vaccines for several parasitic infections in animals, based on attenuated or killed parasites, have been developed during the last 30 years and are used widely. Of these, some are very effective, inducing the desired immunity against challenge with virulent organisms and having few unwanted side effects or problems of administration. An example is the vaccine against lungworms of cattle and sheep, *Dictyocaulus* spp. This vaccine was developed from the work of Jarrett *et al.* (1960) and Jarrett and Sharp (1963) and consists of two doses of 1,000 larvae attenuated by irradiation. Since this pioneering research, millions of cattle have been protected against disease, with a reduction in mean worm burden of 95–98% (Urquhart, 1980, 1985). Vaccinated

345

calves do not develop total sterile immunity and some larvae may infect vaccinated animals after natural challenge. This may be advantageous, since the boost that animals receive naturally each year removes the need for further vaccination. Other killed or attenuated vaccines against theileriosis, babesiosis, and anaplasmosis in cattle and coccidiosis in poultry have been produced and used in various countries. These vaccines vary in their efficacy.

Theileria annulata, a protozoan parasite transmitted by ticks, causes serious disease of cattle in North Africa, the Middle East, and India. A safe and reliable vaccine has been used for many years, consisting of attenuated, macroschizont-infected lymphoblastoid cells (Pipano, 1977). A similar vaccine induces protective immunity against sheep theileriosis caused by *T. hirci* (Hooshmand-Rad, 1985). In contrast, similar approaches with *T. parva* were unsuccessful; cell culture-derived *T. parva* schizonts transferred slowly from donor to recipient cells and recipient animals rejected incompatible donor cells (Dolan, 1987). Therefore, large numbers of living cells were required to infect animals and immunization results were unpredictable (Brown, 1981). A vaccination method is, nevertheless, available for *T. parva*. This consists of infection of cattle with sporozoites followed by drug treatment to control the infection (Radley, 1981). Besides inconvenience, the disadvantages of this method include the antigenic variability of field strains, with occasional breakthrough infections on challenge, and induction of the carrier state (persistent tick-transmissible infections) by immunization (Radley, 1981).

Live vaccines based on attenuation of *Babesia bovis* and *B. bigemina* by serial passage through calves have been used in Australia since 1897 (Callow, 1979), but not extensively in other countries. The reasons for this limited use (Wright and Riddles, 1986) include:

1. Limited shelf life of 5–7 days at 5°C.
2. The vaccine itself may cause post-vaccination mortality of about 1% despite follow-up and treatment of sick animals.
3. Vaccine donor calves may be silently infected with other parasites (*Anaplasma, Theileria, Eperythrozoon*) and growing importance has been attributed recently to latent viral and bacterial diseases.
4. Perpetuation of the protozoan in the environment by induction of a carrier state.
5. In many countries the means do not exist for rapid transport of vaccine from production site to the field.
6. The vaccine contains a high ratio of bovine protein to immunizing

organisms, which can induce hemolytic anemia in newborn calves (Dimmock and Bell, 1970).

In Israel, frozen vaccine is used which has a shelf life of several years and allows testing of donor calves for silent infections (Pipano, 1978). However, the survival rate of *Babesia* after freezing and thawing is low and large numbers of parasites must be administered. This increases the amount of bovine protein inoculated and the cost of the vaccine. Recent attempts to attenuate parasites by *in vitro* culture (Levy and Ristic, 1980) may remove some, but not all of the above obstacles to general use (Buening *et al.*, 1986; Yunker *et al.*, 1987).

Similar problems are associated with an attenuated *Anaplasma* vaccine (Henry *et al.*, 1983). In addition, differentiation of vaccinated from naturally *Anaplasma*-infected animals is not possible with current diagnostic tests. A killed *Anaplasma* vaccine is available in the United States (Norman, 1973) which consists of lyophilized infected red cells reconstituted in an oil adjuvant. Yearly booster doses are recommended. The vaccine can again lead to isoerythrolysis when newborn calves suckle their vaccinated mothers, because of sensitization to red cell antigens in the immunogen (Dennis *et al.*, 1970).

Vaccines are commercially available against *Eimeria* infections of poultry. Parasite infection induces an immune response that renders the host totally or partially resistant to reinfection with the homologous organism (Rose, 1985). The immunity is species-specific. For this reason the vaccine in commercial use consists of a mixture of live oocysts of different species. This vaccine may be administered in combination with drugs to control the infection. The method is not ideal, as *Eimeria* species not present previously may be introduced into a flock (Ryley, 1980). Improvements have been made recently in administration of live *Eimeria* parasites for vaccination purposes. Constant exposure of flocks to low doses of parasites ("trickle" immunization) avoids some of the pathogenic effects of single-dose vaccines while inducing comparable immunity (Davis *et al.*, 1985).

B. MODERN VACCINE TECHNOLOGY

Despite the disadvantages of the vaccines described above, the encouraging fact remains that varying degrees of immunity *can* be engendered and that there are management conditions where attenuated or killed parasite vaccines are practically beneficial. The first goal of new methods of vaccine technology is to develop comparable or better immunity to infection but avoid problems such as: (1) the risk of introduction of parasite species or strains into new areas (a common problem of attenuated vaccines) or (2) immunopathology associated with antigens present in the vaccine but irrelevant to protection (a common problem of killed vaccines). A second and no less important goal is to provide low-cost vaccines that are stable in different environments and readily distributed and administered.

The assumptions often implicit in new approaches to parasite vaccines are:

1. The host normally responds to many antigens from intact and dying parasites; not all of these responses are protective and some may be harmful to the host.

2. It is possible to focus the immune response on a small number of antigens from one or more stages of the life cycle and prevent parasite survival.

3. The significant antigens are often located on the outer surface of the parasite.

4. Methods of protein biochemistry and immunochemistry allow one to identify surface antigens and to select those which do not vary in structure during infection or between different parasite isolates.

5. If antigens vary in structure, there may be regions which do not vary and against which an immunoprotective response can be induced. Such regions may have an essential function in the parasite, for example binding to a receptor molecule on a host cell.

6. Methods in recombinant DNA and synthetic peptide chemistry can provide a convenient source of individual proteins, glycoproteins, or protein fragments for protection.

7. Suitable adjuvants and methods to present synthetic or recombinant antigens in a form resembling the native molecule will be available. Where necessary, both antibody and cell-mediated immunity will be induced.

8. Quality control, distribution, and administration of synthetic or recombinant vaccines will be improved over conventional vaccines. This is because they will be of defined structure and stable compared to attenuated, living, parasites.

9. Modern vaccines will readily be integrated with new techniques for diagnosis using (a) recombinant proteins and serology, or (b) recombinant nucleic acid probes. Use of different proteins for vaccination and serological diagnosis, for example, would enable differentiation of vaccinated from infected animals.

10. This approach is also compatible with modern epidemiology, using the same techniques as in assumption 9 to identify and eliminate reservoirs of infection in host animals and vectors.

Of the above assumptions, good evidence exists for 1–4, 6, 8, 9, 10, and less for 5 and 7, although much progress has been made in antigen presentation, e.g., using virus vectors to induce both antibody and cell-mediated immunity (Moss and Flexner, 1987) and in strategies for identifying T-cell epitopes (Livingstone and Fathman, 1987). The major problems foreseen with molecular vaccines derive from the restricted antigens presented to the host immune system and the variability of host responses expected in a genetically diverse population. If the majority of individuals can be sensitized to an antigen, eventually parasites may be selected that have lost or changed the required structure (reviewed in Mitchell, 1984). This clearly occurs in infections with African trypanosomes (Turner, 1985) and some (Klotz *et al.*, 1987; Handunnetti *et al.*, 1987), but not all (Ferreira *et al.*, 1987), surface antigens of *Plasmodium*; research on many other parasites has not yet progressed to the point where the question can be answered.

A detailed review on vaccination against malaria will not be presented here (the reader is referred to the following excellent reviews: Howard, 1982, 1987; Nussenzweig and Nussenzweig, 1984; Anders *et al.*, 1985; Newbold, 1985); however, in view of the consider- able knowledge accumulated on malaria it is important to consider what problems remain for a subunit vaccination strategy. Antigens of each stage of the life cycle of several different species of mouse and primate malaria have been identified, cloned, sequenced, and ex- pressed in *E. coli,* yeast, and vaccinia systems. This research has revealed that many different *Plasmodium* proteins contain tandemly repeated peptides of varying length. Repeat peptides have been found in other prokaryotic (*e.g.,* streptococcal M protein, Beachey *et al.*, 1978; Scott *et al.*, 1986) and eukaryotic (e.g. *Trypanosoma cruzi,* Peterson *et al.,* 1986; *Schistosoma mansoni,* Bobek *et al.,* 1986) organisms, but the extent of repeats in *Plasmodium* appears unusual. This has provoked the argument as to whether these structures have essential functions for the parasite or are the normal result of unequal crossovers between DNA segments not maintained by natural selection (Smith, 1976). Surface-exposed repeated peptides are considered by some to be suitable targets for a protective immune response (Nussenzweig and Nussenzweig, 1984) and by others to cause cross-reactions that actu- ally impair the development of protective immunity (Anders, 1986). The optimistic viewpoint is supported (for the sporozoite stage of the life cycle) by data showing that vaccination with irradiated *Plasmo-dium* sporozoites induces protective immunity *in vivo* (Nussenzweig *et al.*, 1969). Circumsporozoite surface proteins containing repetitive epitopes were identified that were presumed to have a role in the development of this immunity. Antibodies to these proteins neutralized infectivity of sporozoites *in vitro* (Yoshida *et al.*, 1980) or in passive transfer experiments (Potocnjak *et al.*, 1980) and inhibited invasion of human hepatoma cells *in vitro* (Aley *et al.*, 1986). Moreover, repetitive epitopes of the circumsporozoite surface protein were conserved in nine different isolates of *Plasmodium falciparum* and in six isolates of *P. vivax*, confirming these proteins as major targets for vaccine development (Nussenzweig and Nussenzweig, 1984). The pessimistic viewpoint is supported especially by recent observations that a recombinant surface protein or synthetic repeated epitope of *P. berghei* circumsporozoites induced greater humoral responses than irradiated sporozoites in mice but provided far less protection against challenge infection (Egan *et al.*, 1987). Adoptive transfer of spleen cells from mice immunized with irradiated sporozoites was protective whereas transfer of spleen cells from mice immunized with the subunit vaccines was not (Egan *et al.*, 1987). The critical role for cell-mediated immunity and especially $CD8^+$ T cells has also been recently demonstrated in *P. yoelii* infections (Mogil *et al.*, 1987; Weiss *et al.*, 1988). The observations suggest that both humoral and cell-mediated immunity are necessary for efficient protection *in vivo* and that requisite cell-mediated immunity was not induced by the subunit vaccines tested. Current investigations center on defining *Plasmodium* epitopes inducing T-cell protection (Good, 1988; Good *et al.*, 1988a) and potential problems caused by polymorphism in major T-cell domains of circumsporozoite surface proteins (Good *et al.*, 1988b).

The lesson for development of vaccines in other diseases is that, where possible, *in vivo* challenge experiments should be performed at an early stage to identify the parasite molecules which are suitable vaccine components. Reliance should not be placed totally on correlates of immunity such as *in vitro* neutralization or protection by passive transfer. Research on vaccines for veterinary diseases is important for discovery of the most effective ways to present subunit immunogens to the host. In veterinary diseases one may perform immunization and challenge experiments with the natural host–parasite combination rather than with animal models of human disease. Although much information has been obtained from model systems, there may be differences in virulence and pathogenicity which influence the results of vaccination and challenge. In the *P.*

berghei/AJ mouse model, for example, sporozoite infectivity is only 2% compared with 45% in the natural host (Vanderberg *et al.*, 1968).

Despite problems still to overcome in the production of new antiparasite vaccines, one may be encouraged by recent advances that provide novel methods for the presentation of antigens, e.g., the development of live vectors (this volume, Chapters 6–8), new immunostimulants (e.g., ISCOMs; Morein *et al.*, 1984) and adjuvants (e.g., murabutide; Audibert and Chédid, 1984), and the coupling of antigen to anti-class II MHC antibodies (Carayanniotis and Barber, 1987). Protection against certain parasites by subunit vaccines has been achieved with currently available adjuvants. For example, cattle were protected by immunization with a purified surface protein against homologous and heterologous challenge with virulent *Anaplasma marginale* (Palmer *et al.*, 1986a; also see Section II). *Aotus* monkeys were completely protected against *P. falciparum* challenge by immunization with merozoite surface coat precursor protein (Siddiqui *et al.*, 1987). In humans limited but significant protection was obtained against *P. falciparum* with a recombinant sporozoite vaccine (Ballou *et al.*, 1987).

The focus of this review will be recent progress made in the development of defined subunit vaccines against selected parasites of significance in veterinary medicine. Examples of parasitism considered vary from a rickettsia, through hemoparasitic and intestinal protozoa, to helminths. Each parasite system has unique problems to be considered before an effective vaccine can be produced.

II. Vaccines for Hemoparasites

A. *Babesia*

Babesiosis is an arthropod-borne protozoan disease of domestic animals and a major deterrent to livestock production in many countries. Significant losses occur world-wide due to reduced meat and milk production, and restriction of cattle movement to and from enzootic areas. Introduction of the sporozoite stage into cattle by ticks initiates the cycle of erythrocyte invasion, multiplication to produce merozoites and lysis, resulting in clinical disease.

Recently, there have been many vaccine trials against *Babesia* parasites of cattle. These have involved attenuated and killed merozoites and merozoite antigens varying from poorly defined fractions to single proteins. Statistically significant protection against virulent challenge was obtained with purified parasite antigens but, where comparisons were made, the degree of protection was less than with attenuated parasite vaccines. In some instances of partial protection, the results are difficult to assess because animals immunized with adjuvant and an unrelated protein were not included as a control. Immunostimulants have produced nonspecific protection against *Babesia* in mice (Clarke *et al.*, 1976, 1977), and, although this was not confirmed in *Babesia divergens* infection of cattle (Brocklesby and Purnell, 1977), this may be due to the size of the dose administered. Freund's adjuvant and ovalbumin provide a low level of protection against *Anaplasma* infections in cattle (Palmer *et al.*, 1986a; G. H. Palmer, unpublished). When considering the variability in response to challenge infection obtained in animals not highly inbred, and the small numbers generally available for cattle experiments, it would seem prudent to reduce all possible sources of variation to a minimum.

A major contribution to *Babesia* research was the development of *in vitro* culture systems for continuous growth of the merozoite (Erp *et al.*, 1978, 1980; Levy and Ristic, 1980; Vega *et al.*, 1985). Parasite antigens were found in the supernatant of *B. bovis* cultures which provided partial protection against homologous and heterologous challenge (Montenegro-James and Ristic, 1985), but less than the protection obtained by immunization with attenuated parasites (Kuttler *et al.*, 1982). Culture supernatants contained several parasite proteins (James, 1984); those essential for protection were not defined. Cultures provide a useful experimental source of *Babesia* but may be inconvenient for routine vaccine production; also, culture-derived vaccines are likely to be more expensive than *Babesia* proteins produced and delivered by recombinant DNA methods. Another problem is standardization of the quantity of immunoprotective *B. bovis* proteins required to be in culture supernatants and the maximum quantity of nonimmunoprotective proteins that can be tolerated. Further analysis is required of the amount and composition of antigens present in *Babesia* culture media under different growth conditions, and of the protection afforded by individual components.

An alternative approach toward vaccination against *B. bovis* was taken by Goodger, Wright, and colleagues. A monoclonal antibody (15B1) was used as an immunoadsorbent to isolate a protein of 44 kD from *Babesia bovis*-infected erythrocytes (Wright *et al.*, 1983). Partial protection was conferred by this protein against *B. bovis* challenge. Control and vaccinated animals developed parasitemias and showed temperature rise and changes in packed cell volume. However, there were statistically significant differences between the groups, indicative of protection by the purified protein. Except for one vaccinated animal which died 4 days after the last control animal, vaccinates were less clinically affected than controls. Interestingly, the same monoclonal antibody (15B1) later was used to isolate a protein of 29 kD from infected erythrocytes which was also partially immunoprotective in cattle (Wright *et al.*, 1985). The structural relationship between the two proteins was not defined. The authors considered, but did not clearly establish, that the 44-kD protein was a single polypeptide chain; one possibility is that the 29-kD molecule was a proteolytic cleavage product. If the 44-kD molecule was a complex of more than one polypeptide, a second possibility is that this was dissociated by the more denaturing gel system (0.1% sodium dodecyl sulfate and 0.5 *M* urea) used in the second study, producing the 29-kD molecule and other polypeptides. The 29-kD molecule contained the epitope reactive with monoclonal antibody. This molecule is a candidate to include in a recombinant vaccine.

Novel proteins associated only with the *Babesia*-infected erythrocyte have been demonstrated (Howard *et al.*, 1980a,b); these were of 118, 115, and 60 kD in *B. bovis* infections. It is not known whether these proteins are protective. Complementary DNA libraries have now been prepared in the bacteriophage expression vector λ gt11-amp3 from *B. bovis* mRNA (Gill *et al.*, 1987); therefore recombinant analogs of the above proteins should be available shortly for testing. Thus far, a protein fragment identified in the above library by screening with sera from infected cattle appears to derive from an intact *B. bovis* protein of at least 220 kD; no structural relationship with known immunoprotective proteins was described.

In *B. divergens,* research toward a subunit vaccine has progressed by the demonstration of partial protection afforded by antigen fractions of increasing purity (Taylor *et al.*, 1984, 1986a,b; Winger *et al.*, 1987). The successful experiments have included homologous and heterologous merozoite and sporozoite challenge of immunized cattle and Mongolian gerbils. Effective parasite antigen fractions were an acidic fraction of *B. divergens* merozoites isolated by isoelectric focusing (Taylor *et al.*, 1984), the non-Concanavalin A binding portion of the acidic fraction (Taylor *et al.*, 1986b), and, finally, an affinity-purified protein of approximately 50 kD (Winger *et al.*, 1987). In the latter study, the major surface protein eluted from free merozoites by a saline wash was identified and a monoclonal antibody was isolated that bound to this protein. The antibody reacted strongly with intact merozoites in immunofluorescence but only weakly with merozoites that lacked the 50-kD protein, and it inhibited merozoite invasion of erythrocytes *in vitro*. Moreover, the isolated protein conferred protection on Mongolian gerbils to homologous challenge with live *B. divergens*. One awaits with interest the results of homologous and heterologous challenge experiments in cattle using this protein and defined structural analogs as immunogens.

Babesia bigemina is a major disease of cattle in tropical and subtropical climates. Progress was made toward vaccination against this parasite recently with the development of an immunofluorescence assay for live merozoites (McElwain *et al.*, 1987a). Surface-reactive monoclonal antibodies were identified that immunoprecipitated radio-labeled merozoite proteins of 72, 58, 55, 45, and 36 kD. Homologous and heterologous sera from recovered cattle recognized the same five proteins. Preliminary immunization trials have been performed with the isolated proteins in cattle and suggest that the most protective immunogen is 45 kD (Bp 45). Statistically significant, but only partial, protection was achieved. In vaccinated animals there was reduction in mean peak parasitemia and maximum temperature rise. Moreover, four of five ovalbumin-immunized calves and zero of five Bp 45-immunized calves were hemoglobinuric during the experiment (McElwain *et al.*, 1987b).

The above data on various *Babesia* species suggest that although protection is obtained with defined antigens it is not yet optimal. This may result from the limited number of different antigens tested (mostly from the merozoite stages) or from the methods used for antigen presentation. Most purification methods result in changes in protein conformation from that on the surface of the infective parasite. Probably, molecules that resemble the native epitopes more closely will, in the future, be produced and delivered by synthetic or recombinant methods. It remains to be seen whether acceptable levels of immunity will result. As a further caution, there is evidence in *B. rodhaini* that a membrane protein of the parasite shares an epitope with a protein in uninfected mouse red blood cells (Snary and Smith, 1986). This cross-reaction could be fortuitous, or a contributing factor to parasite pathogenicity or evasion of the host immune response.

B. *Anaplasma*

Anaplasmosis is a hemoparasitic disease of cattle and other ruminants caused by a rickettsia, *Anaplasma marginale*. The disease occurs worldwide, including several regions in the United States, and severely affects meat, milk, and fiber production. The organism is transmitted by arthropod vectors or blood-contaminated fomites. After a prepatent period of 20–40 days there is an acute phase during which erythrocytic parasitemia increases geometrically and severe anemia occurs. The intraerythrocytic inclusion is composed of a host-derived membrane limiting two to eight ovoid "initial bodies."

Progress has been made recently toward a defined subunit vaccine against this parasite, by applying the methods of protein biochemistry and immunochemistry. Two important advances were a structural analysis of the organism following metabolic radiolabeling in short-term *in vitro* culture, and isolation of viable *A. marginale* initial bodies from infected erythrocytes (Barbet *et al.*, 1983; Palmer and McGuire, 1984). Since the mature erythrocyte does not synthesize proteins, the composition of the parasite was analyzed without interference from contaminating erythrocyte proteins (Barbet *et al.*, 1983). Moreover, surface labeling of isolated initial bodies and immunoprecipitation with neutralizing antisera defined those proteins accessible to the host immune response (Palmer and McGuire, 1984). Five surface proteins of 105, 86, 61, 36, and 31 kD were identified. A panel of monoclonal antibodies was produced and clones which bound various proteins of *A. marginale* were isolated. Of the entire panel of antibodies, none bound to *A. ovis*, *Babesia bovis*, *B. bigemina*, *Trypanosoma brucei*, or *T. congolense*. The antibodies did distinguish between isolates of *A. marginale* in immunofluorescence but no differentiation antigens were observed in sequential daily smears taken during infection with a single isolate (McGuire *et al.*, 1984). Monoclonal antibodies were identified that bound to the 105- and 36-kD surface proteins. Antibodies 15D2 and 22B1 (to the 105-kD surface protein) neutralized infectivity of isolated initial bodies *in vitro* and bound to twelve different geographical isolates of *A. marginale* and an isolate of *A. centrale* (Palmer *et al.*, 1986a, 1988). The 105-kD protein (Am 105) was isolated from infected bovine erythrocytes by affinity chromatography on an antibody 15D2-Sepharose column, and found to be a closely spaced doublet on sodium dodecyl sulfate–urea gels. Calves immunized with the isolated protein developed high titers of antibody to *A. marginale*, compared to control ovalbumin-immunized calves, and were significantly protected from challenge. Control calves developed 4–5% parasitemia and clinical anaplasmosis. In contrast, two of five Am 105-immunized calves did not show any parasitized erythrocytes in stained blood smears and the other three calves had <0.01% peak parasitemia. The three Am 105 calves that were transiently infected did not develop clinical disease (Palmer *et al.*, 1986a). The significant protection obtained in this experiment and conservation of a neutralization-sensitive epitope between isolates (and present in tick stages of *A. marginale*; Palmer *et al.*, 1985) suggested that Am 105 was a candidate to include in a subunit vaccine.

Subsequent efforts were directed toward obtaining a convenient source of the Am 105 immunogen via recombinant DNA methods. Although purification of the native protein in milligram amounts was possible from infected bovine erythrocytes, the method was cumbersome and would be inconvenient and expensive for field trials and routine vaccine production. Genomic libraries of *A. marginale* DNA were constructed in *E. coli* and colonies identified that reacted with rabbit and monoclonal anti-Am 105 sera on nitrocellulose immunoblots. On characterization of the recombinant proteins and coding genes, it was discovered that the polypeptide doublet purified by monoclonal antibody chromatography and used to immunize calves was a complex of two structurally and antigenically distinct polypeptides. To date, one of these polypeptides has been expressed as a complete recombinant polypeptide of 105 kD in *E. coli* (Barbet *et al.*, 1987). Part of the second polypeptide (56 kD), containing the neutralization-sensitive epitope in a tandemly repeated 29 amino acid peptide, was expressed in the plasmid vector pUC9 (A. F. Barbet, T. C. McGuire, D. R. Allred, T. M. Harkins, and G. H. Palmer, unpublished). Construction and expression of the complete protein complex is in progress.

There is still considerable research necessary and problems to overcome before a recombinant vaccine against bovine anaplasmosis could be marketed. One problem is an acceptable method of antigen presentation to induce the most effective response (discussed earlier). A second potential problem is structural variation in Am 105. Although the epitope recognized by neutralizing monoclonal antibodies 22B1 and 15D2 is conserved between isolates, there is evidence for allelic polymorphism (Allred *et al.*, 1987) and for amino acid sequence variation in other regions of the molecule (Oberle, 1988). Certainly, cross-protection experiments with previous vaccines (Kreier and Ristic, 1963; Carson *et al.*, 1970; Kuttler and Todorovic, 1973) and structural analysis (Barbet *et al.*, 1983) suggest that variation in protein antigens of *A. marginale* occurs. It is not clear whether variation is sufficiently extensive between isolates to cause problems for a carefully engineered subunit vaccine. An encouraging result was successful protection of calves by Florida isolate Am 105 against challenge with Florida or Washington state *A. marginale* (G. H. Palmer, A. F. Barbet, T. F. McElwain, and T. C. McGuire, unpublished). It is likely that in anaplasmosis, as in other parasite vaccines, there will be several generations of products, involving different peptide combinations and methods of presentation, seeking to obtain the most effective immunity at the lowest cost. The use of Am 105 as a first-generation subunit vaccine in combination with a diagnostic test based on a second polypeptide (e.g., Am 86; Palmer *et al.,* 1986b) or a DNA probe (Goff *et al.,* 1988) is an attractive proposition.

III. Vaccines for Other Protozoan Parasites

A. *Eimeria*

The strong protective immunity which is engendered by most coccidial infections (Rose, 1982) has suggested that an effective subunit vaccine could be manufactured. In *Eimeria* infections of poultry, the practical requirements imposed on a subunit vaccine are stringent compared to many other parasite vaccines (Long, 1984). Due to the intensive methods of production, a vaccine must be very inexpensive to manufacture and easy to deliver. A method for vaccinating flocks would be superior to a vaccine requiring manipulation of individual birds. Also, the vaccine should be effective against at least six species of *Eimeria*. For this reason, subunit vaccine strategies have strong competition from chemoprophylaxis and methods to attenuate parasites by embryo-adaptation or selection for "precociousness" (Jeffers, 1985; abbreviated life cycle due to reduction or elimination of a schizont generation). Stable attenuated parasites of the economically important species of chicken coccidia are now available (Jeffers, 1985; McDonald *et al.,* 1985) and viable oocysts could be administered in the drinking water or feed in a "trickle dose" regimen (Joyner and Norton, 1973). Administration of a multivalent subunit vaccine in a viable recombinant vector could, however, compete with attenuated vaccines without risk of reversion to virulence or spread of *Eimeria* species to new geographic locations.

Progress toward this goal has been hampered by the complex life cycle of the parasite and delineation of those stages and antigens susceptible to immune attack. Different species and stages of the life cycle of *Eimeria* vary in their immunogenicity (Rose, 1985). Immunity induced by infection occurs in large part as a result of development of the asexual stages (Rose, 1982). The first and second generations of schizogony in *Eimeria tenella* are highly immunogenic (Johnson *et al.,* 1979; McDonald *et al.,* 1986). Sporozoites also probably contain protective antigens as their develement is inhibited in solidly immune animals (Rose *et al.,* 1984). Also, anti-sporozoite serum produced by infection and drug treatment inhibits penetration of sporozoites into chicken kidney cells (Bhanushali and Long, 1985). The immunogenicity of different stages observed during infection is likely dependent on the relative numbers of parasites stimulating the immune response and shared versus stage-specific exposed epitopes, among other variables. An effective recombinant vaccine may include antigens from both sporozoites (to immunize against initial invasive stages) and merozoites (to protect against asexual multiplicative stages arising from sporozoites escaping destruction). Most experiments to date have been directed toward analysis of sporozoite proteins.

In *E. tenella* experiments showed that extracts of sporulated oocysts conferred protection on chickens against cecal lesion development (Murray *et al.*, 1985). Chickens were vaccinated immediately after hatching, and immunity was apparent by 3 weeks of age and persisted for the life of the broiler (7 weeks). Interestingly, protection was obtained against several isolates of *E. tenella* and, an *E. acervulina* antigen extract protected against both *E. tenella* and *E. maxima*. Monoclonal antibodies were produced which neutralized *E. tenella* sporozoites *in vitro* and *in vivo* (Danforth, 1985; Crane *et al.*, 1986). In general, surface reactivity of monoclonal antibodies was a necessary, but not sufficient, criterion for activity in neutralization assays. Active antibodies were species and stage specific and recognized proteins of 5–8, 22, and 28 kD in immunoblots (Danforth, 1985).

Surface radiolabeling as an alternative method for identifying exposed proteins of the sporozoite for possible inclusion in a vaccine has been applied to various *Eimeria* species. The major polypeptides labeled by ^{125}I in *E. tenella, E. maxima, E. acervulina,* and *E. nieschulzi* were of 47, 26, 21, and <18 kD (Wisher, 1986), but significant label was incorporated into many other polypeptides. It was not clear whether labeling of minor polypeptide components was a result of (1) many different exposed polypeptides; (2) proteolysis of exposed polypeptides during excystation in medium containing trypsin and bile salts, or (3) low-level incorporation of ^{125}I into nonexposed polypeptides of any sporozoites present in the preparation. In another study of *E. acervulina* sporozoite and merozoite surface antigens, greater than 15 protein bands on sodium dodecyl sulfate gels contained radiolabel (Jenkins and Dame, 1987). The predominant labeled bands were of 14, 15, 21, 23, 24, 34, and 44 kD. In both studies many of the surface antigens were bound by sera from infected chickens in immunoprecipitation and immunoblot assays. Interestingly, the molecular weights of major surface labeled proteins of *E. acervulina* sporozoites and merozoites were different but there were not major changes between second- and third-generation merozoites (Jenkins and Dame, 1987). In contrast to the results with chicken *Coccidia,* in *E. bovis* of cattle only one polypeptide of merozoites and three of sporozoites were radiolabeled significantly by lactoperoxidase catalyzed surface iodination (Reduker and Speer, 1986). The merozoite polypeptide was 15–18 kD and the sporozoite polypeptides 28, 77, and 183 kD; all but the 183 kD were recognized by sera from infected cattle. Each labeled polypeptide corresponded to a stained protein band present in parasites but not in a normal calf intestinal cell lysate.

Experiments to clone and express recombinant analogs of *Eimeria* proteins are in progress; expression libraries of *E. tenella* genomic and complementary DNA have been made in bacteriophage λgt11 and derivatives (Clarke *et al.*, 1987; Danforth, 1985). One recombinant protein from these libraries (Danforth, 1985) has shown evidence of partial protection. Another recombinant surface protein of *Eimeria tenella* sporozoites was expressed in the plasmid vector pWHA63. The recombinant protein was a single polypeptide of 25 kD and contained the sequence information present in two *Eimeria* surface polypeptides of 17 kD and 8 kD recognized by neutralizing monoclonal antibodies. The recombinant polypeptide was not processed identically by *E. coli* and contained important immunological differences compared to the native polypeptides (Brothers *et al.*, 1988). It is unfortunate that because of the economic importance of this disease (worldwide sales of anticoccidials approaching $200 million/year), the problem of drug-resistant parasites (Long, 1984) and the interest of pharmaceutical companies in an effective vaccine, much research on producing and analyzing potential protective antigens is not published. Preliminary data has been presented which reveals the amount of interest in this area (see UCLA symposium on Molecular Strategies of Parasite Invasion, *Journal of Cellular Biochemistry, Suppl.* 10A, 1986); the study of future patents may be the best source of data on practical progress that has resulted.

B. *Toxoplasma*

Toxoplasma gondii is one of the most common protozoan diseases of man and domestic animals. As more efficient diagnostic methods are developed there is increasing realization of the importance of the organism as a pathogen in human and veterinary medicine. As many as 500 million people worldwide show serological evidence of infection (H. P. Hughes, 1985). Although most infections in man are avirulent or subclinical, in immunocompromised hosts the infection is often fatal. The organism may persist without clinical manifestations (Frenkel, 1973) so that animals or humans with inapparent infections are at risk of recrudescence. Congenital toxoplasmosis is a severe disease problem in many species including humans (Hartley and Marshall, 1957; Harding et al., 1961; Chowdhury, 1986). Protective immunity to *T. gondii* is both antibody and cell mediated; although antibody can protect against moderate challenge and does lyse extracellular *Toxoplasma* (Endo and Kobayashi, 1976), there is agreement that cell-mediated immunity is required for efficient protection (Reyes and Frenkel, 1987; Brinkmann et al., 1987) probably via activation of macrophages by γ-interferon (Suzuki et al., 1988).

Research toward a vaccine against *T. gondii* has at times produced surprising results that question some of the assumptions made in modern vaccine technology (see Section I,B). Several groups of investigators have characterized the surface membrane proteins of different strains of *T. gondii* (Handman et al., 1980; Kasper et al., 1982; Johnson et al., 1983). Generally, surface radioiodination of the tachyzoite stage reveals four major labeled proteins in the 14- to 45-kD range on SDS gel electrophoresis. Handman et al. (1980) found labeled proteins of 43, 35, 27, and 14 kD with the lactoperoxidase method in the C37, RH, and C56 strains of the parasite. Monoclonal antibodies were produced that recognized these radiolabeled molecules; two antibodies, 3E6 and 2G11, consistently immunoprecipitated the 35- and 14-kD proteins together. Johnson et al. (1983) obtained similar results, except that a 21-kD protein was found instead of the 27-kD molecule. In the latter study monoclonal antibody 2G11 immunoprecipitated both the 21- and 14-kD proteins. The structural relationship between the 35-, 21-, 27-, and 14-kD proteins was not clear. Monoclonal antibodies were obtained to the 35- and 14-kD surface proteins that, on passive transfer, conferred protection on mice against challenge (Johnson et al., 1983). Protection was not total, since all mice eventually died from highly virulent challenge and developed brain cysts on challenge with an isolate of moderate virulence. Immunization with partially purified *Toxoplasma* proteins containing possibly the same 35- and 14-kD molecules conferred partial protection on mice against challenge (Araujo and Remington, 1984). In a separate series of experiments, a surface protein of 22 kD was found by Kasper et al. (1982) in a cloned derivative of the RH strain, which may be the same as the 21-kD polypeptide observed by Johnson et al. (1983). The principle iodinatable surface protein found by Kasper et al. (1983) was 30 kd. This protein may contain repetitive epitopes although sequence information is not yet available (Rodriguez et al., 1985; Santoro et al., 1986). The 30-kD surface protein was purified to homogeneity by immunoaffinity chromatography, shown to be an integral membrane protein by charge-shift electrophoresis, and used as an immunogen. The surprising result was *enhanced* mortality in immunized mice (Kasper *et al.*, 1985).

A second unexpected result was the observation that monoclonal antibody F_3G_3 conferred significant protection on mice against *Toxoplasma* (Sharma *et al.*, 1984). This antibody recognized a cytoplasmic but *not* cell-surface antigen as determined by agglutination and immunofluorescence assay of living and formalin-fixed tachyzoites (Handman and Remington, 1980). The antigen recognized by monoclonal antibody F_3G_3 was purified by immunoaffinity chromatography and used as an immunogen. Complete protection by antigen in adjuvant against 5×10^6 tachyzoites of the C56 strain was obtained over a 40-day period; all control mice died in 15 days (Sharma *et al.*, 1984). Interestingly, considering the specificity of the monoclonal antibody, sera from mice immunized with the purified antigen *were* agglutinating and positive in the Sabin–Feldman dye test. This test reveals antibodies that lyse extracellular parasites (Endo and Kobayashi, 1976). Surface-accessible regions may, therefore have been present in the purified antigen.

There are both stage- and strain-specific surface antigens of *T. gondii* which may complicate vaccination attempts. Surface proteins of 67 and 25 kD were present on oocyst/sporozoites but not on tachyzoites (Kasper *et al.*, 1984; Kasper and Ware, 1985). In tachyzoites of RH, P, and C strains the apparent molecular weights of the major iodinatable surface proteins were similar, but there were differences in minor labeled components (Ware and Kasper, 1987). Perhaps more important was the observation that parasiticidal monoclonal antibodies against the RH strain varied in their ability to kill parasites of the P and C strains. Mutants of *T. gondii* were obtained which lacked a surface protein of 22 kD (Kasper *et al.*, 1982); disappearance of the protein was associated with resistance to killing by a 22-kD reactive monoclonal antibody. These observations suggest that selection of resistant parasites could accompany use of a recombinant vaccine based on a single surface protein.

Current vaccination attempts center on cloning and expression of *Toxoplasma gondii* outer membrane proteins and development of immunogenic but nonpathogenic and nonpersistent mutants. *Toxoplasma gondii* messenger RNA was purified and used to program *in vitro* synthesis of proteins. More than 11 proteins were recognized by both mouse and human immune serum (Johnson *et al.*, 1986). Recombinant analogs of outer membrane proteins currently are being tested (see UCLA symposium on Molecular Strategies of Parasite Invasion,

Journal of Cellular Biochemistry, Suppl. 10A, 1986). As in *Eimeria* infections, recombinant strategies have competition from the use of attenuated parasites. Mutant parasite populations were developed that did not produce brain cysts, elicited high antibody titers, and did not persist beyond 2 months in normal mice (Waldeland *et al.*, 1983). Athymic mice, however, developed severe lesions. Extensive research on these strains and possible methods of application would be required to avoid any possibility of pathogenic effects in immunosuppressed subjects.

IV. Vaccines for Helminth Parasites

Vaccination strategies against helminths must take into consideration the greater complexity of the parasites, the variety of different stages of the life cycle and the range of host immunological effector mechanisms which may be active *in vivo*. Unlike protozoa, helminths present to the host a large surface which is not subject to phagocytosis. For this reason, different arms of the immune system may be responsible for parasite killing. Helminth infections are characterized by a pronounced elevation of both specific and nonspecific IgE (Jarrett and Miller, 1982). Various helminth allergens have been purified which will induce reaginic antibodies when administered in a specific way; however, the purified molecules often are not substantially more allergenic than other proteins, such as ovalbumin, when administered in similar doses and by similar routes (Jarrett, 1978). Therefore, the specific IgE response may depend more on an adjuvant effect of the intact worm. Another notable observation in helminth infections is the increased number of circulating, activated eosinophils with the capacity to kill parasite targets *in vitro* (Basten *et al.*, 1970; Butterworth, 1984). These data have suggested that one efficient method of host cell defense is the cross-linking of IgE bound to mast cell receptors, causing degranulation and release of mediators which attract eosinophils to the location of the invading helminth. The eosinophils then adhere to the surface of the worm and degranulate, releasing substances such as major basic protein and eosinophil cationic protein, which damage the parasite membrane (Butterworth, 1984). An *in vitro* assay making use of this phenomenon is monoclonal antibody-mediated eosinophil adherence. For example, a monoclonal antibody to a surface antigen of *Trichinella spiralis* mediated the attachment of eosinophils to living newborn larvae, which killed the worms (Ortega-Pierres *et al.*, 1984a). Eosinophils are not the only effector cells against helminths; in some situations neutrophils (Dean *et al.*, 1974) and activated macrophages (Capron *et al.*, 1975) may be equally or more active. Cytotoxic lymphocytes have generally been found inactive (Butterworth, 1984).

The primary methods for control of helminth infections are efficient management techniques and administration of effective antihelminthic drugs. However, in the swine industry for example, losses in the United States due to helminth infection have been estimated at $385 million annually (Stewart *et al.*, 1985). Therefore, there is a clear need for improved antihelminthic vaccines.

A. *Trichinella*

Trichinosis has a wide distribution, occurring in both tropical and temperate climates. The causative agent, *Trichinella spiralis,* is infective to humans and many domestic and wild animal species. The different stages of the life cycle include: four (enteric) larval stages and the adult worms living in the intestinal villi, migrating newborn larvae produced following sexual reproduction of the adults, and intracellular muscle larvae. Resistance to reinfection develops in many hosts (Ruitenberg and Steerenberg, 1976; Despommier, 1977; James *et al.*, 1977; Murrell, 1985) which suggests that an effective vaccine could be developed. Host resistance appears to be due to several different mechanisms: rapid expulsion of infectious larvae immediately after their entry into the small intestine, immunity against preadult and adult worm stages, reduction in fecundity and specific immunity to newborn larvae (Denham and Martinez, 1970; Despommier *et al.*, 1977; Lee and Best, 1983; Urban, 1986).

In immune rats considerable data suggested that anaphylactic reactions in the gut following exposure to *Trichinella* antigens caused structural changes in the intestinal epithelium, immediate expulsion of undamaged infective larvae (Russell and Castro, 1979; Hessel *et al.*, 1982), and subsequent expulsion of adults. This rapid expulsion phenomenon eliminated 80–95% of a challenge infection within 24 hr (Bell and McGregor, 1980; Russell and Castro, 1985) and was associated with alteration in epithelial physiology and ion transport caused by mast cell mediators (Bell *et al.*, 1979; Harari *et al.*, 1987). In pigs expulsion of adult worms on secondary challenge occurred, but took significantly longer than in rats and mice. Also, the fecundity of female worms from immune pigs was reduced 75% compared to controls, and the development of newborn larvae was inhibited (Murrell, 1985). A marked eosinophilia is observed in *T. spiralis* infections, and it is known that rat and mouse eosinophils damage newborn larvae in the presence of antibody (Mackenzie *et al.*, 1981; Kazura and Grove, 1978). Evidence for this effect *in vivo* was obtained by Dessein *et al.*, (1981), who demonstrated that depletion of IgE in rats led to a reduction in eosinophils around the muscle-stage larvae and increased the numbers of larvae recovered. Clearly, the development of a vaccine must take into account this complex immune response induced against the different life-cycle stages of *T. spiralis*.

The surface antigens exposed on different stages of the life cycle have been analyzed using standard radioiodination techniques (Philip *et al.*, 1980; Parkhouse *et al.*, 1981; Clark *et al.*, 1982). Different molecules were labeled on each stage: 64, 58, 34, and 30 kD on newborn larvae; 105, 90, 55, and 47 kD on infective larvae and 40, 33, and 20 kD on adult worms. In addition, there were changes in the surface antigen profile during development of the same stage of the life cycle. On newborn larvae only the 64 kD molecule was labeled; 6–8 hr after release from the adult female the other components became accessible (Jungery *et al.*, 1983). The surface reorganization of newborn larvae observed by surface radiolabeling correlated with differences in immunofluorescent staining using a monoclonal antibody (Ortega-Pierres *et al.*, 1984b). Analysis of the surface-labeled molecules of infective larvae by peptide mapping and lectin binding suggested that they contained common amino acid sequences and that the 47- and 90-kD components were glycosylated (Parkhouse *et al.*, 1981; Clark *et al.*, 1982). One monoclonal antibody immunoprecipitated all four labeled polypeptides (Ortega-Pierres *et al.*, 1984b). The variation in surface antigens between and within different stages of the life cycle may be a mechanism by which the parasite evades a developing immune response; by the time the response has matured, the antigens have changed (Almond and Parkhouse, 1985).

The antibody response to surface-labeled *Trichinella spiralis* antigens in sensitive (C3H) and resistant (NIH) mice was examined by Almond and Parkhouse (1986). An interesting observation was that sensitive mice failed to produce detectable IgA antibody to any stage of the parasite. In contrast, resistant mice did produce IgA antibody and the timing of antibody production to adult worms correlated with their expulsion from the gastrointestinal tract. The significance of this observation for protection and direct demonstration of cause and effect remain to be demonstrated.

Monoclonal antibodies were produced recognizing different surface and secreted antigens of the parasite: 105-, 90-, 57-, and 47-kD surface antigens of infective larvae; 48- to 55-kD secreted antigens of infective larvae and 40- and 20-kD surface antigens of adult worms (Ortega-Pierres *et al.*, 1984a,b, 1986; Silberstein and Despommier, 1984;

Gamble and Graham, 1984; Gamble, 1985). The location of the antigens in the parasites was investigated by immunocytochemical techniques; monoclonal antibodies immunoprecipitating surface label of infective larvae also reacted with secretory stichocyte cells and gut lining (McLaren et al., 1987), as did monoclonal antibodies against the 48- to 55-kD secreted polypeptides. Interestingly, one, but not all, monoclonal antibodies precipitating the 40- and 20-kD surface proteins of adult worms intensely stained the copulatory bell of male parasites (Ortega-Pierres et al., 1986). Antigens isolated by affinity hromatography using monoclonal antibodies to the infective larval surface antigens and the 48- to 55-kD secreted antigens were partially protective in mice against challenge infection (Silberstein and Despommier, 1984, 1985; Gamble, 1985; McLaren et al., 1987). Immunization with the 48- to 55-kD secreted proteins resulted in accelerated expulsion of adult worms and reduced fecundity of adult females. The immunity induced by these antigens could be accounted for entirely by effects on adult worms (Silberstein and Despommier, 1985), even though the antigens were apparently not expressed by adults. It has been suggested, however, that larval stichosome antigens could be present in reduced quantity in the adult stichosome (McLaren et al., 1987), which may account for the specificity of the observed immunity. Partial immunity in rats and mice has also been induced by other T. spiralis antigens of varying degrees of purity (Gamble and Zarlenga, 1986; Grencis et al., 1986), including an allergen of 45 kD (Durham et al., 1984).

Preparation of recombinant analogs of immunoprotective proteins has begun with the isolation of T. spiralis messenger RNA and demonstration of efficient in vitro translation in rabbit reticulocyte lysates (Gamble and Zarlenga, 1986). However, it is likely that extensive basic research into methods of antigen presentation and delivery will be required before an effective vaccine is produced. It appears that several secreted stichocyte antigens, or shed surface antigens, could induce an allergenic response resulting in worm expulsion. The problem will be to induce an immune response of long duration, effective against different stages of the parasite, and without pathogenic effects in the host animal. Novel live bacterial or virus vectors (this volume, Chapters 6–8), capable of delivering a combination of parasite antigens to mucosal surfaces, may provide the desired immunity.

B. *Fasciola*

The liver fluke *Fasciola hepatica* infects a wide range of mammals including man and causes extensive economic losses, especially in sheep and cattle. When environmental conditions are favorable, animals may be exposed to extreme challenge doses resulting in acute infections and high mortality. Chronic fascioliasis occurs with less severe challenge, and is characterized by loss in body weight and reduced milk yield (Haroun and Hillyer, 1986). Mammalian hosts vary in their ability to develop resistance to infection with *F. hepatica*. There is little evidence that a primary infection of sheep stimulates resistance to reinfection (Rushton, 1977), but cattle do develop resistance, characterized by a decrease in the size and number of flukes recovered on challenge infection (Doyle, 1971, 1973). Susceptibility of laboratory animals to *F. hepatica* also varies: rats consistently exhibit resistance to reinfection (Hayes *et al.*, 1972; Oldham and Hughes, 1982), whereas different mouse strains do not develop resistance (Chapman and Mitchell, 1982). Cattle and rats eventually eliminate a primary fluke infection, unlike most other hosts (D. L. Hughes, 1985). These differences suggest a cautious interpretation of vaccination and challenge experiments, and of the use of model systems in this disease.

Various mechanisms have been suggested to account for resistance to reinfection. Migrating flukes of a primary infection may cause extensive liver fibrosis, which presents a physical barrier at the bile duct wall to challenge infections (Sinclair and Joyner, 1974; Hughes and Harness, 1975). However, in rats, resistance may be transferred by immune serum and by cells (Armour and Dargie, 1974; Corba *et al.*, 1971). In sensitized rats eosinophils rapidly coat newly excysted juvenile flukes and degranulate on the surface of the worm (Davies and Goose, 1981); however, attempts to reproduce this *in vitro* were unsuccessful (Duffus and Franks, 1980; Doy and Hughes, 1982).

There has been extensive research on ways to induce resistance with antigens of *F. hepatica* of varying degrees of purity, and the results are variable and conflicting. For example, there are reports of both successful (Lang and Hall, 1977; Rajasekariah *et al.*, 1979) and unsuccessful (Lehner and Sewell, 1979; Burden *et al.*, 1982) vaccination attempts using antigens that may be secretory/excretory products of the fluke. Resistance has been produced in rats by implantation of mature flukes in diffusion chambers, perhaps releasing these antigens (Haroun *et al.*, 1980). Generally, even the successful experiments did not result in sterile immunity (Haroun and Hillyer, 1986). The variability in the results obtained can probably be traced to a lack of molecular definition of the antigens employed and of the surface/secretory/excretory antigens on different stages of the parasite. Methods to characterize these antigens precisely are now available and have been employed recently, although this work is at an early stage in *Fasciola hepatica*.

During parasite development, different tegumental cells were observed by electron microscopy, which were associated with morphologically distinct granules termed T0, T1, and T2 (Bennett and Threadgold, 1975). The immunofluorescence reaction of flukes with cattle and sheep antisera obtained at different times during infection suggested that antibodies were produced to these granules and that the T2 granules were antigenically distinct from T0/T1 granules (Hanna, 1980). A series of monoclonal antibodies was prepared using spleen cells of mice infected with metacercariae. Of 87 clones producing antibody to *F. hepatica,* six different cell lines were identified producing antibody that reacted with T1 granules. These antibodies had unusual characteristics. All six monoclonal antibodies reacted with the same subset of polypeptides on immunoprecipitation and gel electrophoresis: a major component of 50 kD and minor components of 25–40 kD. In inhibition assays, each antibody was capable of blocking and being blocked by each other antibody, suggesting recognition of identical epitopes and structural uniformity in the T1 antigen (Hanna and Trudgett, 1983). In other systems these characteristics have often been associated with repeated sequences (Nussenzweig and Nussenzweig, 1984). Monoclonal antibodies bound primarily to T1 and T0 granules of juvenile flukes and metacercariae with much less intense immunofluorescence labeling of adult flukes. In juveniles and adults, however, gut and excretory systems were also labeled. The significance of the T1/T0 antigens for immunoprotection remains to be established.

Other investigators have attempted to define biochemically the surface and excretory/secretory antigens of *F. hepatica* as potential vaccine targets. The surface of newly excysted juvenile flukes appeared complex, with at least 13 different polypeptides accessible to surface radiolabeling and recognized by sera from infected cattle and goats (Reddington *et al.,* 1984). Juvenile flukes have been cultured *in vitro* and incorporated radioactive amino acids (Irving and Howell, 1982). Radioactive proteins also appeared in the culture medium which were recognized by infected sheep serum. The major polypeptides recognized were 23, 24, and 26 kD. In a subsequent study, the Concanavalin A-reactive glycoproteins of immature and mature flukes were analyzed (Dalton *et al.,* 1985). Two-dimensional gel electrophoresis resolved approximately 12 glycoproteins that were released into the culture medium by immature flukes and recognized by sera from infected rabbits. The major components had molecular weights in the range of 25–38 kD. These components may include some of the same secretory/excretory antigens identified previously by Irving and Howell (1982). The immunoreactive glycoproteins released *in vitro* by immature and mature flukes differed markedly (Dalton *et al.,* 1985).

This data may correlate with earlier observations that antigens released from immature stages were generally more effective in protecting rats than extracts of mature flukes (Rajasekariah *et al.*, 1979; Burden and Hammet, 1980; Burden *et al.*, 1982; Oldham, 1983). Interestingly, the glycoproteins recognized by rat, rabbit, cow, mouse, and sheep antisera were not significantly different (Dalton *et al.*, 1985), suggesting that the varying resistance to reinfection found in these different hosts cannot be correlated with antibody recognition of particular glycoproteins. The possibility remains that different *epitopes* rather than *antigens* are recognized.

Messenger RNA was isolated from *F. hepatica* and used to program synthesis of parasite proteins in rabbit reticulocyte lysates (Dalton *et al.*, 1985; Irving and Howell, 1986). The major proteins synthesized were 20–35 kD and were recognized by sera from infected sheep, rabbits, or sheep vaccinated with excretory/secretory antigens. A 30-kD protein comigrated on gels with a native polypeptide identified as a secretory/excretory protein by biosynthetic labeling (Irving and Howell, 1986). Also, a minor *in vitro* synthesized (unglycosylated) polypeptide component of 64 kD was recognized by rat but not by sheep antiserum. Complementary DNA libraries were prepared from fluke mRNA and recombinant plasmids used to transform mouse cells (Beardsell and Howell, 1987). Transformants were detected which expressed *F. hepatica* proteins and were recognized in immunofluorescence assays by infected sheep serum. To date, it is not known which of the surface or excretory/secretory proteins identified would provide the most efficient protection against disease. The availability of cloned genes and recombinant excretory/secretory proteins should provide this answer.

V. Conclusion

The previous discussion reveals that in many parasitic diseases more information is required to identify those proteins that should be included in a subunit vaccine. This is especially true for those parasites having many stages with different antigens, each inducing a complex immune response. Often the required step which has proven difficult to accomplish in the past is purification of antigens from parasites for testing. The methods of recombinant DNA technology now allow this obstacle to be overcome readily by overexpression in prokaryotic or eukaryotic systems, or even to be totally by-passed using viable recombinant vectors for immunization rather than purified antigens. One may be encouraged that in some diseases, such as malaria, anaplasmosis, and babesiosis, parasite antigens which are immunoprotective *have* been purified. The protection engendered, although significant, has not always been as effective as using viable parasites. In these diseases the main challenge is to develop optimal methods of antigen presentation to induce cell-mediated and humoral immunity as necessary. Cloning of genes for these immunoprotective proteins now allows testing of the most effective methods of presentation, which could be considered the second stage of vaccine development. The availability of live bacterial and viral vectors offers exciting possibilities for combining the advantages of live vaccines with those of single, purified antigens. One may look forward to the time when diagnostic tests enable rapid identification and elimination of reservoirs of infection and a single immunization protects against several parasitic diseases.

REFERENCES

Aley, S. B., Bates, M. D., Tam, J. P., and Hollingdale, M. R. (1986). *J. Exp. Med.* **164,** 1915–1922.
Allred, D. R., Oberle, S., Barbet, A. F., Palmer, G., and McGuire, T. (1987). *J. Cell Biol.* (abstr.) **105,** 155a.
Almond, N. M., and Parkhouse, R. M. (1985). *Curr. Top. Microbiol. Immunol.* **120,** 173–203.
Almond, N. M., and Parkhouse, R. M. (1986). *Parasite Immunol.* **8,** 391–406.
Anders, R. F. (1986). *Parasite Immunol.* **8,** 529–539.
Anders, R. F., Brown, G. V., Coppel, R. L., Stahl, H. D., Bianco, A. E., Favaloro, J. M., Crewther, P. E., Culvenor, J. G., and Kemp, D. J. (1985). *Dev. Biol. Stand.* **62,** 81–89.
Araujo, F. G., and Remington, J. S. (1984). *Infect. Immun.* **45,** 122–126.
Armour, J., and Dargie, J. D. (1974). *Exp. Parasitol.* **35,** 381–388.
Audibert, F., and Chédid, L. (1984). In "Vaccines '84: Modern Approaches to Vaccines" (R. M. Chanock and R. A. Lerner, eds.), pp. 397–400. Cold Spring Harbor Lab., Cold Spring Harbor, New York.
Ballou, W. R., Hoffman, S. L., Sherwood, J. A., Hollingdale, M. R., Neva, F. A., Hockmeyer, W. T., Gordon, D. M., Schneider, I., Wirtz, R. A., Young, J. A., Wasserman, G. F., Reeve, P., Diggs, C. L., and Chulay, J. D. (1987). *Lancet* **1,** 1277–1281.
Barbet, A. F., Anderson, L. W., Palmer, G. H., and McGuire, T. C. (1983). *Infect. Immun.* **40,** 1068–1074.
Barbet, A. F., Palmer, G. H., Myler, P. J., and McGuire, T. C. (1987). *Infect. Immun.* **55,** 2428–2435.
Basten, A., Boyer, M. H., and Beeson, P. B. (1970). *J. Exp. Med.* **131,** 1271–1287.
Beachey, E. H., Seyer, J. M., and Kang, A. H. (1978). *Proc. Natl. Acad. Sci. U.S.A.* **75,** 3163–3167.
Beardsell, P. L., and Howell, M. J. (1987). *Int. J. Parasitol.* **17,** 1057–1061.
Bell, R. G., and McGregor, D. D. (1980). *Infect. Immun.* **29,** 186–193.

Bell, R. G., McGregor, D. D., and Despommier, D. D. (1979). *Exp. Parasitol.* **47**, 140–157.
Bennett, C. E., and Threadgold, L. T. (1975). *Exp. Parasitol.* **38**, 38–55.
Bhanushali, J. K., and Long, P. L. (1985). *In* "Research in Avian Coccidiosis" (L. R. McDonald, L. P. Joyner, and P. L. Long, eds.), pp. 526–534. University of Georgia, Athens.
Bobek, L., Rekosh, D. M., van Keulen, H., and LoVerde, P. T. (1986). *Proc. Natl. Acad. Sci. U.S.A.* **83**, 5544–5548.
Brinkmann, V., Remington, J. S., and Sharma, S. D. (1987). *Infect. Immun.* **55**, 990–994.
Brocklesby, D. W., and Purnell, R. E. (1977). *Nature (London)* **265**, 343.
Brothers, V. M., Kuhn, I., Paul, L. S., Gabe, J. D., Andrews, W. H., Sias, S. R., McCaman, M. T., Dragon, E. A., and Files, J. G. (1988). *Mol. Biochem. Parasit.* **28**, 235–248.
Brown, C. G. D. (1981). *In* "Advances in the Control of Theileriosis" (A. D. Irvin, M. P. Cunningham, and A. S. Young, eds.), pp. 104–119. Martinus Nijhoff, The Hague.
Buening, G. M., Kuttler, K. L., and Rodriguez, S. D. (1986). *Vet. Parasitol.* **22**, 235–242.
Burden, D. J., and Hammet, N. C. (1980). *Vet. Parasitol.* **7**, 51–57.
Burden, D. J., Harness, E., and Hammet, N. C. (1982). *Vet. Parasitol* **9**, 261–266.
Butterworth, A. E. (1984). *Adv. Parasitol* **23**, 143–235.
Callow, L. L. (1979). *J. S. Afr. Vet. Assoc.* **50**, 353–356.
Capron, A., Dessaint, J. P., Capron, M., and Bazin, H. (1975). *Nature (London)* **253**, 474–475.
Carayanniotis, G., and Barber, B. H. (1987). *Nature (London)* **327**, 59–61.
Carson, C. A., Adams, L. G., and Todorovic, R. A. (1970). *Am. J. Vet. Res.* **31**, 1071–1078.
Chapman, C. B., and Mitchell, G. F. (1982). *Int. J. Parasitol.* **12**, 81–91.
Chowdhury, M. N. (1986). *J. Med. (Westbury, N.Y.)* **17**, 373–396.
Clark, N. W., Philipp, M., and Parkhouse, R. M. (1982). *Biochem. J.* **206**, 27–32.
Clarke, I. A., Allison, A. C., and Cox. F. E. G. (1976). *Nature (London)* **259**, 309–311.
Clarke, I. A., Cox, F. E. G., and Allison, A. C. (1977). *Parasitology* **74**, 9–15.
Clarke, L. E., Messer, L. I., Greenwood, N. M., and Wisher, M. H. (1987). *Mol. Biochem. Parasitol.* **22**, 79–87.
Corba, J., Armour, J., Roberts, R. J., and Urquart, G. M. (1971). *Res. Vet. Sci.* **12**, 292–295.
Crane, M. S., Norman, D. J., Gnozzio, M. J., Tate, A. C., Gammon, M., and Murray, P. K. (1986). *Parasite Immunol.* **8**, 467–480.
Dalton, J. P., Tom, T. D., and Strand, M. (1985). *Parasite Immunol.* **7**, 643–657.
Danforth, H. D. (1985). *In* "Research in Avian Coccidiosis" (L. R. McDonald, L. P. Joyner, and P. L. Long, eds.), pp. 574–590. University of Georgia, Athens.
Davies, C., and Goose, J. (1981). *Parasite Immunol.* **3**, 81–86.
Davis, P. J., Barratt, M. E. J., Morgan, M., and Parry, S. H. (1985). *In* "Research in Avian Coccidiosis" (L. R. McDonald, L. P. Joyner, and P. L. Long, eds.), pp. 618–633. University of Georgia, Athens.
Dean, D. A., Wistar, R., and Murrell, K. D. (1974). *Am. J. Trop. Med. Hyg.* **23**, 420–428.
Denham, D. A., and Martinez, A. R. (1970). *J. Helminthol.* **44**, 357–363.
Dennis, R. A., O'Hara, P. J., Young, M. F., and Dorris, K. D. (1970). *J. Am. Vet. Med. Assoc.* **156**, 1861–1869.
Despommier, D. D. (1977). *Am. J. Trop. Med. Hyg.* **26**, 68–75.
Despommier, D. D., Cambell, W. C., and Blair, L. S. (1977). *Parasitology* **74**, 109–119.
Dessein, A. J., Parker, W. L., James, S. L., and David, J. R. (1981). *J. Exp. Med.* **153**, 423–436.
Dimmock, C. K., and Bell, K. (1970). *Aust. Vet. J.* **46**, 44–47.
Dolan, T. T. (1987). *Parasitol. Today* **3**, 4–10.

Doy, T. G., and Hughes, D. L. (1982). *Res. Vet. Sci.* **32,** 118–120.

Doyle, J. J. (1971). *Res. Vet. Sci.* **12,** 527–534.

Doyle, J. J. (1973). *Res. Vet. Sci.* **14,** 97–103.

Duffus, W. P., and Franks, D. (1980). *Clin. Exp. Immunol.* **41,** 430–440.

Durham, C. P., Murrell, K. D., and Lee, C. M. (1984). *Exp. Parasitol.* **57,** 297–306.

Egan, J. E., Weber, J. L., Ballou, W. R., Hollingdale, M. R., Majarian, W. R., Gordon, D. M., Maloy, W. L., Hoffman, S. L., Wirtz, R. A., Schneider, I., Woollett, G. R., Young, J. F., and Hockmeyer, W. T. (1987). *Science* **236,** 453–456.

Endo, T., and Kobayashi, A. (1976). *Exp. Parasitol* **40,** 170–178.

Erp, E. E., Gravely, S. M., Smith, R. D., Ristic, M., Osorno, B. M., and Carson, C. A. (1978). *Am. J. Trop. Med. Hyg.* **27,** 1061–1064.

Erp, E. E., Smith, R. D., Ristic, M., and Osorno, B. M. (1980). *Am. J. Vet. Res.* **41,** 1141–1142.

Ferreira, A., Morimoto, T., Altszuler, R., and Nussenzweig, V. (1987). *J. Immunol.* **138,** 1256–1259.

Frenkel, J. K. (1973). *In* "The Coccidia: *Eimeria, Isospora, Toxoplasma* and Related Genera" (D. M. Hamond and P. L. Long, eds.), pp. 343–410. University Park Press, Baltimore, Maryland.

Gamble, H. R. (1985). *Exp. Parasitol* **59,** 398–404.

Gamble, H. R., and Graham, C. E. (1984). *Am. J. Vet. Res.* **45,** 67–74.

Gamble, H. R., and Zarlenga, D. S. (1986). *Vet. Parasitol.* **20,** 237–250.

Gill, A., Timms, P., and Kemp, D. J. (1987). *Mol. Biochem. Parasitol.* **22,** 195–202.

Goff, W., Barbet, A., Stiller, D., Palmer, G., Knowles, D., Kocan, K., Gorham, J., and McGuire, T. C. (1988). *Proc. Natl. Acad. Sci. U.S.A.* **85,** 919–923.

Good, M. F. (1988). *J. Immunol.* **140,** 1715–1716.

Good, M. F., Berzofsky, J. A., and Miller, L. H. (1988a). *Ann. Rev. Immunol.* **6,** 663–688.

Good, M. F., Pombo, D., Maloy, W. L., De La Cruz, V. F., Miller, L. H., and Berzofsky, J. A. (1988b). *J. Immunol.* **140,** 1645–1650.

Grencis, R. K., Crawford, C., Pritchard, D. I., Behnke, J. M., and Wakelin, D. (1986). *Parasite Immunol.* **8,** 587–596.

Handman, E., and Remington, J. S. (1980). *Immunology* **40,** 579–588.

Handman, E., Goding, J. W., and Remington, J. S. (1980). *J. Immunol.* **124,** 2578–2583.

Handunnetti, S. M., Mendis, K. N., and David, P. H. (1987). *J. Exp. Med.* **165,** 1269–1283.

Hanna, R. E. (1980). *Exp. Parasitol.* **50,** 155–170.

Hanna, R. E., and Trudgett, A. G. (1983). *Parasite Immunol.* **5,** 409–425.

Harari, Y., Russell, D. A., and Castro, G. A. (1987). *J. Immunol.* **138,** 1250–1255.

Harding, J. D., Beverley, J. K., Shaw, I. G., Edwards, B. L., and Bennett, G. H. (1961). *Vet. Rec.* **73,** 3–6.

Haroun, E. M., and Hillyer, G. V. (1986). *Vet. Parasitol.* **20,** 63–93.

Haroun, E. M., Hammond, J. A., and Sewell, M. M. (1980). *Res. Vet. Sci.* **29,** 310–314.

Hartley, W. J., and Marshall, S. C. (1957). *N. Z. Vet. J.* **5,** 119–124.

Hayes, T. J., Bailer, J., and Mitrovic, M. (1972). *J. Parasitol.* **58,** 1103–1105.

Henry, E., Norman, B. B., Fly, D. E., Wichmann, R. W., and York, S. M. (1983). *J. Am. Vet. Med. Assoc.* **183,** 66–69.

Hessel, J., Ramaswamy, K., and Castro, G. A. (1982). *J. Parasitol.* **68,** 202–207.

Hooshmand-Rad, P. (1985). *Dev. Biol. Stand.* **62,** 119–127.

Howard, R. J. (1982). *Immunol. Rev.* **61,** 67–107.

Howard, R. J. (1987). *Int. J. Parasitol.* **17,** 17–29.

Howard, R. J., Rodwell, B. J., Smith, P. M., Callow, L. L., and Mitchell, G. F. (1980a). *J. Protozool.* **27,** 241–247.

Howard, R. J., Smith, P. M., and Mitchell, G. F. (1980b). *Parasitology* **81**, 251–271.
Hughes, D. L. (1985). *Curr. Top. Microbiol. Immunol.* **120**, 241–260.
Hughes, D. L., and Harness, E. (1975). *Eur. Multicolloquy Parasitol.* **18**, 60–61.
Hughes, H. P. (1985). *Curr. Top. Microbiol. Immunol.* **120**, 105–139.
Irving, D. O., and Howell, M. J. (1982). *Parasitology* **85**, 179–188.
Irving, D. O., and Howell, M. J. (1986). *Mol. Biochem. Parasitol.* **19**, 45–50.
James, E. R., Maloney, A., and Denham, D. A. (1977). *J. Parasitol.* **63**, 720–723.
James, M. A. (1984). *Vet. Parasitol.* **14**, 231–237.
Jarrett, E. E. (1978). *Immunol. Rev.* **41**, 52–76.
Jarrett, E. E., and Miller, H. R. (1982). *Prog. Allergy* **31**, 178–233.
Jarrett, W. F. H., and Sharp, N. C. (1963). *J. Parasitol.* **49**, 177–189.
Jarrett, W. F. H., Jennings, F. W., McIntyre, W. I. M., Mulligan, W., and Urquart, G. M. (1960). *Immunology* **3**, 145–151.
Jeffers, T. K. (1985). *In* "Research in Avian Coccidiosis" (L. R. McDonald, L. P. Joyner, and P. L. Long, eds.), pp. 482–501. University of Georgia, Athens.
Jenkins, M. C., and Dame, J. B. (1987). *Mol. Biochem. Parasitol.* **25**, 155–164.
Johnson, A. M., McDonald, P. J., and Neoh, S. H. (1983). *J. Protozool.* **30**, 351–356.
Johnson, A. M., McDonald, P. J., and Illana, S. (1986). *Mol. Biochem. Parasitol.* **18**, 313–320.
Johnson, J., Reid, W. M., and Jeffers, T. K. (1979). *Poult. Sci.* **58**, 37–41.
Joyner, L. P., and Norton, C. C. (1973). *Parasitology* **67**, 333–340.
Jungery, M., Clark, N. W., and Parkhouse, R. M. (1983). *Mol. Biochem. Parasitol.* **7**, 101–109.
Kasper, L. H., and Ware, P. (1985). *J. Clin. Invest.* **75**, 1570–1577.
Kasper, L. H., Crabb, J. H., and Pfefferkorn, E. R. (1982). *J. Immunol.* **129**, 1694–1699.
Kasper, L. H., Crabb, J. H., and Pfefferkorn, E. R. (1983). *J. Immunol.* **130**, 2407–2412.
Kasper, L. H., Bradley, M. S., and Pfefferkorn, E. R. (1984). *J. Immunol.* **132**, 443–449.
Kasper, L. H., Currie, K. M., and Bradley, M. S. (1985). *J. Immunol.* **134**, 3426–3431.
Kazura, J. W., and Grove, D. I. (1978). *Nature (London)* **274**, 588–589.
Klotz, F. W., Hudson, D. W., Coon, H. G., and Miller, L. H. (1987). *J. Exp. Med.* **165**, 359–367.
Kreier, J. P., and Ristic, M. (1963). *Am. J. Vet. Res.* **24**, 688–696.
Kuttler, K. L., and Todorovic, R. A. (1973). *In* "Proceedings of the Sixth National Anaplasmosis Conference" (E. W. Jones, ed.), pp. 106–112. Heritage Press, Stillwater, Oklahoma.
Kuttler, K. L., Levy, M. G., James, M. A., and Ristic, M. (1982). *Am. J. Vet. Res.* **43**, 281–284.
Lang, B. Z., and Hall, R. F. (1977). *J. Parasitol.* **63**, 1046–1049.
Lee, C. M., and Best, Y. (1983). *J. Natl. Med. Assoc.* **75**, 565–570.
Lehner, R. P., and Sewell, M. M. (1979). *Vet. Sci. Commun.* **2**, 337–340.
Levy, M. G., and Ristic, M. (1980). *Science* **207**, 1218–1220.
Livingstone, A. M., and Fathman, C. G. (1987). *Annu. Rev. Immunol.* **5**, 477–501.
Long, P. L. (1984). *Poult. Sci.* **25**, 3–18.
McDonald, V., Shirley, M. W., and Chapman, H. D. (1985). *Res. Vet. Sci.* **39**, 328–332.
McDonald, V., Rose, M. E., and Jeffers, T. K. (1986). *Parasitology* **93**, 1–7.
McElwain, T. F., Perryman, L. E., Davis, W. C., and McGuire, T. C. (1987a). *J. Immunol.* **138**, 2298–2304.
McElwain, T. F., Perryman, L. E., Davis, W. C., and McGuire, T. C. (1987b). *Proc. Int. Congr. Malaria Babesiosis, 3rd*, p. 261.
McGuire, T. C., Palmer, G. H., Goff, W. L., Johnson, M. I., and Davis, W. C. (1984). *Infect. Immun.* **45**, 697–700.

Mackenzie, C. D., Jungery, M., Taylor, P. M., and Ogilvie, B. M. (1981). *J. Pathol.* **133,** 161–175.

McLaren, D. J., Ortega-Pierres, G., and Parkhouse, R. M. (1987). *Parasitology* **94,** 101–114.

Mitchell, G. F. (1984). *Parasite Immunol.* **6,** 493–498.

Mogil, R. J., Patton, C. L., and Green, D. R. (1987). *J. Immunol.* **138,** 1933–1939.

Montenegro-James, S., and Ristic, M. (1985). *Vet. Parasitol.* **18,** 321–337.

Morein, B., Sundquist, B., Hoglund, S., Dalsgaard, K., and Osterhaus, A. (1984). *In* "Vaccines '84: Modern Approaches to Vaccines" (R. M. Chanock and R. A. Lerner, eds.), pp. 363–367. Cold Spring Harbor Lab., Cold Spring Harbor, New York.

Moss, B., and Flexner, C. (1987). *Annu. Rev. Immunol.* **5,** 305–324.

Murray, P. K., Bhogal, B. S., Crane, M. S., and MacDonald, T. T. (1985). *In* "Research in Avian Coccidiosis" (L. R. McDonald, L. P. Joyner, and P. L. Long, eds.), pp. 564–573. University of Georgia, Athens.

Murrell, K. D. (1985). *Exp. Parasitol.* **59,** 347–354.

Newbold, C. I. (1985). *Curr. Top. Microbiol. Immunol.* **120,** 69–104.

Norman, B. B. (1973). *In* "Proceedings of the Sixth National Anaplasmosis Conference" (E. W. Jones, ed.), pp. 103–106. Heritage Press, Stillwater, Oklahoma.

Nussenzweig, R. S., and Nussenzweig, V. (1984). *Philos. Trans. R. Soc. London, Ser. B* **307,** 117–128.

Nussenzweig, R. S., Vanderberg, J. P., and Most, H. (1969). *Mil. Med., Suppl.* **134,** 1176–1182.

Oberle, S. M., Palmer, G. H., Barbet, A. F., and McGuire, T. C. (1988). *Infect. Immun.* **56,** 1567–1573.

Oldham, G. (1983). *Res. Vet. Sci.* **34,** 240–244.

Oldham, G., and Hughes, D. L. (1982). *Exp. Parasitol.* **54,** 7–11.

Ortega-Pierres, G., Chayen, A., Clark, N. W., and Parkhouse, R. M. (1984b). *Parasitol-* **6,** 275–284.

Ortega-Pierres, G., Chayen, A., Clark, N. W., and Parkhouse, R. M. (1984b). *Parasitology* **88,** 359–369.

Ortega-Pierres, G., Clark, N. W., and Parkhouse, R. M. (1986). *Parasite Immunol.* **8,** 613–617.

Palmer, G. H., and McGuire, T. C. (1984). *J. Immunol.* **133,** 1010–1015.

Palmer, G. H., Kocan, K. M., Barron, S. J., Hair, J. A., Barbet, A. F., Davis, W. C., and McGuire, T. C. (1985). *Infect. Immun.* **50,** 881–886.

Palmer, G. H., Barbet, A. F., Davis, W. C., and McGuire, T. C. (1986a). *Science* **231,** 1299–1302.

Palmer, G. H., Barbet, A. F., Kuttler, K. L., and McGuire, T. C. (1986b). *J. Clin. Microsc.* **23,** 1078–1083.

Palmer, G. H., Barbet, A. F., Musoke, A. J., Katende, J. M., Rurangirwa, F., Shkap, V., Pipano, E., Davis, W. C., and McGuire, T. C. (1988). *Int. J. Parasitol.* **18,** 33–38.

Parkhouse, R. M., Philipp, M., and Ogilvie, B. M. (1981). *Parasite Immunol.* **3,** 339–352.

Peterson, D. S., Wrightsman, R. A., and Manning, J. E. (1986). *Nature (London)* **322,** 566–568.

Philipp, M., Parkhouse, R. M., and Ogilvie, B. M. (1980). *Nature (London)* **287,** 538–540.

Pipano, E. (1977). *In* "Theileriosis" (J. B. Henson and M. Campbell, eds.), pp. 55–65. Int. Dev. Res. Cent., Ottawa.

Pipano, E. (1978). *In* "Tick-borne Diseases and Their Vectors" (J. K. H. Wilde, ed.), pp. 389–390. University of Edinburgh, Edinburgh.

Potocnjak, P., Yoshida, N., Nussenzweig, R. S., and Nussenzweig, V. (1980). *J. Exp. Med.* **151,** 1504–1513.

Radley, D. E. (1981). In "Advances in the Control of Theileriosis" (A. D. Irvin, M. P. Cunningham, and A. S. Young, eds.), pp. 227–237. Martinus Nijhoff, The Hague.

Rajasekariah, G. R., Mitchell, G. F., Chapman, C. B., and Montague, P. E. (1979). Parasitology 79, 393–400.

Reddington, J. J., Leid, R. W., and Wescott, R. B. (1984). Vet. Parasitol. 14, 209–229.

Reduker, D. W., and Speer, C. A. (1986). J. Parasitol. 72, 901–907.

Reyes, L., and Frankel, J. K. (1987). Infect. Immun. 55, 856–863.

Rodriguez, C., Afchain, D., Capron, A., Dissous, C., and Santoro, F. (1985). Eur. J. Immunol. 15, 747–749.

Rose, M. E. (1982). In "The Biology of the Coccidia" (P. L. Long, ed.), pp. 330–371. University Park Press, Baltimore, Maryland.

Rose, M. E. (1985). Curr. Top. Microbiol. Immunol. 120, 7–17.

Rose, M. E., Lawn, A. M., and Millard, B. J. (1984). Parasitology 88, 190–210.

Ruitenberg, E. J., and Steerenberg, P. A. (1976). J. Parasitol. 62, 164–166.

Rushton, B. (1977). Res. Vet. Sci. 22, 133–134.

Russell, D. A., and Castro, G. A. (1979). J. Infect. Dis. 139, 304–312.

Russell, D. A., and Castro, G. A. (1985). Immunology 54, 573–579.

Ryley, J. F. (1980). Parasitology 80, 189–209.

Santoro, F., Charif, H., and Capron, A. (1986). Parasite Immunol. 8, 631–639.

Scott, J. R., Hollingshead, S. K., and Fischetti, V. A. (1986). Infect. Immun. 52, 609–612.

Sharma, S. D., Araujo, F. G., and Remington, J. S. (1984). J. Immunol. 133, 2818–2820.

Siddiqui, W. A., Tam, L. Q., Kramer, K. J., Hui, G. S. N., Case, S., Yamaga, K. M., Chang, S. P., Chan, E. B., and Kan, S. (1987). Proc. Natl. Acad. Sci. U.S.A. 84, 3014–3018.

Silberstein, D. S., and Despommier, D. D. (1984). J. Immunol. 132, 898–904.

Silberstein, D. S., and Despommier, D. D. (1985). Science 227, 948–950.

Sinclair, I. J., and Joyner, L. P. (1974). Res. Vet. Sci. 16, 320–327.

Smith, G. P. (1976). Science 191, 528–535.

Snary, D., and Smith, M. A. (1986). Mol. Biochem. Parasitol. 20, 101–109.

Stewart, T. B., Batte, G., Connell, H. E., Corwin, R. M., Ferguson, D. L., Gamble, H. R., Murrell, K. D., Prestwood, A. K., Stuart, B. P., Tromba, F. G., and Wheat, B. E. (1985). Am. J. Vet. Res. 46, 1029–1033.

Suzuki, Y., Orellana, M. A., Schreiber, R. D., and Remington, J. S. (1988). Science 240, 516–518.

Taylor, S. M., Kenny, J., Mallon, T., and Elliot, C. T. (1984). Vet. Parasitol. 16, 235–242.

Taylor, S. M., Elliot, C. T., and Kenny, J. (1986a). J. Comp. Pathol. 96, 101–107.

Taylor, S. M., Elliot, C. T., and Kenny, J. (1986b). Vet. Parasitol. 21, 99–105.

Turner, M. J. (1985). Curr. Top. Microbiol. Immunol. 120, 141–158.

Urban, J. R. (1986). Vet. Clin. North Am.: Food Anim. Pract. 2, 765–778.

Urquart, G. M. (1980). Vet. Parasitol. 6, 217–239.

Urquart, G. M. (1985). Dev. Biol. Stand. 62, 109–112.

Vanderberg, J. P., Nussenzweig, R. S., and Most, H. (1968). J. Parasitol. 54, 1009–1016.

Vega, C. A., Buening, G. M., Green, T. J., and Carson, C. A. (1985). Am. J. Vet. Res. 46, 416–420.

Waldeland, H., Pfefferkorn, E. R., and Frenkel, J. K. (1983). J. Parasit. 69, 171–175.

Ware, P. L., and Kasper, L. H. (1987). Infect. Immun. 55, 778–783.

Weiss, W. R., Sedegah, M., Beaudoin, R. L., Miller, L. H., and Good, M. F. (1988). Proc. Natl. Acad. Sci. U.S.A. 85, 573–576.

Winger, C. M., Canning, E. U., and Culverhouse, J. D. (1987). Parasitology 94, 17–27.

Wisher, M. H. (1986). Mol. Biochem. Parasitol. 21, 7–15.

Wright, I. G., and Riddles, P. W. (1986). "Expert Consultation on Biotechnology for Livestock Production and Health." Food Agric. Organ. U. N., Rome.

Wright, I. G., White, M., Tracey-Patte, P. D., Donaldson, R. A., Goodger, B. V., Waltisbuhl, D. J., and Mahoney, D. F. (1983). *Infect. Immun.* **41**, 244–250.

Wright, I. G., Mirre, G. B., Rode-Bramanis, K., Chamberlain, M., Goodger, B. V., and Waltisbuhl, D. J. (1985). *Infect. Immun.* **48**, 109–113.

Yoshida, N., Nussenzweig, R. S., Potocnjak, P., Nussenzweig, V., and Aikawa, M. (1980). *Science* **207,** 71–73.

Yunker, C. E., Kuttler, K. L., and Johnson, L. W. (1987). *Vet. Parasitol.* **24,** 7–13.

Vaccines against Tumor Antigens

RALPH B. ARLINGHAUS

Department of Molecular Pathology, The University of Texas System Cancer Center at Houston, M.D. Anderson Hospital and Tumor Institute, Houston, Texas

I. Introduction

Cancer is a disease characterized by uncontrolled growth of abnormal cells at the site of the initial tumor and at other sites in the human body. The ability of a tumor cell to grow at tissue locations other than its site of origin (known as a metastatic tumor or metastasis) is directly responsible for the devastating effects of cancer. The tumor can be fast or slow growing, but in either case the cells of the tumor have escaped normal growth regulation. Cancer is a multistage process that is still poorly understood. This lack of knowledge is understandable, given the extreme complexity of macromolecular mechanisms ongoing in normal and cancer cells.

The events leading up to the development of a typical cancer might be described as follows: an abnormal cell arises in a tissue; the cell fails to respond to the many regulatory factors present in its microenvironment. The initiating event (or events) provides a growth advantage over its neighbors. A small tumor develops; after some time the tumor becomes vascularized to allow continued expansion of the tumor. Events then occur that allow the tumor to shed viable cells which spread to local and distant regions of the body. It is this last event that makes cancer so deadly.

It is widely believed that tumor cells or even small tumors arise in animals and humans but fail to progress to the malignant state necessary for the lethal spread of the tumor. The body's immune system, both its humoral (antibodies) and cell-mediated components (cytotoxic T cells), plays a role in destroying tumor cells. The key to immune destruction of the tumor is the degree of recognition of the tumor cell surface by the components of the immune system. The tumor cell surface, if viewed as nonself, will elicit an immune response that destroys the tumor.

II. Immune Surveillance

A battery of general defense mechanisms counteracts foreign antigens (Fig. 1). These defense mechanisms include cytokines such as the interferons, immunocompetent cells such as natural killer cells, cytotoxic T lymphocytes, and antibodies produced by B lymphocytes. Antibodies bound to tumor cells can trigger the binding and action of the complement system as well as the binding of antibody-dependent cytotoxic T cells.

The cell-mediated immune system also employs blood cells such as macrophages that play roles in tumor cell destruction.

T lymphocytes are unable to recognize antigens unless presented as a complex with a member of the major histocompatibility complex (MHC) group of surface proteins. In other words, all T cell activities require the presentation of tumor antigens as surface MHC-tumors antigen complexes.

The MHC class 1 antigens are expressed in virtually all cell types and play a role in the immune presentation of cells bearing foreign antigens (Zinkernagel and Doherty, 1979). The absence of class 1 molecules from the surface of tumor cells would likely afford protection against immune recognition, allowing cells to escape destruction. Thus, many natural tumors of epithelial derivation, including embryonal carcinomas (Jacob, 1977), small cell carcinomas of the lung (Doyle *et al.*, 1985), neuroblastomas (Trowsdale *et al.*, 1980), and many others (Hayashi *et al.*, 1985) either do not express or display greatly

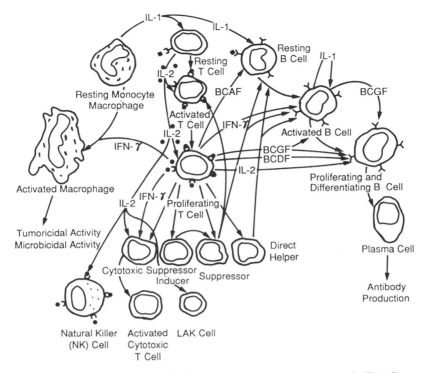

FIG. 1.   Schematic diagram of the human immunoregulatory network. This diagram was taken from Fauci *et al.* (1987). IL, Interleukin; IFN, interferon; LAK, lymphokine-activated killer cell; BCGF, B-cell growth factor; BCDF-B, cell differentiation factor; BCAF, B-cell-activating factor. ■, antigen; ●, IL-2.

reduced levels of class 1 MHC antigens on their cell surfaces. Such an alteration may be essential for malignancy.

Evidence that suppression of class 1 antigens in tumor cells is a critical determinant for their malignant growth state comes from recent experiments that show that expression of a transfected class 1 gene can abrogate the tumorigenicity of different malignant cell lines (Hui *et al.*, 1984; Tanaka *et al.*, 1985; Wallich *et al.*, 1985). These studies demonstrate that conversion of a normal cell to a tumor cell alone is often insufficient to induce malignancy and suggest that immunoselection of those tumor cells that have lost the expression of their class 1 MHC surface proteins is responsible for their escape from host surveillance and destruction (Hayashi *et al.*, 1985). These findings again emphasize the tremendous complexity involved in generating a malignant tumor.

III. Immunotherapy

Established cancers are very difficult to eradicate. Successful therapy requires radical procedures such as radiation treatment, surgery, and chemotherapy. Attempts to use immunotherapy have, in general, not met with much success. Most immunotherapies for human cancer have used nonspecific stimulants or tumor cell-derived preparations to stimulate endogenous anti-tumor specific immunity in the cancer patient (Terry, 1982). These approaches were ineffective and have largely been abandoned. However, recent attempts at treating patients with lymphocyte-activated killer cells in conjunction with interleukin-2 (IL-2) appear have met with some success (S. Rosenberg, in Fauci *et al.*, 1987). Positive responses have been observed in colorectal cancer (4 of 17), melanoma (6 of 14), and renal cell cancer (9 of 10) patients. Nevertheless, the treatment is limited by substantial dose-limited toxicity. As judged from animal models, minimal disease should be more responsive than advanced disease, where the tumors are large and disseminated. Thus, lymphokine-activated killer cell and IL-2 therapy as an adjuvant to surgery in patients with resected tumors has begun (S. Rosenberg, in Fauci *et al.*, 1987).

IV. Anti-idiotype Antibodies

Niels Jerne proposed his network theory of the immune system in 1974. It constitutes the theoretical basis for the construction of idiotype vaccines (Nisonoff and Lamoyi, 1981). In this theory as described by UytdeHaag et al. (1986), Jerne hypothesized a mutual recognition of idiotopes in the immune system during a normal "nonimmune state," resulting in a permanent communication between the elements of the system. Antibody produced in response to external or internal stimuli (Ab1) is regulated by antibody (Ab2) recognizing idiotype specificities of Ab1. Experiments using a cascade of immunizations (Ab1, Ab2, Ab3, etc.) support the concept that idiotypes may function as targets for regulatory signals (Urbain *et al.*, 1977; Cazenave, 1977; Bona *et al.*, 1981).

Two types of anti-idiotype Ab2 antibodies can be distinguished. They are termed Ab2α and Ab2β. Ab2β is believed to resemble the antigen, and for obvious reasons, such antibodies have vaccine potential. For a variety of reasons, such vaccines should be composed of several monoclonal antibody antidiotypes.

V. Vaccines against Tumor Viruses

An emerging group of carcinogens are tumor viruses such as the hepatitis B virus and several members of the retrovirus and herpes virus families of viruses. However, it should be possible to produce safe and effective vaccines against these tumor-inducing viruses and so prevent their infection of the host.

A successful vaccine for Marek's disease in chickens, caused by a herpes virus, has been employed for some time (Purchase *et al.,* 1972). The symptoms of Marek's disease include a generalized lymphomatosis involving lymphocytic invasion of nerve trunks and subsequent paralysis of the bird (Zur Hausen, 1980). Vaccines against tumor-causing retroviruses are also being developed, and one is currently on the market (Leukocell[tm], Norden Laboratories, Lincoln, NE). This vaccine is claimed to prevent feline leukemia virus (FeLV) infection in domestic house cats. However, the vaccine was reported to provide little protection against a laboratory challenge of cats with the feline leukemia virus (Pederson *et al.,* 1985; Gilbert *et al.,* 1987). Effective vaccines also exist for the hepatitis B virus, thought to be a major factor in the cause of primary liver cancer in the world.

The involvement of both DNA and RNA tumor viruses in cancers of animals and humans has been clearly demonstrated. Given the success achieved in preventing infection of the host by vaccines derived from tumor viruses, I have elected to review several important examples of these types of viruses, including FeLV, hepatitis B virus, and the recently discovered human T-cell leukemia virus. Space limitations limit my coverage of other tumor viruses [see Zur Hausen (1980) for a review of oncogenic herpes viruses, and Phillips (1983) for oncogenic DNA viruses].

VI. Feline Leukemia Virus Vaccines

FeLV is a horizontally transmitted oncogenic retrovirus of cats. It induces a variety of diseases in domestic cats, ranging from immunosuppression and wasting to leukemia or lymphoma (Hardy *et al.,* 1980). Like all retroviruses it makes a DNA copy from its RNA genome. The double-stranded DNA copy is then inserted into the chromosomal DNA of the host cell. The integrated DNA, termed the provirus, is structured much like that shown for murine leukemia viruses (MLV), as shown in Fig. 2. The surface of this virus contains

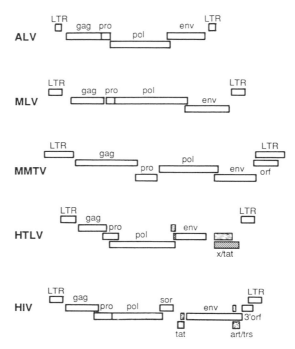

Fig. 2.   Genome schematics of retroviral genomes. ALV, Avian leukosis virus; MLV,
murine leukemia virus; MMTV, mouse mammary tumor virus; HTLV, human T-cell
leukemia virus; HIV, human immunodeficiency virus. HTLV-2 is used as an example of
HTLV, and HTLV-3/LAV is used as an example of HIV. Boxes indicate LTR (long
terminal repeat sequences) and coding sequences, including core protein gene (*gag*),
protease gene (*pro*), reverse transcriptase (*pol*), envelope gene (*env*), open reading frame
(*orf*), *trans*-acting transcriptional activator (*tat*), short open reading frame (*sor*), anti-
repression *trans*-activator (*art*), and *trans*-acting regulator for splicing (*trs*). (Taken from
the back cover of the abstract book from the 1987 Cold Spring Harbor meeting on RNA
Tumor Viruses.)

two different virus-coded proteins that are embedded in the lipid
envelope of the virus. They are identified as a 70,000 mol. wt.
glycoprotein (gp70) and a nonglycosylated protein of 15,000–18,000
mol. wt. (p15E, the E is for envelope). These two proteins are derived
from a common intracellular precursor protein termed gp85; is trans-
lated from a spliced messenger RNA encoded by sequences in the 3'
third of the viral genome.

Virus-neutralizing antibody is believed to be mediated by antibodies
against gp70. Experiments using polyclonal anti-gp70 antibodies have
been successful in demonstrating protection against FeLV. Polyclonal

antibody to gp70 with *in vitro* neutralization activity was shown to be protective in cats upon administration through the colostrum (Hoover *et al.*, 1977), or after systemic inoculation, provided that the antibody is administered within 6 days of virus exposure (De Noronha *et al.*, 1977; Cotter *et al.*, 1980; Haley *et al.*, 1985).

The success with passive immunization employing polyclonal antibodies prompted a study with monoclonal antibodies with high-titer neutralization activity (Weijer *et al.*, 1986). A mixture of two virus-neutralizing monoclonal antibodies directed against the same epitope on gp70 was inoculated into 10 SPF (pathogen-free) cats previously infected on day 0 with FeLV. The antibodies were administered every 2 days starting at various times after infection (days 0–40). Surprisingly, no protection was achieved. Early anti-idiotypic response by cat antibody to the inoculated mouse monoclonal antibody strongly suggests that anti-FeLV antibody was rapidly cleared from the circulation.

Anti-idiotypic antibodies, particularly those that resemble the virus-neutralizing epitopes, are thought to be useful vaccine candidates. Antibody 2 (the antibody raised against a neutralizing monoclonal antibody elicited an antibody 3 response under certain conditions. However, antibody 3 produced within weeks after the initial inoculation of cats failed to bind to FeLV in enzyme-linked immunosorbent assays (ELISAs); but after 20 weeks some recognition of the virus was achieved (UytdeHaag *et al.*, 1986). Whether this response is a neutralizing one has not yet been reported.

Several methods have been considered for active vaccination of cats against FeLV infection—these include live or inactivated whole virus or virus-producing cells (Jarrett *et al.*, 1975; Yohn *et al.*, 1976; Olsen *et al.*, 1977; Grant *et al.*, 1980; Schaller *et al.*, 1977; Pederson *et al.*, 1979; Mathes *et al.*, 1982; Lewis *et al.*, 1981; Salerno *et al.*, 1978). Earlier attempts at achieving complete protection have not been successful (Jarrett *et al.*, 1975; Yohn *et al.*, 1976; Olsen *et al.*, 1977; Grant *et al.*, 1980; Schaller *et al.*, 1977; Pederson *et al.*, 1978). Subunit vaccines were only partially protective when relatively high doses and Freund's complete adjuvant were used.

In a more recent study, induction of protective immunity was demonstrated by a subunit vaccine consisting of a gp70/85 complexed to a glycoside known as Quil A (Osterhaus *et al.*, 1985). In micelle form, Quil A has regions accessible for hydrophobic interaction with membrane proteins. The resulting structure can be highly immunogenic even when presenting poorly immunogenic membrane antigens. These structures are known as ISCOMS, or immunostimulating complexes. In this study, eight cats were vaccinated with a gp70/85 ISCOM and compared to six unvaccinated control cats. After virus challenge, three of the control cats (50%) developed viremia. At 10 weeks following challenge, none of the vaccinated cats developed viremia.

The results obtained with this method of protection offer promise for the development of a safe and effective vaccine against FeLV. The level of antigen used was quite low (2–3 μg) and no adjuvant (e.g., Freund's adjuvant) was necessary. Further tests with larger numbers of cats must be performed to prove the efficacy of this approach. In addition, the preparation was contaminated with a variety of other proteins (Osterhaus et al., 1985).

Recombinant vaccinia virus poses a potentially useful and practical method of delivering surface antigens from infectious agents to populations in need of a vaccine. Recently (Gilbert et al., 1987), a recombinant vaccinia virus encoding the envelope gene of the Gardner–Arnstein strain of FeLV subgroup B was prepared and shown to express and process the FeLV envelope protein. The mature gp70 protein was shown to be transported to and accumulate at the surface of the recombinant virus-infected cells. Surprisingly, although animals mounted a typical virus-neutralizing antibody response to the vaccinia virus vector, the investigators were unable to detect antibodies against FeLV gp70 in any of the vaccinated animals. Subsequent "booster" immunization with killed FeLV was unable to elicit evidence of immunologic priming by the recombinant virus. However, cats vaccinated with such a recombinant were not challenged with virulent virus. Therefore, it remains to be shown whether this approach could provide protection through cell-mediated responses. These results appear to be manifestations of the complexities involved in the development of vaccines to protect against retrovirus infections.

VII. Hepatitis B Vaccines and Liver Cancer

The incidence of primary liver cancer (hepatocellular carcinoma or hepatoma) varies with race, age, sex, and geographical location. It is relatively uncommon in the United States and Europe (about 6,000 cases per year), but it is the most frequent cancer of males in many areas of Africa and Southeast Asia (Melnick, 1983). Annual mortality rates of up to 100 per 100,000 have been reported. In Taiwan alone (population 17 million), about 10,000 people die of hepatoma each year. Worldwide, some 500,000 people are estimated to die each year from liver cancer.

It is now clear that persistent or past infection with hepatitis B virus (HBV) is a common feature of hepatoma, especially in endemic areas. However, only a few patients give a history of having had an acute bout of hepatitis. Thus, the original HBV infection must have been subclinical in most patients who develop hepatoma (Kew *et al.,* 1974; Vogel *et al.,* 1970).

As mentioned above, epidemiologic studies have shown a distinct correlation between the incidence of chronic HBV infection and the prevalence of hepatocellular carcinoma (HCC) (Szmuness, 1978). In addition, human chronic HBV carriers have an increased risk of HCC (Beasley *et al.,* 1981).

HBV is a complex, double-shelled particle with an approximate diameter of 45 nm. It contains a 28-nm core surrounded by a lipoprotein envelope. The core contains a circular, double-stranded DNA molecule composed of one strand of fixed length and a shorter strand of variable length. A viral DNA polymerase fills in the variable single-stranded region forming a 3,200-bp DNA.

The surface envelope of the virus contains three forms of related proteins (p25/gp28, p33/gp36, and p39/gp42) that exist either as glycosylated (gp28) or unglycosylated (p25) viral proteins (Fig. 3). The p25 protein is encoded by the S gene beginning at the third possible translational initiation site of a larger open reading frame; this ATG is preceded in frame by 174 codons (in the case of the *adw* subtype) designated the pre-S region (Tiollais *et al.,* 1981). The large open reading frame of the S gene terminates at a single stop codon but can initiate at three possible start codons, which define the pre-S(1), pre-S(2), and S regions, yielding p39, p33, and p25, respectively. All

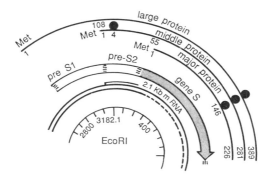

FIG. 3. Genetic organization of the hepatitis B virus surface antigens. (Taken from Tiollais *et al.,* 1985.) See text for details. The large filled circles represent glycosylation sites.

three polypeptides share the 226 amino acid residues of the S region (p25); p33 consists of the p25 sequence plus an amino-terminal 55 residues [pre-S(2)], and p39 consists of p33 plus an amino-terminal 119 residues [pre-S(1)].

The presence and integration of HBV DNA into the host genome of patients with HCC were demonstrated by Marion *et al.* (1980) and at other laboratories (Brechot *et al.*, 1980, 1982; Chen *et al.*, 1982; Shafritz and Kew, 1981; Yaginuma *et al.*, 1987). The woodchuck hepatitis virus, a hepadnavirus with similar properties to HBV (Cote *et al.*, 1986), induces HCC as a sequel to chronic infection by the virus, and the viral DNA is also integrated into chromosomal DNA (Ogston *et al.*, 1982). Thus, HBV plays a major role in HBV-associated human HCC, and integration of the viral genome is often associated with development of the cancer.

Lack of a normal cell system for propagating the virus has required that vaccines be prepared from plasma of infected individuals. This type of vaccine (Heptavax-B, Merck Sharp & Dohme, West Point, PA) is composed of highly purified surface antigen. Safety considerations include the possible presence of not only live HBV in the vaccine but also of other live viruses that might have been present in the blood of the donor samples at the time the plasma was collected. Another vaccine has now been developed. It is a recombinant DNA-generated preparation composed of partially purified surface antigen produced in yeast (Ward, 1986; McAleer *et al.*, 1984). Both the plasma-derived and the yeast recombinant preparations are essentially composed of the p25 HBV surface antigen. These vaccines have proved to be quite effective in stimulating useful levels of neutralizing antibody to the HBV surface antigen. However, a wide range of antibody responses are observed in vaccinated populations, suggesting that better vaccines should be developed.

Future generations of vaccines that will also prevent HBV infection are being developed (Milich *et al.*, 1986). These vaccines will in all likelihood include not only the S antigen but also the pre-S regions of the HBV surface antigen (Milich *et al.*, 1985, 1986).

Milich and colleagues (1985, 1986) have examined in mice the T- and B-cell immune responses generated against short peptides from the pre-S(1), pre-S(2), and S gene products. Regarding the pre-S(1), a number of conclusions were reached, including: the pre-S(1) region is immunogenic at the T- and B-cell levels; anti-pre-S(1)-specific antibody production is regulated by H-2-linked genes and can be independent of anti-S and anti-pre-S(2) antibody production; immunization with surface antigen particles containing all of pre-S(1) can bypass nonresponsiveness to the S and pre-S(2) regions in terms of antibody production; synthetic peptides (e.g., residues 32–53, 94–117) can define murine and human antibody binding sites on the pre-S(1) region; pre-S(1)-specific T cells can be ellicited in the S and pre-S(2) region of nonresponder mice and provide functional help for S-, pre-S(2), and pre-S(1)-specific antibody production; and finally a T-cell recognition site in the pre-S(1) region, amino acid residues 12–32, was identified.

The results described by Milich *et al.* (1986) provide evidence that the immune response to one region of the HBV surface antigen can influence the responses to other regions. This observation was made possible by the study of variably nonresponsive mouse strains. Thus, immunization of the S and pre-S(2) region-nonresponder B10.M strain with the p39 surface antigen elicited S- and pre-S(2)-specific antibody responses as well as pre-S(1)-specific antibody and T-cell responses. A similar situation was observed for the pre-S(2) region (Milich *et al.,* 1985). The fact that production of antibody to the three regions of HBV surface antigen is independently H-2 restricted and yet exhibits overlapping regulatory mechanisms suggests the influence of region-specific T-cell recognition of the surface antigen, which could function to help B-cell clones responsive to all three regions of the HBV surface antigen. Thus, Milich *et al.* (1986) showed the B10.M strain of mice (a nonresponder to S and pre-S(2) region antigens) primed with the p39 antigen stimulated T-cell recognition of only the pre-S(1) region, whereas this strain produced antibodies against all three regions after immunization with p39. However, qualitative and quantitative differences are detected in the antibody responses from homologous and nonhomologous T cell help situations, in that T-cell response of one region gives higher antibody responses in that same region compared to antibody responses in other regions.

The cumulative results of the studies of Milich *et al.* (1986) on pre-S(1) and the other HBV surface antigens have important implications in terms of future HBV vaccine development. Their previous work identified an unexpectedly low number of T-cell recognition sites (in mice) on the p25 S antigen in spite of its particulate nature and the large size of the antigen (226 amino acids). This was clearly manifested in the identification of nonresponder mouse strains after p25 immunization. In contrast, a nonresponder mouse strain resulting from p39 antigen immunization has yet to be identified. Therefore, inclusion of pre-S antigen sequences in the plasma-derived p25 surface antigen vaccine or the recombinant DNA yeast-produced p25 antigen vaccine should decrease the incidence of genetic nonresponsiveness, and possibly provide a more immunogenic surface antigen vaccine. Milich *et al.* (1986) proposed that the spectrum of clinical manifestations of HBV infection may correlate with the genetic ability of the host to mount an appropriate T-cell response to a single or viral antigenic region or a group of them. It seems clear from these studies that the surface polypeptides of HBV present an array of T-cell determinants that the host can recognize, and the specificity of this recognition process can be influenced by the MHC-linked genes.

VIII. Human T-Cell Lymphotropic Retroviruses

Two structurally different human retroviruses have been isolated and identified in recent years, namely HTLV-like viruses (HTLV-1, or human T-cell leukemia virus 1) and HIV-like viruses (HIV-1, or human immunodeficiency virus, type 1). Their proviral DNA structure is listed in Fig. 2 in comparison with type C and type B animal retrovirus proviruses. The complexity of the gene products generated by the viruses increases from the type C viruses, which produce *gag-*, *pol-*, and *env*-encoded gene products as well as protease (*pro*, Crawford and Goff, 1985) and integrase (*int*) functions (Fig. 2, Kopchick *et al.*, 1981; Hagino-Yamagishi *et al.*, 1987), to the HTLV and HIV viruses, which encode a variety of other gene products some of which are involved in controlling virus protein expression and inducing the transcription of important cellular genes. For example, in the case of HTLV, the genes for IL-2 and its receptor are thought to be activated by virus-encoded gene products.

IX. Human T-Cell Leukemia Virus

This virus i· the first human retrovirus whose identity was well established (Poiesz *et al.*, 1980; Yoshida *et al.*, 1982). It is associated with a unique T-cell malignancy known as adult T-cell leukemia (ATL) (Uchiyama *et al.*, 1977). It is likely that studies on HTLV-1 will provide strategies for diagnosis, treatment, and prevention of ATL.

Even now, as a result of these studies, novel and new mechanisms of leukemogenesis have been uncovered. ATL, described first by Takatsuki and his colleagues (Uchiyama *et al.*, 1977), affects mostly adults and is frequently associated with hypercalcemia and skin lesions. The malignant cells in most cases are T cells with a highly lobulated nucleus and they express the receptor for IL-2.

ATL is endemic in southwestern Japan, the West Indies, and central Africa. HTLV-1 was first isolated from American patients with T-cell lymphoma (Poiesz *et al.*, 1980, 1981) and later from Japanese patients with ATL (Yoshida *et al.*, 1982). The etiological association of HTLV-1 with ATL has been established firmly (Yoshida and Seiki, 1987). Viral infection is thought to be by means of close contact with an infected individual, probably requiring transfer of living infected cells from virus carriers to recipients. Sera-positive people are mostly over 20 years of age, and the proportion increases with age. Only a small proportion of the infected population develops leukemia, and these do so after a long latent period.

The HTLV-1 genome contains the usual replication genes required for virus replication. However, the unique feature of this virus (Fig. 2) is an unusual sequence termed the pX (or *tat*) region, which is located between the *env* gene and the 3' long terminal repeat (LTR) (Seiki *et al.*, 1983). This sequence is not a typical oncogene derived from cellular genomic sequences, and its presence has established HTLV-1 as a member of a new retrovirus group. It is now a common marker for the HTLV family including simian (STLV-1) and bovine (BLV) retroviruses.

A crucial question is whether a viral function is involved in the mechanism of leukemogenesis in ATL. Tumor cells of all ATL patients contain the integrated form of the viral DNA. Furthermore, analysis of the viral–cellular junction sequences showed that the primary tumor cells were monoclonal (Yoshida and Seiki, 1987). The presence of the provirus and the monoclonality of the tumor with respect to the provirus' position in the cellular genome argue strongly that the virus plays a causative role in the development of ATL at the single-cell level.

Two types of mechanisms are known to induce tumors in retrovirus-infected animals. In one a cellular proto-oncogene is acquired by the virus and in the other the integrated proviral LTR activates an adjacent cellular proto-oncogene. The first mechanism is unlikely for HTLV-1 since the virus does not code for a typical oncogene. The second mechanism is also ruled out because different patients with ATL have proviral DNA in different chromosomes. The current model relates to *trans*-acting viral functions. The pX sequence is thought to be involved in the *trans* activation of other cellular genes, and it is this *trans* activation that leads to the development of the ATL.

Figure 4 illustrates a scheme for pX gene arrangements in the HTLV-1 genome and the mechanism of expression of the pX genes and their function as proposed originally by Yoshida and his colleagues

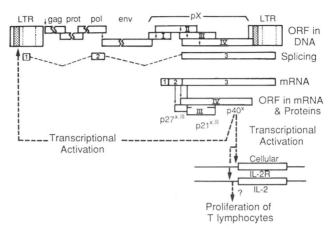

FIG. 4. Model for pX gene expression and function in the HTLV-1 genome. (Taken from Yoshida and Seiki, 1987.) In the ORF (open reading frame for protein coding) in the DNA sequences, the first translation initiation codon (ATG) in each ORF is identified by a small vertical arrow (↓), and AUG initiation codons (longer vertical arrow) in the messenger RNAs represent the beginning of the translational open reading frame. Two AUGs for p40^X and p27^{X-III}, located in exon 2, thus originate from the very 3' region of the *pol* gene. An AUG for p21^{X-III} is derived from ORF III in DNA sequence. Shaded regions in two LTRs represent an enhancer that consisted of three direct repeats of 21 nucleotides which respond to the p40X-mediated *trans*-activation process.

(Yoshida and Seiki, 1987). In this model, a gene product of the pX region (p40^x, a nuclear protein) activates the promoter of the cellular receptor for IL-2 and the factor itself. This induces the proliferation of T lymphocytes. A possible mechanism of progression of the initial virus-infected cell to the acute phase of ATL has also been proposed by Yoshida and colleagues (Yoshida and Seiki, 1987), as shown in Fig. 5. Briefly, the progression involves a carrier state in which virus-infected cells free of expressed viral structural proteins at their cell surface are selected by immunological means. Viral antigen-negative cells with abnormal growth properties develop, forming an intermediate pre-malignant stage. After a number of years, the acute phase of the disease sets in, resulting in death of the patient.

Recent evidence has demonstrated a synergistic aberrant activation of the IL-2 autocrine loop by HTLV-1-encoded p40^x and T3/Ti complex triggering (Maruyama *et al.*, 1987). Ti is the α/β dimer on T cells that recognizes a given antigen (in association with MHC antigens) presented by antigen-presenting cells. T3 is a T-cell surface antigen that forms a complex with Ti. The IL-2 autocrine loop employs the simultaneous expression of both the IL-2 growth factor and the IL-2 receptor

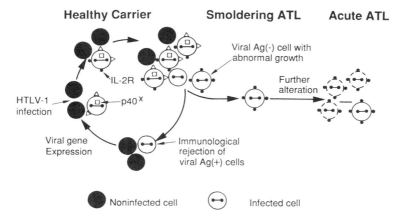

FIG. 5. Possible mechanism of progression of adult T-cell leukemia induced by HTLV-1 infection. ($\square$) p40^x encoded by pX sequence of HTLV-1; ($\triangle$) the envelope glycoprotein of HTLV-1; ($\bullet$) cellular coded IL-2 receptor; ($\bullet$–$\bullet$) integrated viral DNA. This model was taken from Yoshida and Seiki (1987).

genes. In this model, the viral surface antigen encoded by the *env* gene along with p40^x would thus play a role in the early phase of the disease; an important role in retrovirus virus-induced mouse leukemia of viral gp70 (encoded by the *env* gene of the virus) was initially proposed by McGrath and Weissman (1984).

How can this deadly disease be prevented? The answer must lie in priming the humoral and cellular immune systems of the individuals at risk with envelope antigens of the virus. The immune defense systems must prevent the initial infection of the host cell caused by either infectious virus alone or by exposure of the recipient to live infected cells from the infected donor. The immune systems must be capable of effectively lysing not only the virus but virus-infected cells.

Obviously then, the surface envelope proteins of the virus would be the target for vaccine candidates. The approaches used to prevent FeLV infection should be applicable. These approaches would include use of ISCOMS, recombinant DNA-produced envelope proteins, and synthetic peptides whose composition would be predicted from the sequence of the envelope proteins. It is clear from the best available information that once the virus has been allowed to infect the T cell through many cycles of replication, the activation of the IL-2 receptor and growth factor genes will occur at some point. The fact that the HTLV-1 protein p40^x, a nuclear protein, is implicated in this process and the proposal that a viral antigen-negative cell is selected as an intermediate in tumor development clearly indicate that vaccines against p40ˣ will be useless in preventing the disease. Furthermore, once the disease has progressed to the intermediate stage, the tumor cell lacks the usual viral antigens on its cell surface, thereby preventing effective antiviral immunotherapy directed at viral antigens.

X. Human Immunodeficiency Virus

Human immunodeficiency virus (HIV) also produces a complex set of gene products in infected cells. These include products of the *sor, tat, trs,* and a 3′ open reading frame (Fig. 2 of Gallo, 1987). Some of these genes encode proteins that are involved in regulating viral gene expression, namely *tat* and *trs.* These proteins appear to be *trans* activators that regulate viral gene expression (Knight *et al.,* 1987).

The *tat* protein is thought to provide the virus with a positive feedback loop through which a viral product can amplify the production of new virions. The *tat* protein is 86 amino acids in length with a cluster of positively charged amino acids and is thought to affect the synthesis of other viral proteins by binding to critical regulatory sequences at the 5′ end of viral messenger RNA. Employing the same messenger RNA that codes for the *tat* protein, but using a different reading frame, the *art* or *trs* gene of HIV produces a different small (116 amino acids), positively charged protein, which is thought to function as a second essential *trans*-acting factor in viral replication (Mitsuya and Broder, 1987). In the absence of this regulatory factor, *gag*- and *env*-encoded protein synthesis is severely diminished.

HIV is thought to infect T4-positive cells, principally T helper cells. In addition, it is thought to infect monocyte/macrophage cells (Fauci *et al.,* 1987). In the Fauci review (Fauci *et al.,* 1987) Dr. H. C. Lane proposed a hypothetical model in which the antigen-presenting monocyte/macrophage serves as a source of infectious virus; he also proposed that during the process of T4 activation by a given antigen, HIV particles are released by the antigen-presenting macrophage, causing the infection of the interacting T helper cell. The subsequent amplification of the memory T-cell clone is prevented by the cell killing effect of the HIV gene products. (I would propose that HIV-encoded *tat* and *trs* might play a role in blocking translation of certain messenger RNAs required for expansion of the T cell clone.)

The tumor-causing effects of HIV are under study but as yet unclear. The predominant theory is that immunosuppression by the virus allows endogenous herpes viruses to induce B-cell lymphomas (Gallo, 1987).

A vaccine against such an unusual virus as HIV will be difficult to produce. Again as in HTLV-1, both cellular and humoral entities of the immune systems must be optimally primed so as to produce a thorough attack on the infecting virus. Vaccines of choice will probably include recombinant DNA-generated *env*-encoded proteins and possibly synthetic peptides either alone or in combination with rDNA produced proteins. A key point of attack by the vaccine will be to prevent infection of the monocyte/macrophage and or T4 helper cell.

XI. Summary

Effective vaccines against tumor antigens have not yet been produced. However, immunomodulators hold much promise in cancer therapy. Such treatments will probably involve using combinations of various immunomodulators together with activated killer cells. Development of vaccines against tumor-causing viruses seems to be a rational approach to preventing the onset of virus-induced cancers. It seems that efficient vaccines have already been developed for hepatitis B virus; such vaccines have the potential to decrease the incidence of its associated hepatoma. However, successful vaccines against RNA-containing tumor viruses have yet to be developed, although they hold much promise.

REFERENCES

Beasley, R. P., Hwang, L. Y., Lin, C. C., and Chien, C. S. (1981). *Lancet* **2**, 1129–1133.
Bona, C. A., Heber-Katz, E., and Paul, W. E. (1981). *J. Exp. Med.* **153**, 951–960.
Brechot, C., Pourcel, C., Louis, A., Rain, B., and Tiollais, P. (1980). *Nature (London)* **286**, 533–535.
Brechot, C., Pourcel, C., Hadchouel, M., Dejean, A., Louise, A., Scotto, J., and Tiollais, P. (1982). *Hepatology* **2**, 27S–34S.
Cazenave, P. A. (1977). *Proc. Natl. Acad. Sci. U.S.A.* **74**, 5122–5126.
Chen, D.-S., Hoyer, B. H., Nelson, J., Pourcel, R. H., and Gerin, J. L. (1982). *Hepatology* **2**, 42S–46S.
Cote, P. J., Shapiro, M., Engle, R. E., Papper, H., Purcell, R. H., and Gerin, J. L. (1986). *J. Virol.* **60**, 895–901.
Cotter, S. M., Essex, M., McLane, M. F., Grant, C. K., and Hardy, W. D., Jr. (1980). *Dev. Cancer Res.* **4**, 219–226.
Crawford, S., and Goff, S. (1985). *J. Virol.* **53**, 899–907.
De Noronha, F., Baggs, R., Schafer, W., and Bolognesi, D. P. (1977). *Nature (London)* **267**, 54–56.
Doyle, A., Martin, W. J., Funa, K., Gazdar, A., Carney, D., Martin, S. E., Lennoila, I., Cutletta, F., Mulshere, J., Bunn, P., and Menna, J. (1985). *J. Exp. Med.* **161**, 1135–1151.

Fauci, A. S., Rosenberg, S., Sherwin, S. A., Dinarello, C. A., Longo, D. L., and Lane, C. H. (1987). *Ann. Intern. Med.* **106**, 421–433.

Gallo, R. C. (1987). *Sci. Am.* **256**, 47–56.

Gilbert, J. H., Pederson, N. C., and Nunberg, J. H. (1987). *Virus Res.* **7**, 49–67.

Grant, C. K., de Noronha, F., Tusch, C., Michalek, M. T., and McLane, M.-F. (1980). *JNCI, J. Natl. Cancer Inst.* **65**, 1285.

Hagino-Yamagishi, K., Donehower, L. A., and Varmus, H. E. (1987). *J. Virol.* **61**, 1964–1971.

Haley, P. J., Hoover, E. A., Quackenbush, S. L., Gasper, P. W., and Macy, D. W. (1985). *JNCI, J. Natl. Cancer Inst.* **74**, 821–827.

Hardy, W. D., Jr., Essex, M., and McClelland, A. J., eds. (1980). "Feline Leukemia Virus." Elsevier/North-Holland, New York.

Hayashi, H., Tanaka, K., Jay, F., Khourz, G., and Jay, G. (1985). *Cell (Cambridge, Mass.)* **43**, 263–267.

Hoover, E. A., Schaller, J. P., Mathes, L. E., and Olsen, R. G. (1977). *Infect. Immun.* **16**, 54–59.

Hui, K., Grosveld, F., and Festenstein, H. (1984). *Nature (London)* **311**, 750–752.

Jacob, F. (1977). *Immunol. Rev.* **33**, 3–32.

Jarrett, W., Jarrett, O., Mackey, L., Laird, H., Hood, C., and Hay, D. (1975). *Int. J. Cancer* **16**, 134.

Jerne, N. K. (1974). *Ann. Immunol. (Paris)* **125C**, 373–387.

Kew, M. C., Geddes, E. W., Macnab, G. M., and Bersohn, I. (1974). *Cancer (Philadelphia)* **34**, 539–541.

Knight, D. M., Flomerfeld, F. A., and Ghrayeb, J. (1987). *Science* **236**, 837–840.

Kopchick, J., Harless, J., Gesisser, B. S., Kellman, R., Hewitt, R. R., and Arlinghaus, R. B. (1981). *J. Virol.* **37**, 274–283.

Lewis, M. G., Mathes, L. E., and Olsen, R. G. (1981). *Infect. Immun.* **34**, 888.

McAleer, W. J., Buynak, E. B., Maigetter, R. Z., Wampler, D. E., Miller, W. J., and Hilleman, M. R. (1984). *Nature (London)* **307**, 178–180.

McGrath, M. S., and Weissman, I. L. (1984). In "Human T-cell Leukemia/Lymphoma Viruses" (R. C. Gallo *et al.,* eds.), pp. 205–215. Cold Spring Harbor Lab., Cold Spring Harbor, New York.

Marion, P. L., Salazar, F. H., Alexander, J. J., and Robinson, W. S. (1980). *J. Virol.* **33**, 792–802.

Maruyama, M., Shibuya, H., Harada, H., Hatakeyama, M., Seiki, M., Fujita, T., Inoue, J-I., Yoshida, M., and Taniguchi, T. (1987). *Cell (Cambridge, Mass.)* **48**, 434–350.

Mathes, L. E., Lewis, M. G., and Olsen, R. G. (1982). In "Advances in Comparative Leukemia Research" (D. S. Yohn and J. R. Blakeslee, eds.), p. 217. Elsevier/North Holland, New York.

Melnick, J. L. (1983). In "Viruses Associated with Human Cancer" (L. O. Phillips, ed.), pp. 337–367. Dekker, New York.

Milich, D. R., Thornton, G. B., Neurath, A. R., Kent, S. B., Michel, M.-L., Tiollais, P., and Chisari, F. V. (1985). *Science* **228**, 1195–1199.

Milich, D. R., McLachlan, A., Chisari, F. V., Kent, S. B., and Thornton, G. B. (1986). *J. Immunol.* **137**, 315–322.

Mitsuya, H., and Broder, S. (1987). *Nature (London)* **26**, 773–778.

Nisonoff, A., and Lamoyi, E. (1981). *Clin. Immunol. Immunopathol.* **21**, 397–410.

Ogston, C. W., Jonak, G. J., Rogler, C. E., Astrin, S. M., and Summers, J. (1982). *Cell (Cambridge, Mass.)* **29**, 385–394.

Olsen, R. G., Hoover, E. A., Schaller, J. P., Mathes, L. E., and Wolff, L. H. (1977). *Cancer Res.* **37**, 2082.

Osterhaus, A., Weijer, K., UytdeHaag, F., Jarrett, O., Sundquist, B., and Morlin, B. (1985). *J. Immunol.* **135,** 591–596.

Pederson, N. C., Theilen, G. H., and Werner, L. L. (1979). *Am. J. Vet. Res.* **40,** 1120.

Pederson, N. C., Johnson, L., and Ott, R. L. (1985). *Feline Pract.* **15,** 7–20.

Phillips, L. (1983). *In* "Viruses Associated with Human Cancer" (L. O. Phillips, ed.), pp. 3–368. Dekker, New York.

Poiesz, B. J., Ruscetti, F. W., Gazdar, A. F., Bunn, P. A., Minna, J. D., and Gallo, R. C. (1980). *Proc. Natl. Acad. Sci. U.S.A.* **77,** 7451–7419.

Poiesz, B. J., Ruscetti, F. W., Reitz, M. S., Kalyanaraman, V. S., and Gallo, R. C. (1981). *Nature (London)* **294,** 268.

Purchase, H. G., Okazaki, W., and Burmester, B. R. (1972). *Avian Dis.* **16,** 59–68.

Salerno, D. A., Lehman, F. D., Casson, U. M., and Hilleman, M. R. (1978). *JNCI, J. Natl. Cancer Inst.* **61,** 1487.

Schaller, J. P., Hoover, E. A., and Olsen, R. G. (1977) *J. Natl. Cancer Inst. (U.S.)* **59,** 1441.

Seiki, M., Hattori, S., Hirayama, Y., and Yoshida, M. (1983). *Proc. Natl. Acad. Sci. U.S.A.* **80,** 3618–3622.

Shafritz, D. A., and Kew, M. C. (1981). *Hepatology* **1,** 1–8.

Szmuness, W. (1978). *Prog. Med. Virol.* **24,** 40–69.

Tanaka, K., Isselbacher, K. J., Khourz, G., and Jay, G. (1985). *Science* **228,** 26–30.

Terry, W. A. (1982). "Immunotherapy of Human Cancer." Elsevier/North-Holland, New York.

Tiollais, P., Charnay, P., and Vyas, G. N. (1981). *Science* **213,** 406.

Tiollais, P., Pourcel, C., and Dejean, H. (1985). *Nature (London)* **317,** 489–495.

Trowsdale, J., Travers, P., Bodmer, W. F., and Patillo, R. A. (1980). *J. Immunol.* **130,** 2471–2478.

Uchiyama, T., Yodoi, J., Sagawa, K., Takatsuki, K., and Uchino, H. (1977). *Blood* **50,** 481–491.

Urbain, J., Wikler, M., Franssen, J. D., and Collignon, C. (1977). *Proc. Natl. Acad. Sci. U.S.A.* **74,** 5126–5130.

UytdeHaag, F. G. C. M., Bunschoten, H., Weiger, K., and Osterhaus, A. D. M. E. (1986). *Immunol. Rev.* **90,** 93–110.

Vogel, C. L., Anthony, P. P., Mody, N., and Barker, L. F. (1970). *Lancet* **2,** 621–624.

Wallich, R., Bulbue, N., Hammerling, G. J., Katsar, S., Segal, S., and Feldman, M. (1985). *Nature (London)* **315,** 301–305.

Ward, R. (1986). *Nature (London)* **324,** 506.

Weijer, K., UytdeHaag, F. G. C. M., Jarrett, O., Lutz, H., and Osterhaus, A. D. M. E. (1986). *Int. J. Cancer* **38,** 81–87.

Yaginuma, K., Kobayashi, H., Kobayashi, M., Morishima, T., Matsuyama, K., and Koike, K. (1987). *J. Virol.* **61,** 1808–1813.

Yohn, D. S., Olsen, R. G., Schaller, J. P., Hoover, E. A., Mathes, L. E., Heding, L., and Davis, G. W. (1976). *Cancer Res.* **36,** 646.

Yoshida, M., and Seiki, M. (1987). *Annu. Rev. Immunol.* **5,** 451–559.

Yoshida, M., Miyoshi, I., and Hinuma, Y. (1982). *Proc. Natl. Acad. Sci. U.S.A.* **79,** 2031–2035.

Zinkernagel, R. M., and Doherty, P. C. (1979). *Adv. Immunol.* **27,** 51–77.

Zur Hausen, H. (1980). *In* "DNA Tumor Viruses" (J. Tooze, ed.), 2nd ed., Part 2, pp. 747–795. Cold Spring Harbor Lab., Cold Spring Harbor, New York.

Human Immunodeficiency Virus: An Agent That Defies Vaccination

NEAL NATHANSON AND FRANCISCO GONZALEZ-SCARANO

Departments of Microbiology and Neurology, University of Pennsylvania Medical Center, Philadelphia, Pennsylvania

I. Introduction
    A. Pathogenesis
    B. Immunobiology
II. Infection with HIV
    A. Natural History of HIV Infection
    B. Acquisition of Infection and Passive Immunity
    C. Persistence and the Immune Response
III. Immune Response
    A. Neutralizing Antibody
    B. Antigenic Variation
    C. Cell-Mediated Immunity
IV. Experimental Vaccines
    A. Preparation of Antigens
    B. Immune Response to Candidate Antigens
    C. Passive Immunization
    D. Active Immunization
V. Discussion and Commentary
    A. Why a Conventional Vaccine Is Unlikely to Protect
    B. Alternative Approaches to Preventing AIDS
    C. Conclusion
    References

I. Introduction

Classical viral vaccines were developed to protect against acute infectious disease, and were formulated with relatively little information about the molecular biology of the responsible agent. It is a more

397

subtle task to design a vaccine for a persistent virus that causes chronic disease. Rational design of such a vaccine must consider the goals of immunization, the molecular biology of the virus, and the pathogenesis and immunobiology of the infection.

The goals that must be defined for a new vaccine include: (1) Is the successfully immunized subject to be protected against infection or just against disease, and for what period after immunization? (2) Is immunization to be targetted on subjects not yet infected? This is the usual situation with most existing vaccines, except rabies, but human immunodeficiency virus (HIV) represents an instance in which post-infection immunization is a potential target. (3) What is the minimum efficacy acceptable for a vaccine? What is the maximum acceptable frequency and severity of immunization complications? (4) What are the practical parameters for a vaccine? How many doses must be administered and at what intervals? What is the cost per dose or per immunized subject?

A. PATHOGENESIS

The descriptive aspects of pathogenesis include all of the individual steps that occur between the portal of entry of an infectious agent and dysfunction of the target cells or tissue. Before a successful vaccine can be formulated, some critical questions must be answered. What is the mechanism of transmission and what cells are infected initially? Does the infection disseminate through the blood and, if so, is there a plasma or cell-assocated viremia? What are the target cells, and are specific virus receptors involved in initiating cellular infection? Is disease mediated through cellular destruction or dysfunction, or indirectly through the immune response or release of toxins? What viral genes determine virulence and do they vary among strains? What host determinants, genetic, immunological, or other, influence pathogenesis?

B. IMMUNOBIOLOGY

In spite of recent major advances in the molecular biology and genetics of the immune response, the relative contribution of cellular and humoral responses to the protection afforded by vaccines is still far from clear. The viral proteins and epitopes which are involved in neutralization and in recognition by cytolytic T cells (CTLs) are distinct. In addition, specific elements of the immune response can enhance viral infection or can mediate viral disease.

Vaccine efficacy is usually measured by antibody response because antibody is easy to assay, can neutralize virus in cell culture, and often protects when administered to animals prior to infection. However, antibodies against specific viral epitopes may either fail to neutralize, enhance infection, act as autoantibodies, or initiate immune complex disease.

Cellular immune responses, particularly CTL responses, are very difficult to apply to large groups of human subjects and are infrequently used in assessing immune responses to vaccines. However, the CTL response may play a central role in clearance of infected cells. Cellular responses may also mediate virus-initiated pathological lesions.

Finally, the relative contribution of the two arms of the immune response may differ depending upon the context of immunization. Antibody is effective prior to initial challenge with viruses which disseminate through plasma viremia, but cellular immunity may be crucial to contend with an ongoing or persistent infection.

II. Infection with HIV

A. Natural History of HIV Infection

There are three principal modes of transmission of HIV, i.e., sexual, blood or blood products, and maternal–child. It is likely that in most instances virus-infected cells carry the infection from donor to recipient, although cell-free virus is involved when blood products are the source of infection. The identity of the infected cells which transmit infection is unknown, but monocytes and T lymphocytes are probably responsible (Ho *et al.*, 1987; Fauci, 1988).

After entry of infected donor cells, virus is presumably transmitted to recipient cells. The mode of viral spread is not well defined but may be accomplished by cell-to-cell contact since virus is usually isolated from cells and not from cell-free plasma in viremic individuals (Fauci and Lane, 1987; Fauci, 1988; Ho *et al.*, 1987).

Isolation studies suggest that the monocyte may be a target early in the course of HIV infection (Gartner and Popovic, 1988; Gendelman *et al.*, 1988; Roy and Wainberg, 1988). Laboratory data indicate that proliferating macrophages are more permissive than nonproliferating, nonreplicating macrophages (Crowe *et al.*, 1987; Gendelman *et al.*, 1988). This contrasts with the finding for visna virus that differentiated ovine macrophages produce more infectious virus than freshly purified blood monocytes (Gendelman *et al.*, 1986; Narayan *et al.*, 1982,

1983). However, it is clear that infected monocytes carry the virus into a variety of tissues in the course of their natural trafficking. Macrophages are an important site of HIV infection of brain (Price et al., 1988) and have been reported to be infected in lung, skin, and other tissues (Chayt et al., 1986; Fauci, 1988; Koenig et al., 1986; Levy et al., 1985; Shaw et al., 1985; Tschachler et al., 1987).

The course of infection with HIV can be divided into three stages: (1) an initial stage of modest replication accompanied by a minor transient nondescript illness, (2) a long period of semilatency often lasting many years, and (3) a final stage of increasing clinical illness with frank immunodeficiency or neurological symptoms. The level of viremia in the first few months of infection appears to be higher, as judged by levels of p24 protein in blood (plasma or cellular lysate), and viremia then drops to minimal levels during the latent period (Redfield, cited in Price et al., 1988). This drop may reflect the impact of immune surveillance (Nathanson et al., 1985). The identity of virus-infected cells during the latent period is unknown but may include monocytes and T lymphocytes. The frequency of infected cells in the blood which are actively transcribing the genome is very low, less than 1 : 1000 (Harper et al., 1986; Fauci, 1988).

With the onset of clinical evidence of immunodeficiency, viremia increases, at least as judged by the frequency of isolation from blood (Redfield, cited in Price et al., 1988). At the same time, a drop in absolute number of T4 lymphocytes or a drop in the ratio of T4/T8 cells indicates immune perturbation. Virus can be found by in situ hybridization in blood monocytes, T4 cells, and tissue monocytes (Chayt et al., 1986; Levy et al., 1985; Tschachler et al., 1987). It is likely that virus is also present in some indigenous brain cells, either glia or neurons, and perhaps in a few other cell types (Koenig et al., 1986; Price et al., 1988; Shaw et al., 1985).

Even in advanced stages of disease, the number of infected cells remains low (Chayt et al., 1986; Koenig et al., 1986; Shaw et al., 1985); a similar phenomenon has been seen in ovine visna (Geballe et al., 1985; Haase, 1986; Peluso et al., 1985). One of the enigmas of HIV infection is how a small number of infected cells can initiate such profound reductions in T4 lymphocytes (Fauci and Lane, 1987; Fauci, 1988). A further mystery is why many patients with profound functional immunodeficiency may possess considerable numbers (up to normal limits) of T4 lymphocytes. Likewise, the severe manifestations of AIDS encephalopathy appear excessive in relation to the numbers of infected cells in the brain (Price et al., 1988).

B. Acquisition of Infection and Passive Immunity

The unusual mode of acquisition of HIV infection provides some important observations on passive immunity. Persons who have acquired infection as a result of blood transfusion have received considerable amounts of plasma containing anti-HIV antibodies; yet they become infected. (It should be noted that this differs from transfusion-acquired hepatitis B infection, because hepatitis B carriers have no free antibody against HBsAg, the protective antigen.) Likewise, children infected *in utero* usually are infected during the third trimester in spite of the benefit of prior acquisition of passive antibody during the first two trimesters. At the very least, these observations document the co-existence of antibody and infectious cells. They further suggest that the presence of antibody prior to, or from the time of, infection fails to provide passive protection.

C. Persistence and the Immune Response

Serological studies have shown that essentially all infected persons develop antibody against HIV within 4–8 weeks after infection (Ho *et al.*, 1987; Zarling *et al.*, 1987; Price *et al.*, 1988). Antibody to p24 (the major *gag* or core protein) appears first followed by antibody against gp120, the major surface glycoprotein; this resembles the kinetics of the immune response in ovine visna (Petursson *et al.*, 1976). Both antibodies remain present throughout the latent period, but there appears to be a drop in anti-p24 antibody associated with the clinical phase of infection (Redfield, cited in Price *et al.*, 1988). Low levels of neutralizing activity can be measured in the sera of many infected persons (Clapham *et al.*, 1987; Levy *et al.*, 1987; Weiss *et al.*, 1985). In spite of this antiviral immune response, the infection persists and in a high proportion of infected persons eventually develops into progressive disease. At the least, these observations suggest that the host mounts an immune response long prior to overt immunodepression, but can neither clear infection nor contain it.

III. Immune Response

A. Neutralizing Antibody

A number of different protocols have been employed to measure neutralizing activity (Geffin *et al.*, 1987; McDougal *et al.*, 1985; Putney *et al.,* 1987; Robert-Guroff *et al.,* 1985; Weiss *et al.,* 1985). Most infected persons produce neutralizing antibody, but the titers are not high (Clapham *et al.,* 1987; Levy *et al.,* 1987; Weiss *et al.,* 1985). Whether this reflects the assay method, the immunobiological response to the virus, or the nature of the neutralizing epitopes is not clear. It does appear that the immune response to natural infection, often taken as the benchmark for potential immune response to a viral vaccine, holds only modest promise.

B. Antigenic Variation

Antigenic variation of lentiviruses has been described in seminal studies of visna (Clements *et al.,* 1980; Narayan *et al.,* 1977, 1978, 1981). Antigenic variants are generated during long-term infection and are presumed to be selected by the pressure of antiviral antibody. However, their role in persistence of visna virus has been debated (Lutley *et al.,* 1983; Thormar *et al.,* 1983), since many isolates from long-term infected animals are antigenically similar to the infecting virus. Furthermore, the existence of cells carrying a latent provirus offers another important alternative mechanism to explain persistent escape from immune surveillance.

HIV-1 likewise exhibits considerable variation in several domains of the *env* gene which encodes the surface glycoproteins involved in neutralization (Alizon *et al.,* 1987; Benn *et al.,* 1985; Starcich *et al.,* 1986; Staben *et al.,* 1986; Willey *et al.,* 1986). As yet there has been no systematic classification of the numerous antigenic variants of HIV-1 (Geffin *et al.,* 1987). Infected persons raise antibody which is capable of neutralizing the virus with which they are infected and most other isolates of HIV-1 (Clapham *et al.,* 1987; Levy *et al.,* 1985). However, animals immunized with HIV antigenic constructs or peptides often raise a type-specific response to individual gp120 domains or epitopes (Goudsmit and Meloen, 1988; Ho *et al.,* 1988; Mathews *et al.,* 1986; Putney *et al.,* 1988). It is not yet clear whether antigenic variation might play a role in vaccine efficacy (Mathews *et al.,* 1986).

HIV-2 clearly differs much more from HIV-1 than individual isolates of HIV-1 differ from each other, and the glycoproteins of the two viruses are readily distinguished by human antisera (Clavel *et al.,* 1986, 1987). Presumably any pluripotent vaccine should contain antigens of both viruses.

C. Cell-Mediated Immunity

There have been a number of attempts to develop an assay for cellular immunity to HIV-1 (Eichberg *et al.*, 1987; Hu *et al.*, 1987a; Krohn *et al.*, 1987; Mattinen *et al.*, 1988; Plata *et al.*, 1987; Ruscetti *et al.*, 1986; Zarling *et al.*, 1986, 1987, 1988). Most work has been done with a lymphocyte proliferation assay, rather than the very difficult but more meaningful CTL assay (Plata *et al.*, 1987; Zarling *et al.*, 1987). There are few data on course of cellular responses during the natural history of infection. CTL activity has been found in cells obtained by pulmonary lavage from HIV-infected patients with interstitial pneumonitis (Plata *et al.*, 1987). Chimpanzees produce CTLs specific for glycoproteins after immunization with a vaccinia construct bearing the *env* gene (Zarling *et al.*, 1987). It may be speculated that CTLs could play a crucial role in immune surveillance against HIV-infected cells, and it is likely that CTL response includes clones specific for either envelope or core proteins. Thus, there is an important gap in current knowledge of the immune response during natural HIV infection.

IV. Experimental Vaccines

A. Preparation of Antigens

There is a flurry of developmental activity to produce experimental immunogens for a potential HIV vaccine (Webber, 1987). Most efforts have involved recombinant DNA technology, with the development of clones which represent the *env* gene product (gp160) or the two constituent proteins, gp120 and gp41, or domains within these proteins (Hu *et al.*, 1987a,b; Kieny *et al.*, 1987; Krohn *et al.*, 1987; Putney *et al.*, 1987; Steimer *et al.*, 1987; Webber, 1987). Much of the effort has focussed on the use of different expression systems for production of viral protein with attention to processing (glycosylation and charge), solubility, secretion, and conformation of the protein. In addition, some laboratories have synthesized peptides (Goudsmit and Meloen, 1988; Ho *et al.*, 1988; Kennedy *et al.*, 1987; Putney *et al.*, 1988) as potential immunogens which can also contribute to the dissection of epitope structure of the glycoprotein.

B. Immune Response to Candidate Antigens

Almost all trials of candidates immunogens have utilized a wide variety of experimental animals. The limited published data indicate that, as expected, recombinant HIV *env* proteins and synthetic peptides are potentially immunogenic (Benn *et al.*, 1985; Hu *et al.*, 1987a, 1988; Kennedy *et al.*, 1987; Krohn *et al.*, 1987; Lafrado *et al.*, 1988; Putney *et al.*, 1986, 1987, 1988; Robey *et al.*, 1986; Webber, 1987; Zagury *et al.*, 1987). Responses often are most marked when the immunizing antigen is used as the recorder antigen in a serological assay. Immunized animals that develop antibody responses often exhibit neutralizing activity, assuming the immunizing peptide includes neutralizing domains of gp120 or gp41.

C. Passive Immunization

A classical approach to evaluating the potential efficacy of a viral vaccine is the passive immunization of an appropriate experimental animal with antiviral antibody, followed by challenge with the virus. This provides information on protection afforded by antibody alone, and permits quantitation of the required titer of antibody (Bodian, 1952; Nathanson and Bodian, 1962).

A limited number of such studies have been conducted, followed by HIV challenge. In one study (Prince *et al.*, 1988) the immunized chimpanzees received a dose of 1 ml of human globulin per kilo, with a neutralizing titer of 2,000 which should have conferred on the recipients a titer of about 20–40 (Nathanson and Bodian, 1962). In a subsequent study a much larger dose of globulin was used (Prince and Eichberg, cited as Kolata, 1988). However, the immunized chimpanzees were not protected against infection, although there are no data on eventual disease since these animals have not developed immunodeficiency in studies reported to date (Eichberg *et al.*, 1987; Zarling *et al.*, 1987).

D. Active Immunization

To date there have been a very limited number of trials of active immunization of chimpanzees or monkeys followed by challenge with HIV or simian immunodeficiency virus (SIV) (Arthur *et al.*, 1988; Fultz *et al.*, 1986, 1987; Hu *et al.*, 1987a,b 1988; Kennedy *et al.*, 1987; Kannagi *et al.*, 1986; Letvin *et al.*, 1985, 1987). The published results indicate that immunized animals developed antibody and cellular immune responses (Zarling *et al.*, 1987), but failed to resist infection upon challenge.

These preliminary trials cannot be considered an exhaustive test of the potential of active immunization. Possibly a more effective immunogen, a smaller virus challenge, or challenge by a more physiological route will yield more promising results. However, the available date do not augur well.

V. Discussion and Commentary

A. WHY A CONVENTIONAL VACCINE IS UNLIKELY TO PROTECT

A conventional vaccine would be designed to protect uninfected persons against HIV infection or, at least, against AIDS. The observations sketched above provide evidence regarding the potential efficacy of a vaccine.

1. Pathogenesis

It appears likely that virus is transmitted by infected white blood cells, either T lymphocytes or monocytes, which enter the tissues or the circulation of the uninfected recipient. Isolation studies indicate that free infectious HIV rarely is found in the plasma of viremic individuals. In fact, special protocols must be used to transmit the viral genome from infected white blood cells (WBCs) to indicator T lymphocytes maintained with interleukin-2 (IL-2) and phytohemagglutinin (PHA) in a coculture system. Most successful viral vaccines protect the immunized individual against challenge with free infectious virus. It is much more difficult to protect against infected cells.

Infected cells often carry a latent genome, presumably as a provirus, with little or no production of virus or viral proteins or viral mRNA. Immune surveillance mechanisms cannot attack such latently infected cells, since they express no viral antigens. Such cells can harbor the provirus for their full lifespan, providing an optimal mechanism for prepetuation of the viral genome.

Transmission of HIV from infected to uninfected cells can probably occur by cell-to-cell contact as well as via cell free virus. The very strong binding of the viral glycoprotein gp120 to the CD4 cellular receptor, with subsequent fusion of the cellular membranes, provides a ready mechanism for direct transmission of the genome (McDougal *et al.*, 1986). This mechanism could permit spread of infection in the presence of antibody, just as measles, another enveloped virus, spreads from cell to cell in the presence of hypernormal levels of neutralizing antibody in the brains of patients with subacute sclerosing panencephalitis.

2. Immunobiology

The genome of HIV is plastic, with hypervariable regions in the *env* gene. Since a number of the neutralizing domains fall within the hypervariable regions of the *env* gene, variation in some of the viral epitopes is common, leading to alterations in the neutralization profile of different strains of HIV. In some instances of experimental ovine lentivirus infection, variation in antigenic profile is sufficient so that variants can escape the host's antibody response, even when that response can contain the initial infecting virus (Narayan *et al.*, 1977, 1978, 1981; Lutley *et al.*, 1983; Thormar *et al.*, 1983).

Passive immunization occurs in many instances where infection is transmitted. Recipients of blood receive a considerable amount of antibody from the infected donor at the time of infection. Fetuses probably are exposed to maternal antibody prior to infection. In neither instance is there evidence of protection.

During the long latent period, infected persons raise an active immune response, both humoral and cellular. During this period, the virus burden is minimal, since the proportion of cells in the circulation which are transcribing viral RNA is less than 1 : 1,000, and there are relatively few hybridization-positive cells in tissues. However, immune surveillance is incapable of clearing these few infected cells.

Finally, preliminary trials of candidate immunogens in chimpanzees have failed to demonstrate evidence of protection against HIV (Hu *et al.*, 1987a).

Current successful humans viral vaccines include those against poliovirus, measles, mumps, rubella, smallpox, yellow fever, and hepatitis B. In each instance, the spread of infection involves a phase of cell-free plasma viremia, when the virus is readily susceptible to neutralization. In these infections, it has been shown by passive immunization experiments, that antibody alone, at modest levels, is capable of preventing viremia and aborting infection before it produces clinical disease (Bodian, 1952; Francis *et al.*, 1957; Nathanson and Bodian, 1962). Under these circumstances, a conventional vaccine, given as preexposure prophylaxis, can be highly effective.

HIV infection presents a significantly different and more difficult challenge, for the reasons summarized above. It is highly questionable whether a conventional vaccine, even one employing recombinant DNA methodology, will be capable of preventing AIDS.

B. ALTERNATIVE APPROACHES TO PREVENTING AIDS

We believe that HIV and AIDS present a unique challenge which requires pioneering approaches to viral disease prevention. The following discussion is necessarily speculative and must be read with caution.

We begin with several premises:

1. No conventional vaccine given to uninfected persons will be able to prevent HIV infection. (Also, we predict that such an immunogen will be unacceptable to many uninfected individuals because of the stigma of a positive serological test.)

2. The target population for AIDS prophylaxis should be those already infected (Salk, 1987). Infected persons are at highest risk of AIDS, and they are healthy and immunoresponsive for long periods prior to onset of immunodeficiency. (Also, we predict that this population will be much more willing to participate in trials of preventive measures, and that it will be ethically acceptable to test unconventional methods of bioprophylaxis in this group.)

3. Neither cellular nor humoral immune responses, even if stimulated to higher levels than occur during unmanipulated HIV infection, will clear existing infection or protect against progression from latency to AIDS. (We do, however, support vigorous efforts to test this proposition, in animal models and in humans.)

4. The goal of prophylaxis should be the protection of a sufficient number of key target cells (such as T4 lymphocytes) rather than the eradication of an existing HIV infection.

We believe that, if these premises are correct, we are forced to consider two approaches to prophylaxis of infected persons: (1) Development of an antiviral compound that can be used on a long-term basis without excessive complications. This approach falls outside the scope of this chapter, but is a major goal of many research programs. (2) The use of "intracellular vaccination" (Baltimore, 1987), i.e., infection or transfection of uninfected cells to render them resistant to superinfection with HIV. Such an approach could involve the construction of an altered or avirulent strain of HIV (Fisher *et al.*, 1986; Folks *et al.*, 1987), which would establish persistent infection and render infected cells resistant to superinfection with virulent HIV. Alternatively, uninfected cells could be stably transfected with a construct which encoded an RNA transcript capable of interfering with successful replication of HIV, such as an anti-sense *tat* sequence.

These prophylactic treatments might either be applied *in vivo* using viral vectors, or used in cultured cells obtained from infected subjects which would subsequently be reinfused into the donor.

C. CONCLUSION

Vaccines have been successfully developed for prevention of many viral diseases of humans. There are a number of other viral infections that cause diseases worthy of prevention but are more difficult to attack. These include herpes simplex, cytomegalovirus, and varicella zoster, all capable of persisting as latent infections. HIV is perhaps the most difficult to control of all such virus diseases, and certainly the most important on a worldwide basis. We have reviewed HIV as a prototype of those viruses that will probably defy conventional vaccines, and that challenge us to devise new approaches to immunization.

REFERENCES

Alizon, M., Sonigo, P., and Wain-Hobson, S. (1987). *In* "Vaccines '87: Modern Approaches to New Vaccines" (R. M. Chanock, R. A. Lerner, F. Brown, and H. Ginsberg, eds.), pp. 146–153. Cold Spring Harbor Lab., Cold Spring Harbor, New York.

Arthur, I. O., Pyle, S. W., Bess, J. W., Nara, P. L., Kelliher, J. C., Morein, B., Gilden, R. V., and Fischinger, P. J. (1988). *J. Cell. Biochem.* **12B,** 14.

Baltimore, D. (1987). *Am. Soc. Microbiol. News* **53,** 602–603.

Benn, S., Rutledge, R., Folks, T., Gold, J., Baker, L., McCormick, J., Feorino, P., Piot, P., Quinn, T., and Martin, M. (1985). *Science* **230,** 949–952.

Bodian, D. (1952). *Am. J. Hyg.* **56,** 78–88.

Chyat, K. J., Harper, M. E., Marselle, L. M., Lewin, E. B., Rose, R. M., Oleske, J. M., Epstein, L. G., Wong-Staal, F., and Gallo, R. C. (1986). *JAMA J. Am. Med. Assoc.* **256,** 2356–2359.

Clapham, P. R., Weiss, R. A., Dalgleish, A. G., Beverely, P. C. L., Sattentau, Q. J., Lasky, L. A., Berman, P. W., Maddon, P., Axel, R., and McDougal, J. S. (1987). *In* "Vaccines '87: Modern Approaches to New Vaccines" (R. M. Chanock, R. A., Lerner, F., Brown, and H. Ginsberg, eds.), pp. 174–178. Cold Spring Harbor Lab., Cold Spring Harbor, New York.

Clavel, F., Guetard, D., Brun-Vezinet, F., Chamaret, S., Rey, M. A., Santos-Ferriera, M. O., Laurent, A. G., Dauguet, C., Katlama, C., Rouzioux, C., Klatzmann, D., Champalinmaud, J. L., and Montagnier, L. (1986). *Science* **233,** 343–346.

Clavel, F., Guetard, D., Chamaret, S., Favier, V., Alizon, M., Montagnier, L., Frun-Vezinet, F., Klatzmann, D., Santos-Ferriera, M. O., and Champalimaud, J. L. (1987). *In* "Vaccines '87: Modern Approaches to New Vaccines" (R.M. Chanock, R. A. Lerner, F. Brown, and H. Ginsberg, eds.), pp. 179–184. Cold Spring Harbor Lab., Cold Spring Harbor, New York.

Clements, J. E., Pederson, F. S., Narayan, O., and Haseltilne, W. A. (1980). *Proc. Natl. Acad. Sci. U.S.A.* **77,** 4454–4458.

Crowe, S., Mills, J., and McGrath, M. S. (1987). *AIDS Res. Hum. Retroviruses* **3,** 135–145.

Eichberg, J. W., Zarling, J. M., Aler, H. J., Levy, J. A., Berman, P. W., Gregory, T., Lasky, L. A., McClure, J., Cobb, K. E., Moran, P. A., Hu, S. L., Kennedy, R. C., Chanh, T. C., and Dreesman, G. R. (1987). *J. Virol.* **61,** 3804–3808.

Fauci, A. S. (1988). *Science* **239,** 617–622.

Fauci, A. S., and Lane, E. C. (1987). *In* "Vaccines '87: Modern Approaches to New Vaccines" (R. M. Chanock, R. A. Lerner, F. Brown, and H. Ginsberg, eds.), pp. 164–167. Cold Spring Harbor Lab., Cold Spring Harbor, New York.

Fisher, A. G., Ratner, L., Mitsuya, H., Marselle, L. M., Harper, M. E., Broder, S., Gallo, R. C., and Wong-Staal, F. (1986). *Science* **233,** 655–659.

Folks, T. M., Justement, J. S., Powell, D., Kinter, A., Rabson, A., and Fauci, A. S. (1987). *In* "Vaccines '87: Modern Approaches to New Vaccines" (R. M. Chanock, R. A. Lerner, F. Brown, and H. Ginsberg, eds.), pp. 143–145. Cold Spring Harbor Lab., Cold Spring Harbor, New York.

Francis, T., Jr., Napier, J. A., Voigh, R. B., Hemphill, F. M., Wenner, H. A., Korns, R. F., Boisen, M., Tolchinsky, E., and Diamond, E. L. (1957). "Evaluation of the 1954 Field Trial of Poliomyelitis Vaccine," p. 172. Edwards Brothers, Ann Arbor, Michigan.

Fultz, P. N., McClure, H. M., Swenson, R. B., McGrath, C. R., Brodie, A., Getchell, J. P., Jensen, F. C., Anderson, D. C., Broderson, J. R., and Francis, D. P. (1986). *J. Virol.* **58,** 116–124.

Fultz, P. N., Switzer, W., McGrath, N., Srinivasram, A., McClure, H. M., Brodie, A., and Swenson, B. (1987). *In* "Vaccines '87: Modern Approaches to New Vaccines" (R. M. Chanock, R. A. Lerner, F. Brown, and H. Ginsberg, eds.), pp. 205–208. Cold Spring Harbor Lab., Cold Spring Harbor, New York.

Gartner, S., and Popovic, M. (1988). *Lancet* **2,** 916.

Geballe, A. P., Ventura, P., Stowring, L., and Haase, A. T. (1985). *Virology* **141,** 148–154.

Geffin, R., Parks, E. S., Parks, W. P., Hahn, B., and Shaw, G. M. (1987). *In* "Vaccines '87: Modern Approaches to New VAccines" (R. M. Chanock, R. A. Lerner, F. Brown, and H. Ginsberg, eds.), pp. 159–163. Cold Spring Harbor Lab., Cold Spring Harbor, New York.

Gendelman, H. E., Narayan, O., Molneaux, S., Clements, J. E., and Ghotbi, Z. (1985). *Proc. Natl. Acad. Sci. U.S.A.* **82,** 7086–7090.

Gendelman, H. E., Narayan, O., Kennedy-stoskopf, S., Kennedy, P. G. E., Ghotbi, Z., Clements, J. E., Stanley, J., and Pezeshkapour, G. (1986). *J. Virol.* **58,** 67–74.

Gendelman, H. E., Orenstein, J., Martin, M. A., Ferrua, C., Pezeshpour, G. H., Phipps, T., Wahl, L., Fauci, A. S., Burke, D., and Meltzer, M. S. (1988). *J. Exp. Med.* (in press).

Goudsmit, J., and Meloen, R. H. (1988). *J. Cell. Biochem.* **12B,** 34.

Haase, A. T. (1986) *Nature (London)* **322,** 130–136.

Harper, M. E., Marselle, L. M., Gallo, R. C., and Wong-Staal, F. (1986). *Proc. Natl. Acad. Sci. U.S.A.* **83,** 772–776.

Ho, D. D., Pomerantz, R. J., and Kaplan, J. C. (1987). *N. Engl. J. Med.* **317,** 278–286.

Ho, D. D., Alam, M., and Gurney, M. E. (1988). *J. Cell. Biochem.* **12B,** 34.

Hu, S. L., Fultz, P. N., McClure, H. M., Eichberg, J. W., Thomas, E. K., Zarling, J., Singhal, M. C., Kosowski, S. G., Swenson, R. B., Anderson, D. C., and Todaro, G. (1987a). *Nature (London)* **328,** 721–723.

Hu, S. L., Moran, P. A., McClure, J., Kosowski, S. G., Zarling, J. M., and Morton, W.

(1987b). *In* "Vaccines '87: Modern Approaches to New Vaccines" (R. M. Chanock, R. A. Lerner, F. Brown, and H. Ginsberg, eds.), pp. 231–235.

Hu, S. L., Zarling, J. M., Fultz, P. N., Eichberg, J. W., Kinney-Thomas, E., Sridhar, P., Travis, B., and Estin, C. D. (1988). *J. Cell. Biochem.* **12B**, 9.

Kannagi, M., Kiyotaki, M., Desrosiers, R. C., Reimann, K. A., King, N. W., Waldron, L. M., and Letvin, N. L. (1986). *J. Clin. Invest.* **78**, 1229–1236.

Kennedy, R. C., Kanda, P., Dreesman, G. R., Eichberg, J. W., Chanh, T. C., Ho, D. H., and Sparrow, J. T. (1987). *In* "Vaccines '87: Modern Approaches to New Vaccines" (1987). (R. M. Chanock, R. A. Lerner, F. Brown, and H. Ginsberg, eds.), pp. 250–255. Cold Spring Harbor Lab., Cold Spring Harbor, New York.

Kieny, M. P., Rautman, G., Lecocq, J. P., Wain-Hobson, S., Montagnier, L., and Girard, M. (1987). *In* "Vaccines '87: Modern Approaches to New Vaccines" (R. M. Chanock, R. A. Lerner, F. Brown, and H. Ginsberg, eds.), pp. 242–249. Cold Spring Harbor Lab., Cold Spring Harbor, New York.

Koenig, S., Gendelman, H. E., Orenstein, J. M., Dal Canto, M. C., Pezeshpour, G. H., Yungbluth, M., Janotta, F., Aksamit, A., Martin, M. A., and Fauci, A. S. (1986). *Science* **233**, 1089–1093.

Kolata, G. (1988). *N. Y. Times* Feb. 16 p. 1.

Krohn, K., Robey, W. G., Putney, S., Talle, M. A., and Ranki, A. (1987). *In* "Vaccines '87: Modern Approaches to New Vaccines" (R. M. Chanock, R. A., Lerner, F., Brown, and H. Ginsberg, eds.), pp. 225–230. Cold Spring Harbor Lab., Cold Spring Harbor, New York.

Lafrado, L. J., Hunsman, G., Kelliher, J. C., and Hobson, W. C. (1988). *J. Cell. Biochem.* **12B**, 42.

Letvin, N. L., Daniel, M. D., Sehgal, P. K., Desrosiers, R. C., Hunt, R. D., Waldron, L. M., McKey, J. J., Schmidt, D. K., Chalifoux, L. V., and King, N. W. (1985). *Science* **230**, 71–73.

Letvin, N. L., Daniel, M. D., King, N. W., Kiyotaki, M., Kannagi, M., Chalifoux, L. V., Sehgal, P. K., Desrosiers, R. C., Arthur, L. O., and Allison, A. C. (1987). *In* "Vaccines '87: Modern Approaches to New Vaccines" (R. M. Chanock, R. A. Lerner, F. Brown, and H. Ginsberg, eds.), pp. 209–213. Cold Spring Harbor Lab., Cold Spring Harbor, New York.

Levy, J. A., Kaminsky, L. S., Morrow, W. J. W., Steimer, K. S., Luciw, P., Dina, D., Hoxie, J., and Oshiro, L. (1985). *Ann. Intern. Med.* **103**, 694–699.

Levy, J. A., Evans, L., Pan, L. Z., Tateno, M., Reed, M. F., Walker, C., Homsy, J., and Cheng-Mayer, C. (1987). *In* "Vaccines '87: Modern Approaches to New Vaccines" (R. M. Chanock, R. A. Lerner, F. Brown, and H. Ginsberg, eds.), pp. 168–173. Cold Spring Harbor Lab., Cold Spring Harbor, New York.

Lutley, R., Petursson, G., Palsson, P. A., Georgsson, G., Klein, J., and Nathanson, N. (1983). *J. Gen. Virol.* **64**, 1433–1440.

McDougal, J. S., Cort, S. P., Kennedy, M. S., Cabridilla, C. D., Feorino, P. M., Francis, D. P., Hicks, D., Kalyanaraman, V. S., and Martin, L. S. (1985). *J. Immunol. Methods* **76**, 171–183.

McDougal, J. S., Kennedy, M. S., Sligh, J. S., Cort, S. P., Mawle, A., and Nicholson, J. K. A. (1986). *Science* **231**, 382–285.

Mathews, T. J., Langlois, A. J., Robey, W. G., Chang, N. T., Gallo, R. C., Rishinger, P. J., and Bolognesi, D. P. (1986). *Proc. Natl. Acad. Sci. U.S.A.* **83**, 9709–9713.

Mattinen, S., Ranki, A., and Krohn, K. (1988). *J. Cell. Biochem.* **12B**, 43.

Narayan, O., Griffin, D. E., and Chase, J. (1977). *Science* **197**, 376–378.

Narayan, O., Griffin, D. E., and Clements J. E. (1978). *J. Gen. Virol.* **41**, 343–352.

Narrayan, O., Clements, J. E., Griffin, D. E., and Wolinsky, J. S. (1981). *Infect. Immun.* **32**, 1045–1050.

Narayan, O., Wolinsky, J. S., Clements, J. E., Strandberg, J. D., Griffin, D. E., and Cork, L. C. (1982). *J. Gen. Virol.* **59**, 345–356.

Narayan, O., Kennedy-Stoskopf, S., Sheffer, D., Friffin, D. E., and Clements, J. E. (1983). *Infect. Immun.* **41**, 67–73.

Nathanson, N., and Bodian, D. (1962). *Bull. Johns Hopkins Hosp.* **111**, 198–220.

Nathanson, N., Georgsson, G., Palsson, P. A., Najjar, J. A., Lutley, R., and Petursson, G. (1985). *Rev. Infect. Dis.* **7**, 75–82.

Peluso, R., Haase, A. T., Stowring, L., Edwards, M., and Ventura, P. (1985). *Virology* **147**, 231–236.

Petursson, G., Nathanson, N., Georgsson, G., Panitch, H., and Palsson, P. A. (1976). *Lab. Invest.* **35**, 402–412.

Plata, F., Autran, B., Martins, L. P., Wain-Hobson, S., Raphael, M., Mayaud, C., Denis, M., Guillon, J. M., and Debre, P. (1987). *Nature (London)* **328**, 348–353.

Price, R. W., Brew, B., Sidtis, J., Rosenblum, M., Scheck, A. C., and Cleary, P. (1988). *Science* **239**, 586–591.

Prince, A. M., Pascual, D., Kurokawa, D., and Baker, L. (1987). *In* "Vaccines '87: Modern Approaches to New Vaccines" (R. M. Chanock, R. A. Lerner, F. Brown, and H. Ginsberg, eds.), pp. 194–198. Cold Spring Harbor Lab., Cold Spring Harbor, New York.

Prince, A. M., Eichberg, J., Brotman, B., Valinsky, J., Shulman, R., and Horowitz, B. (1988). *J. Cell. Biochem.* **12B**, 44.

Putney, S. D., Mathews, T. J., Robey, W. G., Lynn, D. L., Robert-Gurooff, M., Mueller, W. T., Langlois, A. J., Ghrayeb, J., Petteway, S. R., Weinhold, K. J., Fischingerk, P. J., Wong-Staal, F., Gallo, R. C., and Bolognesi, D. P. (1986). *Science* **234**, 1392–1395.

Putney, S. D., Javaherian, K., Jackson, J., Lynn, D., Rusche, J., Mueller, W. T., Matthews, T., Bolognesi, D., Ghrayeb, J., Chanda, P. K., Rober, W. G., Petteway, S. R., Robert-Guroff, M., Wong-Staal, F., Krohn, K., and Gallo, R. C. (1987). *In* "Vaccines '87: Modern Approaches to New Vaccines" (R. M. Chanock, R. A. Lerner, F. Brown, and H. Ginsberg, eds.), pp. 256–259. Cold Spring Harbor Lab., Cold Spring Harbor, New York.

Putney, S. D., Petro, J., Lynn, D. L., Grimailia, R., Matsushita, M., Robert-Guroff, M., Gallo, R. C., Bolognesi, D. P., Mathews, T. J., and Rusche, J. R. (1988). *J. Cell. Biochem.* **12B**, 5.

Robert-Guroff, M., Brown, M., and Gallo, R. C. (1985). *Nature (London)* **316**, 72–74.

Robey, W. G., Arthur, L. O., Mathews, T. J., Langlois, A., Copeland, T. D., Lerche, N. W., Orozslan, S., Bolognesi, D. P., Gilden, R. V., and Fischinger, P. J. (1986). *Proc. Natl. Acad. Sci. U.S.A.* **83**, 7023–7027.

Roy, S., and Wainberg, M. A. (1988). *J. Leuk. Biol.* **43**, 91–97.

Ruscetti, F. W., Mikovits, M. A., Kalyanaraman, V. S., Overton, R., Stevenson, H., Stromberg, K., Herberman, R. B., Farrar, W. L., and Ortaldo, J. R. (1986). *J. Immunol.* **136**, 3619–3625.

Salk, J. (1987). *Nature (London)* **327**, 473–476.

Shaw, G. M., Harper, M. E., Hahn, B. H., Epstein, L. G., Gajdusek, D. C., Price, R. W., Navia, B. A., Petito, C. K., OHara, C. J., Groopman, J. E., Cho, E. S., Wong-Staal, F., and Gallo, R. C. (1985). *Science* **227**, 177–182.

Staben, C., Stephans, J., Barr, P., Sabin, E., Parkes, D., Luciw, P., Steimer, K., Dina, D., Shimabukuro, J., and Levy, J. (1986). *In* "Vaccines '86" (F. Brown, R. M. Chanock, and R. A. Lerner, eds.), pp. 345–352. Cold Spring Harbor Lab., Cold Spring Harbor, New York.

Starcich, B. R., Hahn, B. H., Shaw, G. M., McNeely, P. D., Modrow, S., Wolf, H., Parks, E. S., and Parks, W. P. (1986). *Cell (Cambridge, Mass.)* **45,** 637–648.

Steimer, K. S., van Nest, G., Dina, D., Barr, P. J., Luciw, P. A., and Miller, E. T. (1987). *In* "Vaccines '87: Modern Approaches to New Vaccines" (R. M. Chanock, R. A. Lerner, F. Brown, and H. Ginsberg, eds.), pp. 236–241. Cold Spring Harbor Lab., Cold Spring Harbor, New York.

Thormar, H., Barshatsky, M. R., and Kozlowski, P. B. (1983). *J. Gen. Virol.* **64,** 1427–1432.

Tschachler, E., Groh, V., Popovic, M., Mann, D. L., Konrad, K., Safai, B., Eron, L., Veronese, F. D., Wolff, K., and Stingl, G. (1987). *J. Invest. Dermatol.* **88,** 233–237.

Webber, (1987). *Am. Soc. Microbiol. News* **53,** 468–469.

Weiss, R. A., Clapham, P. R., Cheinsong-Popov, R., Dalgleish, A. G., Carne, C. A., Weller, I. V. D., and Tedder, R. S. (1985). *Nature (London)* **316,** 69–72.

Willey, R. L., Rutledge, R. A., Dias, S., Folks, T., Theodore, T., Buckler, C. E., and Martin, M. A. (1986). *Proc. Natl. Acad. Sci. U.S.A.* **83,** 5038–5042.

Winters, M. A., Humphres, R. C., Sharma, I. K., Bhatia, G., Smith, S., and Robinson, W. W. (1988). *J. Cell. Biochem.* **12B,** 28.

Zagury, D., Leonard, R., Fouchard, M., Reveil, B., Bernard, J., Ittele, D., Cattan, A., Zirimwabagano, L., Kalumbo, M., Justin, W., Salaun, J., and Goussard, B. (1987). *Nature (London)* **326,** 249–250.

Zarling, J. M., Morton, W., Moran, P. A., McClure, J., Kosowski, S. G., and Hu, S. L. (1986). *Nature (London)* **323,** 344–347.

Zarling, J. M., Eichberg, J. W., Moran, P. A., McClure, J., Sridhar, P., and Hu, S. L. (1987). *J. Immunol.* **139,** 988–990.

Zarling, J. M., Moran, P., Grosmaire, L. S., Hu, S. L., Shriver, K., Eichberg, J. W., Kinney-Thomas, E., and Ledbetter, J. A. (1988). *J. Cell. Biochem.* **12B,** 9.

Animal Virus Infections That Defy Vaccination: Equine Infectious Anemia, Caprine Arthritis-Encephalitis, Maedi-Visna, and Feline Infectious Peritonitis

NIELS C. PEDERSEN

Department of Medicine, School of Veterinary Medicine, University of California, Davis, California

I. Ungulate Lentivirus Infections

A. INTRODUCTION

Lentiviruses are associated with persistent infection and chronic disease in three major species of livestock—horses, sheep, and goats. Another lentivirus named bovine immunodeficiency virus (BIV) recently has been described (Gonda *et al.,* 1987). It is a Visna-like virus that was originally isolated over a decade ago from cattle with persistent lymphocytosis, lymphadenopathy, weakness, emaciation, and central nervous system (CNS) lesions (Van der Maaten *et al.*, 1972). There is very little information on the epidemiology, clinical manifestations, or importance of bovine lentivirus infections, so this section will concern itself mainly with the better characterized lentiviruses of horses, sheep, and goats. A phylogenetic tree showing the possible evolutionary relationship of various animal lentiviruses and human immunodeficiency virus (HIV) of man to each other and to types C and D retroviruses has been recently constructed (Gonda *et al.*, 1987) (Fig. 1). Just how far back in history that the various retroviruses diverged from each other has not been determined.

B. COURSE OF INFECTION

1. Equine Infectious Anemia

Equine infectious anemia virus (EIAV) infects Equidae throughout the world. The disease is characterized by recurrent bouts of fever, anemia, thrombocytopenia, weight loss, and depression. Horses are infected by the transfer of blood between viremic and susceptible animals by biting flies (McGuire *et al.*, 1987), contaminated needles and surgical implements, *in utero* from mares in the clinical stages of illness, and neonatally by the ingestion of virus containing colostrum and milk (Issel and Foil, 1984; McGuire *et al.*, 1987; Stein *et al.*, 1942; Stein and Mott, 1942). Horses are most infectious when they are clinically ill. Horses in the later asymptomatic carrier stage of illness are minimally infectious by all of these routes.

The incubation period ranges from days to several months, depending mainly on the amount of virus that is transferred (McGuire *et al.*, 1987). The appearance of the initial fever corresponds to the primary viremic phase. Viremia declines rapidly as the fever subsides. Viremia and fever recur after periods as short as 2–8 weeks, however. Several recurrent episodes of disease are observed during the first several months of infection. A characteristic anemia begins to appear after the first febrile period. Although the hematocrit tends to improve after each febrile period, horses with frequent and severe febrile episodes usually get progressively more anemic. Clinical signs subside with time; the recurrent febrile episodes become milder and the anemia slowly resolves. Horses that survive this initial clinical phase of illness remain infected for life, but the level of virus in their blood and tissues is very low (Coggins, 1984).

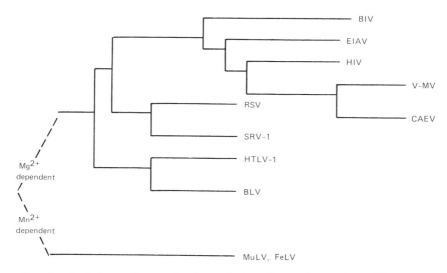

Fig. 1. A phylogenetic tree for the evolution of type C, type D, and lentiviruses based on published amino acid sequences for the polymerase genes. The first major subdivision of retroviruses was based on the requirement of the polymerase enzyme for either Mg^{2+} or Mn^{2+}. BIV, bovine immunodeficiency virus; BLV, bovine leukemia virus; CAEV, caprine arthritis-encephalitis virus; EIAV, equine infectious anemia virus; FeLV, feline leukemia virus; HIV, human immunodeficiency virus; HTLV-1, human T-cell leukemia virus-1; MuLV, murine leukemia virus; RSV, Rous sarcoma virus; SRV-1, simian retrovirus-1; V-MV, visna-maedi virus. [Redrawn from Gonda et al. (1987).]

2. Caprine Arthritis-Encephalitis

Caprine arthritis-encephalitis virus (CAEV) infection is particularly common in milking goats (Narayan et al., 1987). Virtually all milking goat herds in the United States are affected, and an average of 80% of individual animals in these herds are virus carriers. The infection is much less common in nondairy or free-roaming goats (Adams et al., 1984). Kids are infected when they ingest colostrum from their chronically infected mothers (Kennedy-Stoskopf et al., 1985). The virus persists in high levels within macrophages in the synovium and mammary glands and is shed in the milk (Kennedy-Stoskopf et al., 1985). Horizontal transmission between infected and susceptible animals continues to occur throughout life (East et al., 1987). Contaminated teat cups may provide one mode of horizontal infection.

A primary phase of infection has not been recognized (Narayan et al., 1987). A proportion of infected goats develop a chronic rheumatoid-like arthritis and fibrosis of the udder. Encephalitis is an uncommon manifestation of the infection in younger goats. The unrelenting arthritis gradually leads to joint enlargment, deformities, and lameness. As the animals become progressively more lame they are culled from the herd. This may take many years, however, and many infected animals remain in the milking string for a normal lifetime.

3. Ovine Visna-Maedi

Maedi is a chronic fibrosing interstitial pneumonia that was first recognized in Icelandic sheep following the introduction of infected rams from Europe in the 1930s (Sigurdsson, 1954). Visna is a chronic paralytic disorder of sheep (Sigurdsson, et al., 1957). Both diseases are forms of the same virus infection, i.e., visna-maedi virus (V-MV). The North American equivalent of maedi is a disease called ovine progressive pneumonia (OPP). The OPP virus (OPPV) is a variant of V-MV (Takemoto et al., 1971).

The V-MV is shed from body fluids, in particular sputum of animals with chronic pneumonia. Transmission is more efficient, therefore, when affected and susceptible animals are kept together in close confinement. Neonatal transmission through colostrum and milk may also occur, as well as in utero infections (Cutlip et al., 1981).

C. PATHOGENESIS

1. EIAV

EIAV replicates mainly in macrophages in the spleen, lymph nodes, and liver (McGuire et al., 1971). Infection of phagocytic elements is associated with hyperplasia of lymphoid cells and macrophages in the above organs, and interstitial mononuclear cell infiltrates in nonlymphoid tissues such as the kidney, adrenal glands, brain, and heart. Hyperplastic and infiltrative lesions tend to disappear as the horses enter the chronic carrier stage of illness.

The typical anemia of EIAV infection is caused both by a decreased production and increased destruction of red blood cells (reviewed by McGuire et al., 1987). There is a pronounced phagocytosis of red blood cells by macrophages. Immunosuppression does not occur to any extent in EIAV infection. There is a decrease in IgG(T) production in clinically affected horses, but its cause or significance are unknown (McGuire, 1976).

2. CAEV

CAEV replicates mainly in macrophages within the mammary gland and synovium (Narayan and Cork, 1985). Hyperplasia of lymphoid organs is not as prominent as in EIAV infection, but infiltrates in target tissues such as the synovial membrane may be quite pronounced. The clinical signs of arthritis and udder fibrosis result in part from host immune responses to virus-laden macrophages. Central nervous system signs in young goats are usually a result of demyelination with minimal inflammatory changes.

3. V-MV

V-MV and OPP viruses also replicate mainly in macrophages (Narayan and Cork, 1985). The target organ for these viruses appears to be the lungs. Lung lesions are characterized by massive interstitial infiltrates of macrophages and hyperplasia of diffuse lymphoid aggregates (Sigurdsson, 1954). The resulting chronic interstitial pneumonia leads to a chronic cough, and in later stages, to fatigue, dyspnea, and cachexia. CNS lesions are of a demyelinating nature (Sigurdsson et al., 1957).

D. Immune Responses

1. EIAV

Immunity to EIAV is the strongest of the various lentivirus infections of animals (McGuire et al., 1987). The emergence of variant strains of the virus is associated with the rapid production of variant-specific virus-neutralizing antibodies. These antibodies are probably instrumental in eliminating each wave of viremia. Mutants of EIAV appear rapidly and randomly in the blood and not along a predestined mutagenic course (Hussain et al., 1987; Salinovich et al., 1986). Immunity appears to play a key role, however, in selecting for serologically distinct mutants. After the virus goes through a number of mutations, the virus-neutralizing antibodies in the blood also achieve a broad spectrum of specificity. The virus becomes relatively quiescent in macrophages after this time. Infectious virus is very difficult to find in the blood, and large amounts of tissues are required for transmission or virus recovery studies (Coggins, 1984; McGuire et al., 1987). These observations suggest two things: (1) there is a finite number of major serological mutants of EIAV and these mutants arise during the first few months of infection, and (2) immunity, although not completely effective, is nearly capable of eliminating the infection. EIAV infection represents, therefore, the single lentivirus infection of animals that comes closest to responding to host immunity in a conventional manner.

2. CAEV

Goats infected with CAEV develop weak or negligible titers of virus-neutralizing antibodies (Narayan *et al.*, 1987). There are tremendous amounts of anti-envelope antibodies as detectable by other types of assays, however (Johnson *et al.*, 1983; Narayan *et al.*, 1987). It appears, therefore, that either goats fail to respond immunologically to relevant antigens of the virus envelope or that the viral envelope lacks neutralizing epitopes. The former appears to be the case; some rabbits will develop complement-dependent virus-neutralizing antibodies when immunized with CAEV (Anderson *et al.*, 1983). A proportion of goats will produce virus-neutralizing antibodies if immunized with large amounts of viral antigen incorporated with high levels of inactivated *Mycobacterium tuberculosis* (Narayan *et al.*, 1984). The neutralizing activity of such artificially induced antibodies is extremely narrow, reacting only with the immunizing strain and not with other isolates.

Variant strains of CAEV appear in the blood of infected goats (Ellis *et al.*, 1987; Narayan *et al.*, 1987). The selection pressure for such variants is unknown; the lack of strong virus-neutralizing activity suggests that either it is not immunologic or that antibody-mediated selection is by mechanisms other than virus neutralization. Variant strains of the virus coexist in the body with parental strains (Ellis *et al.*, 1987; Narayan *et al.*, 1987).

3. V-MV

Host immunity to V-MV is intermediate between that of EIAV and CAEV. Virus-neutralizing antibodies to the infecting strain appear within a few weeks (Narayan *et al.*, 1987). Variants that fail to react to the initial neutralizing antibodies appear slowly with time (Lutley *et al.*, 1983; Narayan *et al.*, 1978, 1981), and at a lower frequency than with EIAV (Thormar *et al.*, 1983). The appearance of virus-neutralizing antibodies to new serotypes is relatively slow, often taking months or years. Antibody titers to variant viruses are not as high as to the parental infecting strain (Narayan *et al.*, 1987).

Unlike EIAV infection, virus-neutralizing antibodies have a limited effect on decreasing the burden of V-MV in infected sheep. One possible explanation for this phenomena was described by Narayan and co-workers (1987). They found that virus-neutralizing antibodies from infected sheep required 15 min at body temperature to neutralize infectivity, whereas virus binding to infected cells took only 2 min. Theoretically, virus could spread from cell to cell faster than it could be neutralized.

Sheep infected with V-MV never reach a state like EIAV infection, where clinical signs are minimal and/or virus is not easily rescued from blood or tissues by animal inoculation or tissue culture isolation. Variant viruses, when present, appear to coexist with each other (reviewed by Narayan et al., 1987). Distinct serologic variants have been induced in vitro by treating cultures infected with early animal isolates with early immune sera. Viruses resistant to early antibodies appear within several week in vitro. Late isolates grown in the presence of late antisera showed much less tendency to undergo such rapid mutation (Narayan et al., 1987).

E. Experimental Vaccines

1. EIAV

EIA is the only lentivirus infection of animals where vaccination has some immunologic basis. Virus-neutralizing antibodies to various serotypes are strong, and infected horses usually reach a state where the virus is relatively well contained. The problem with variant serotypes, although formidable, is not impossible (Hussain et al., 1987). This optimism is supported by preliminary vaccine studies. Horses inoculated three to eight times with a virulence-attenuated, cloned isolate of the Wyoming strain of EIAV resisted challenge with an antigenically similar but virulent clone of the same strain (Kono et al., 1970). Immunity to other virulent isolates was not induced, however, and vaccinated animals immunized with different strains developed clinical signs of EIA.

2. CAEV

McGuire and co-workers (1986) attempted to immunize goats against CAEV using formalin-inactivated virus with Freund's complete adjuvant. Goats vaccinated several times with the preparation became infected following challenge-exposure with virulent virus. Moreover, vaccinated goats developed more severe arthritis than did unvaccinated control animals.

3. V-MV

Initial studies with inactivated V-MV vaccines have been unsuccessful. Cutlip and associates (1987) prepared heat-, formalin-, or ethyleneimine-inactivated whole virus vaccines and used them without adjuvants, or with alumnium hydroxide or Freund's complete adjuvant. The vaccinated sheep produced virus-precipitating antibodies but were not protected when challenge-exposed with live virus.

Nathanson and co-workers (1981) attempted a post-exposure vaccine experiment. Sheep were infected with V-MV and immediately began on a regimen of immunizations with either detergent-disrupted, gradient-purified virus in Freund's complete adjuvant or living V-MV-infected autochthonous testicular cells. Sheep injected with detergent-disrupted virus tended to have more severe lesions than infected control animals that were not given post-exposure vaccinations. The infected cell immunizations had no influence on the subsequent disease course.

F. DISCUSSION AND COMMENTARY

The prospects of developing effective vaccines against lentivirus infections of sheep and goats appears unlikely. There is some hope that vaccines may be developed against EIAV infection of horses, however. It is interesting to note that preliminary successes or failures to develop lentivirus vaccines have been predictable, given what is known about natural infections in each of these species. Horses respond reasonably well to their infection. After overcoming the initial phase of the illness, which is closely related to the rapid sequential appearance of random serotypic variants, horses are able to damp down the virus. Although they do not appear to be able to eliminate the virus completely from their bodies, the burden of infectious virus that remains is very low. Predictably, attenuated live-virus vaccines against EIAV were effective in preventing disease caused by serotypically similar virulent strains of the virus. Also predictably, this immunity was not strain specific. Attempts to immunize goats and sheep, which seem unable to substantially decrease their virus burden during the course of natural infection, have failed. This is also not surprising. Vaccines mimic the immunologic events that occur in natural infections, and all effective vaccines heretofore developed have been against diseases to which naturally infected individuals develop immunity. Conversely, no effective vaccines have ever been developed for infections against which the host cannot naturally and effectively respond.

There appears to be a great emphasis on the role of humoral immunity, in particular virus-neutralizing antibodies, in immunity to lentivirus infections (McGuire *et al.*, 1987; Narayan *et al.*, 1987). The inability to induce immunity is usually equated either to a failure to develop such antibodies or the emergence of antigenic variants. Such overemphasis on humoral immunity is unfortunate. Virus-neutralizing antibodies appear in the serum of humans infected with HIV and in sheep infected with V-MV. The disease course in these two infections is not substantially different from CAEV, which does not induce virus-neutralizing antibodies. Cellular immunity usually has proven to be the most effective entity in infections involving the cell-associated microorganisms. Why do lentiviruses persist, and even replicate, within infected cells in the face of host immunity (Narayan *et al.*, 1982; Peluso *et al.*, 1985)? Is there a primary failure of cell-mediated immunity to become specifically activated following lentivirus exposure, or do secondary inhibitory factors to cellular immunity arise as a result of infection? Vaccine development will be greatly impeded until these questions can be answered.

II. Feline Infectious Peritonitis

A. Introduction

Feline infectious peritonitis (FIP) is a common viral disease entity of domestic cats. The FIP virus (FIPV) is antigenically similar to canine coronavirus (CCV), transmissible gastroenteritis virus (TGEV) of swine, human coronavirus 229E (HCV-229E), and feline enteric coronavirus (FeCV) (Pedersen, 1983a,b; Pedersen *et al.*, 1978).

FIPV has an interesting interrelationship with the common enteric coronavirus (FeCV) of cats (Pedersen, 1983a). The two viruses are closely related morphologically, antigenically, and genetically (Boyle *et al.*, 1984). In fact, coronaviruses of cats exist as a spectrum that ranges from highly virulent FIP inducers on one extreme to purely enteric pathogens (non-FIP inducers) on the other (Pedersen, 1987). Intermediate strains between these extremes exist in abudnance. Strains of coronaviruses that behave as enteric coronaviruses have even been cloned from stocks of FIPV-inducing viruses (Pedersen, 1987; Pederen and Black, 1983).

The primary difference between FeCV and FIPV isolates lies in their cell tropisms. FeCV isolates have a strong tropism for mature epithelial cells of the small intestine and are difficult to grow in culture

(Pedersen *et al.*, 1981b, 1984) and they can be found within macrophages in the regional mesenteric lymph nodes following infection, but there is no evidence that they actually replicate or persist in such cells (Pedersen *et al.*, 1984). They have very little systemic pathogenicity. Feline enteric coronaviruses cause mainly a localized infection of the gut; following recovery, the virus continues to be shed at some level in the feces of some cats (Pedersen *et al.*, 1981b, 1984). FIPV isolates are less tropic for the intestinal epithelium and have acquired a pronounced ability to replicate in macrophages (Pedersen, 1976). This ability to replicate in macrophages probably accounts for their disease-causing properties. Macrophages not only serve as an important site for replication, but also carry the virus to many other areas of the body (Weiss and Scott, 1981a).

B. COURSE OF INFECTION

FIP occurs mainly in cats between 6 months and 3 years of age. The disease is particularly prevalent among purebred kittens raised in catteries or among animals living in large multiple cat households. Outbreaks of disease tend to be sporadic, seldom involving more than one or two animals at a time. Mortality among clinically affected individuals is virtually 100%. The disease tends to appear, disappear, and reappear at unpredictable intervals among infected populations. many cofactors, including genetic susceptibility, stress, and other concurrent diseases (in particular feline leukemia virus infection) play important roles in the clinical expression of the infection (Pedersen, 1987).

The disease occurs in two basic forms: (1) the effusive or wet form of FIP, and (2) the noneffusive or dry form of FIP. The effusive form is about three to five times more prevalent than the noneffusive form in both natural and experimental infections (Pedersen, 1987). The effusive form of FIP is heralded by the appearance of a chronic fluctuating fever and abdominal and/or pleural fluid effusions. Effusions consist of a characteristic high protein exudate with a rather sticky or mucinous character. Affected individuals usually began to lose weight and become progressively more lethargic. Death ultimately ensues in from 1 to 12 weeks. A fluctuating and persistent fever is also seen in cats with noneffusive FIP. Instead of peritoneal or pleural effusions, cats with this form of the disease tend to develop a disseminated granulomatous disease with a predilection for the central nervous system, eyes, kidneys, mesenteric lymph nodes, and, less commonly, other parenchymatous organs. The clinical course is also one of progressive weight loss, anorexia, and death within 1–6 months.

C. Pathogenesis

The source of FIPV in nature is unknown. A chronic carrier state has been induced experimentally in cats (Pedersen, 1987). Carrier queens will pass the virus to their kittens in the prenatal or neonatal period of life (Pedersen, 1987). It is very difficult to induce FIP in susceptible cats by exposing them to cats that are clinically ill with the disease, however. Susceptible cats exposed to such animals are much more likely to develop an enteric coronavirus infection. This suggests that cats with FIP do not shed a great amount of FIPV; rather they shed FeCV. A second possible source of FIPV is FeCV carriers. FIPV may be a common mutation of the basic enteric coronavirus, and FIP-inducing mutants may be generated during initial FeCV infection or during the proceeding carrier state (Pedersen, 1987). FIPV might be generated *de novo*, therefore, in any cat with acute or chronic FeCV infection. The mutant FIPV could infect the cat in which it originated, or might be shed in the excretions and infect other animals.

The route of infection in nature is unknown. It is either intrinsic as suggested above, or it is extrinsic. Experimental studies mimicking both possibilities have been reported. Following oral or intratracheal infection (extrinsic exposure), the virus infects the mature epithelial cells (Hayashi *et al.*, 1982; Pedersen *et al.*, 1981a). Following intraperitoneal or other parenteral routes (intrinsic exposure), the virus replicates initially in phagocytic cells. Regardless of the initial site of replication, replication within macrophages appears to be central to the disease. Once the virus enters phagocytic cells (directly, or via the gut or respiratory epithelium), virus replication begins in earnest. Macrophages also carry the virus to the various target tissues (Weiss and Scott, 1981a). The main targets are the serosal membranes lining the abdominal and pleural cavities and organs, meninges, and ependyma of brain and spinal cord, and the uveal tract (Pedersen, 1983b). The type of disease that develops is dependent on the type and strength of the immune response resulting during primary infection (Pedersen, 1987).

D. Immune Response

The bulk of experimental evidence supports the notion that FIPV immunity is entirely cellular (Pedersen, 1987). The passive transfer of sera, even from FIPV-immune individuals, makes the recipient more susceptible rather than immune to disease (Pedersen and Boyle, 1980; Weiss and Scott, 1981b). Following infection and spread of the virus to phagocytic cells, both humoral and cellular immunity are triggered. If the cat makes humoral immunity, but fails to develop cellular immunity, the effusive form of FIP ensues (Pedersen, 1987). If the animal makes good cellular immunity, regardless of the humoral immune response, the infection is rapidly contained within macrophages and no clinical signs are observed. If, however, cellular immunity is only partial, the noneffusive form of FIP develops. The noneffusive form of FIP represents, therefore, an intermediate state between complete and minimal immunity. Strong macrophage and T-lymphocyte activation presumably are essential for containment of virus. In contrast, partial cellular immunity will be only partially effective in slowing down the spread and replication of the virus, and thus granulomas develop. The effusive form of FIP is characterized by masses of virus-laden proliferating macrophages around blood vessels in the omentum and serosal surfaces and no cellular immunity. In contrast, the lesions of noneffusive FIP have fewer macrophages, less of the macrophages are infected with virus, and the level of antigen in infected macrophages is lower. Evidence from experimental infection suggests that the effusive form is almost always preceded by a brief episode of effusive disease (Pedersen, 1987). This further supports the importance of stepwise immunity in the pathogenesis of FIP.

Naturally and experimentally infected cats occasionally have recovered spontaneously from the infection. Recovery is either very rapid, with no clinical illness seen following initial infection, or it progresses at a slower pace from the noneffusive form of illness (Pedersen and Black, 1983; Pedersen, 1987).

There is an interesting immunologic relationship between FeCV and FIPV infections. Cats that have previously recovered from FeCV infection, and have cross-reacting antibodies to FIPV, will develop an accelerated form of effusive FIP upon challenge-exposure with FIPV (Pedersen and Boyle, 1980; Pedersen et al., 1981b; Weiss and Scott, 1981b). Effusive FIP in coronavirus antibody-free cats usually occurs from 7 to 14 days following infection with FIPV, which is at the same time that serum antibodies are detectable in the blood (Pedersen et al., 1981a). These cats usually die after a period of 2–4 weeks of illness. If the cats are preinfected with FeCV, however, they will develop effusive FIP within 24–48 hr and die from a more fulminating form of the disease within a week or so (Pedersen et al., 1981b). The accelerated form of the disease can be recreated by passively administering FeCV immune sera to susceptible cats prior to infection with FIPV (Pedersen and Boyle, 1980). It can also be recreated by administering serum from cats with active FIP, or cats that are immune to FIP (Pedersen and Black, 1983). The failure of immune sera to protect cats from FIPV infection, and the acceleration of disease associated with antibodies, is supportive of the idea that humoral immunity is nonprotective and, indeed, harmful.

The accelerated form of effusive FIP occurring in previously FeCV-sensitized cats has strong clinical and immunopathologic similarities to the dengue hemorrhagic shock syndrome of man (Horzinek and Osterhaus, 1979; Pedersen and Boyle, 1980; Weiss and Scott, 1981b). This occurs in people that are primarily sensitized to one serotype of dengue fever virus and subsequently infected with a closely related but different serotype.

E. EXPERIMENTAL VACCINES

Cats immunized with closely related coronaviruses, such as FeCV, CCV, TGEV, or HCV-229E are not protected against FIPV challenge-exposure (Barlough et al., 1984, 1985; Pedersen et al., 1981b; Stoddart et al., 1988; Toma et al., 1979; Woods and Pedersen, 1979). Cats preimmunized with virulence-attenuated live or inactivated FIPV are also hypersensitive to virulent FIPV exposure (Jacobse-Geels et al., 1980; Pedersen and Black, 1983).

Immunity to FIPV has been induced with some difficulty in cats using virulent strains of FIPV. A proportion of cats infected with sublethal doses of highly virulent FIPV will seroconvert and be resistant to subsequent challenge-exposure with massive levels of the same virulent virus (Pedersen and Black, 1983). A similar phenomena has been observed with cats that are infected experimentally with FIPV strains of low virulence (Pedersen, 1987). Cats infected with low-virulence strains will either develop FIP, or seroconvert without illness. If this latter group of animals is challenged with a more virulent strain of FIPV, some will be immune and some will develop accelerated effusive FIPV (Pedersen, 1987).

Kittens born to queens that have been immunized with virulent FIPV will pass on maternal antibodies to their young (Pedersen, 1987). These antibodies will last for only 4 weeks or so. After this time, the kittens undergo an active asymptomatic coronavirus infection, as evidenced by a rise in antibody titers starting at around 4–6 weeks of age (Pedersen, 1987). The queen is the source of this infection. If these kittens are challenge-exposed to a large dose of virulent FIPV between 8 and 10 weeks of age, they will be immune (Pedersen, 1987). If they are not infected until 22 weeks of age, however, some will be immune and others will develop the accelerated form of the disease (Pedersen, 1987).

When FIPV recovered cats are infected with feline leukemia virus (FeLV) between 0 and 4 months after FIPV challenge, they will almost always develop FIP and die within several weeks (Pedersen, 1987). It is apparent, therefore, that FIPV recovered cats still carry the virus for a period of time after initial exposure. If FIPV immune cats are not infected with FeLV until 7–9 months after initial FIPV challenge, FIP cannot be induced (Pedersen, 1987). This suggests either that the FIPV is lost with time from the body, or that the overlying FIPV immunity has gained sufficient strength during the ensuing months to withstand perturbations caused by the FeLV infection. Experiments with the immunity of kittens born to FIPV carrier queens suggests that the former situation is correct. If so, immunity to FIPV involves pre-munition (infection immunity), and immunity is only maintained for as long as the virus persists in the body.

F. DISCUSSION AND COMMENTARY

The likelihood of developing an effective FIPV vaccine given the immunologic vicissitudes of FIPV infection appear slim. Based on what is known about immunity to this virus, the ideal vaccine would be an attenuated live agent that would persist in macrophages for long periods of time without inducing disease. Persistence of the virus would also have to induce protective cellular immunity. Attempts have been made to find just such FIPV isolates (Pedersen, 1987). If they are too attenuated, they will not persist long enough in macrophages to induce immunity. If they are partially attenuated in virulence, they will persist in macrophages and induce immunity in a portion of cats, but will either cause FIP or hypersensitization to FIPV in others.

An ideal killed vaccine would induce strong cellular immunity by mimicking the way virulent FIPV is presented to macrophages. It would also have to induce immunity that would persist for a long epriod of time. At the present time, all killed and avirulent FIPV vaccines have failed to induce protective cellular immunity and have actually sensitized vaccinates to disease. Because virus persistence appears to be essential for immunity, it is unlikely that such an idealized killed virus vaccine could be developed. The same misgivings that apply to inactivated whole virus vaccines could also be echoed for subunit vaccines made up of the viral proteins.

REFERENCES

Adams, D. S., Oliver, R. E., Ameghino, E., DeMartini, J. C., Verwoerd, D. W., Houvers, D. J., Waghela, S., Gorham, J. R., Hyllseth, B., Dawson, M., Trigo, F. J., and McGuire, T. C. (1984). *Vet. Rec.* **115**, 493–495.

Anderson, L. W., Klevjer-Anderson, P., and McGlure, T. C. (1983). *Infect. Immun.* **42,** 845–847.

Barlough, J. E., Stoddart, C. A., Sorresso, G. P., Jacobson, R. H., and Scott, F. W. (1984). *Lab. Anim. Sci.* **34,** 592–597.

Barlough, J. E., Johnson-Lussenburg, C. M., Stoddart, C. A., Jacobson, R. H., and Scott, F. W. (1985). *Can. J. Comp. Med.* **49,** 303–307.

Boyle, J. F., Pedersen, N. C., Evermann, J. F., McKeirnan, A. J., Ott, R. L., and Black, J. W. (1984). *Adv. Exp. Med. Biol.* **173,** 133–147.

Coggins, L. (1984). *J. Am. Vet. Med. Assoc.* **184,** 279–281.

Cutlip, R. C., Lehmkuhl, H. D., and Jackson, T. A. (1981). *Am. J. Vet. Res.* **42,** 1795–1797.

Cutlip, R. C., Lehmkuhl, H. D., Brogden, K. A., and Schmeer, M. J. F. (1987). *Vet. Microbiol.* **13,** 201–204.

East, N. E., Rowe, J. D., Madewell, B. R., and Floyd, K. (1987). *J. Am. Vet. Med. Assoc.* **190,** 182–186.

Ellis, T. M., Wilcox, G. E., and Robinson, W. F. (1987). *J. Gen. Virol.* **68,** 3145–3152.

Gonda, M. A., Braun, M. J., Carter, S. C., Kost, T. A., Bess, J. W., Jr., Arthur, L. O., and Van der Maaten, M. J. (1987). *Nature (London)* **330,** 388–391.

Hayashi, T., Aatabe, Y., Nakayama, H., and Fujiwara. K. (1982). *Jpn. J. Vet. Sci.* **44,** 97–106.

Horzinek, M. C., and Osterhaus, A. D. M. E. (1979). *Arch. Virol.* **59,** 1–15.

Hussain, K. A., Issel, C. J., Schnorr, K. L., Rwambo, P. M., and Montelaro, R. C. (1987). *J. Virol.* **61,** 2956–2961.

Issel, C. J., and Foil, L. D. (1984). *J. Am. Vet. Med. Assoc.* **184,** 293–297.

Jacobse-Geels, H. E. L., Daha, M. R., and Horzinek, M. C. (1980). *J. Immunol.* **125,** 1606–1610.

Johnson, G. C., Barbet, A. F., Klevjer-Anderson, P., and McGuire, T. C. (1983). *Infect. Immun.* **41,** 657–665.

Kennedy-Stoskopf, S., Narayan, O., and Strandberg, J. D. (1985). *J. Comp. Pathol.* **95,** 609–617.

Kono, Y., Kobayashi, K., and Fukunaga, Y. (1970). *Natl. Inst. Anim. Health Q.* **10,** 113–122.

Lutley, R., Petursson, G., Palsson, P. A., Georgsson, G., Klein, J., and Nathanson, N. (1983). *J. Gen. Virol.* **64,** 1433–1440.

McGuire, T. C. (1976). *Immunology* **30,** 17–24.

McGuire, T. C., Crawford, T. B., and Henson, J. B. (1971). *Am. J. Pathol.* **62,** 283–294.

McGuire, T. C., Adams, D. S., Johnson, G. C., Klevjer-Anderson, P., Barbee, D. D., and Gorham, J. R. (1986). *Am. J. Vet. Res.* **47,** 537–540.

McGuire, T. C., O'Rourke, K., and Cheevers, W. P. (1987). *Contrib. Microbiol. Immunol.* **8,** 77–89.

Narayan, O., and Cork, L. C. (1985). *Rev. Infect. Dis.* **7,** 89–98.

Narayan, O., Griffin, D. E., and Clements, J. E. (1978). *J. Gen. Virol.* **41,** 343–352.

Narayan, O., Clements, J. E., Griffin, D. E., and Wolinsky, J. S. (1981). *Infect. Immun.* **32,** 1045–1050.

Narayan, O., Wolinsky, J. S., Clements, J. E., Strandberg, J. D., Griffin, D. E., and Cork, L. C. (1982). *J. Gen. Virol.* **59,** 345–356.

Narayan, O., Sheffer, D., Griffin, D. E., Clements, J. E., and Hess, J. (1984). *J. Virol.* **49,** 349–355.

Narayan, O., Clements, J., Kennedy-Stoskopf, S., Sheffer, D., and Royal, W. (1987). *Contrlb. Microbiol. Immunol.* **8,** 60–76.

Nathanson, N., Martin, J. R., Georgsson, G., Palsson, P. A., Lutley, R. E., and Petursson, G. (1981). *J. Comp. Pathol.* **91,** 185–191.

Pedersen, N. C. (1976). *Am. J. Vet. Res.* **37**, 567–571.

Pedersen, N. C. (1983a). *Feline Pract.* **13**(4), 13–17.

Pedersen, N. C. (1983b). *Feline Pract.* **13**(5), 5–14.

Pedersen, N. C. (1987). *Adv. Exp. Med. Biol.* **218**, 529–550.

Pedersen, N. C., and Black, J. W. (1983). *Am. J. Vet. Res.* **44**, 229–234.

Pedersen, N. C., and Boyle, J. F. (1980). *Am. J. Vet. Res.* **41**, 868–876.

Pedersen, N. C., Ward, J., and Mengeling, W. L. (1978). *Arch. Virol.* **58**, 45–54.

Pedersen, N. C., Boyle, J. F., and Floyd, K. (1981a). *Am. J. Vet. Res.* **42**, 363–367.

Pedersen, N. C., Boyle, J. F., Floyd, K., Fudge, A., and Barker, J. (1981b). *Am. J. Vet. Res.* **42**, 368–377.

Pedersen, N. C., Evermann, J. F., McKiernan, A. J., and Ott, R. L. (1984). *Am. J. Vet. Res.* **45**, 2580–2585.

Peluso, R., Haase, A. T., Stowring, L., Edwards, M., and Ventura, P. (1985). *Virology* **147**, 231–236.

Salinovich, O., Payne, S. L., Montelaro, R. C., Hussain, K. A., Issel, C. J., and Schorr, K. L. (1986). *J. Virol.* **57**, 71–80.

Sigurdsson, B. (1954). *Br. Vet. J.* **110**, 225–270.

Sigurdsson, B., Palsson, P. A., and Grissom, H. (1957). *J. Neuropathol. Exp. Neurol.* **156**, 389–403.

Stein, C. D., and Mott, L. O. (1942). *Vet. Med.* **37**, 370–377.

Stein, C. D., Lotze, J. C., and Mott, L. O. (1942). *Am. J. Vet. Res.* **3**, 183–193.

Stoddart, C. A., Barlough, J. E., Baldwin, C. A., and Scott, F. W. (1988). *Res. Vet. Sci.* (in press).

Takemoto, K. K., Mattern, C. F. T., Stone, L. B., Coe, J. E., and Lavelle, G. (1971). *J. Virol.* **7**, 301–308.

Thormar, H., Barshatsky, M. R., and Kozlowski, P. B. (1983). *J. Gen. Virol.* **64**, 1427–1432.

Toma, B., Duret, C., Chappuis, G., and Pellerin, B. (1979). *Recl. Med. Vet.* **155**, 799–803.

Van der Maaten, M. J., Boothe, A. D., and Seger, C. L. (1972). *J. Natl Cancer Inst. (U.S.)* **49**, 1649–1657.

Weiss, R. G., and Scott, F. W. (1981a). *Am. J. Vet. Res.* **42**, 382–390.

Weiss, R. G., and Scott, F. W. (1981b). *Comp. Immunol. Microbiol. Infect. Dis.* **4**, 175–189.

Woods, R. D., and Pedersen, N. C. (1979). *J. Vet. Microbiol.* **4**, 11–16.

INDEX

B

Babesia, 351–354
  immunostimulants, 352
  vaccine, shelf life, 346–347
Babesia bigemina, 346, 354
Babesia bovis, 346, 352–353
Babesia divergens, subunit vaccine, 353–354
Bacillus, 37–38
Bacillus anthracis, 130
Bacillus Calmette-Guerin, 294–295
  as heterologous antigen carrier, 295–296
Bacillus subtilis, recombinant DNA technologies, 117–118
Bacterial diseases, biosynthetic vaccines, 126
Bacterial immunity, 101–102
Bacterial vaccines, reason for developing, 272
Bacteriodes nodosus, 131–132
B cells
  as antigen-presenting cells, 311
  differentiation and maturation, 95
B-cell stimulatory factor, 98
BCG, 294–295
  as heterologous antigen carrier, 295–296
  vaccine, 41
Biodegradable microcapsules, as vehicles, 321–323
Biosynthetic vaccines, 109–111
  adjuvants and delivery technology, 158
  AIDS, 146–149
  anthrax, 129–130
  bacterial diseases, 126
  Brucellosis, 136–137
  cellular immune response and immunogen choice, 151–154
  definition, 110
  enterotoxigenic *E. coli*, cholera, 126–128
  evoking autoimmune responses, 155
  foot-and-mouth disease, 139–141
  gonococcal infections, 130–131
  hepatitis A, 141
  hepatitis B, 137–139
  herpesvirus infections, 141–146
  immunogen, form and presentation, 155–158
  mycobacterial infections, 133–134

natural pathogen, 112–113
negative immunologic reactions, 154–155
ovine footrot, 131–132
pertussis, 128–129
protective immunity and neutralizing antibody, 149–151
recombinant DNA technologies, 113–125
  Autographa californica nuclear polyhedrosis virus, 119–121
  Bacillus subtilis, 117–118
  common denominators, 113
  E. coli, 114–117
  expression plasmid stability, 115–116
  fungi, 118–119
  gene fusions, 116
  insect cells, 119–121
  mammalian cells, 121–125
  mRNA stability, 115
  prokaryotes, 114–118
  Streptococcal infections, 135–136
  subunit vaccines, 109–111
  syphilis, 132–133
  viral diseases, 137
Black death, 45
Bluetongue virus, 19–20
B-lymphocytes, 95–96
Bordetella, 47–48
Bordetella pertussis, 48, 128
  immunostimulators, 332–333
Bovine coronavirus, 34
Bovine parainfluenza virus, 27–28
Bovine respiratory syncytial virus, 31
Bovine rotavirus, 19
Bovine virus diarrhea virus, 23
Brucella, 48–50
  vaccines, 291–293
Brucella abortus, 49, 292
Brucella melitensis, 49, 292
Brucella ovis, 49–50
Brucellosis, 291
  biosynthetic vaccines, 136–137

C

Caliciviridae, 17–18
Camelpox, 199
Campylobacter, 50

F

Fab fragment, in complex with
neuraminidase, 66
Facultative intracellular pathogens, 273
Fasciola, 365–368
glycoproteins, 367–368
messenger RNA, 368
monoclonal antibodies, 367
resistance, 366
Fasciola hepatica, 365–368
Feline calicivirus, 17–18
Feline coronavirus, immunologic
relationship with feline infectious
peritonitis, 424
Feline infectious peritonitis, 34, 421–422
cellular immunity, 423–424
coronavirus antibody-free cats, 424
course of infection, 422–423
experimental vaccines, 425–426
forms, 422
humoral immunity, 423–424
immune response, 423–425
immunologic relationship with
coronavirus, 424
pathogenesis, 423
Feline leukemia virus vaccines, 33–34,
381
monoclonal and anti-idiotypic
antibodies, 383
Quil A, 383
recombinant vaccinia virus, 384
virus-neutralizing antibody, 382–383
Feline panleukopenia virus, 3
Feline rhinotracheitis virus, 9
Ferritin-anti-Ig conjugates, 311
FHA gene, 129
Fibroma virus vaccines, 199
Flaviviridae, 24
Foot and mouth disease, 14–15
amino acid sequences, 187
antigenic sites, 83–84, 178
antigenic variation, 175, 185–187
biosynthetic vaccines, 139–141
coat protein sequencing, 177–179
cross-neutralization tests, 186
epitopes, 191
first comprehensive vaccination
program, 174–175
fusion proteins with peptide, 180–181
future, 190–192

immunogenicity of inactivated
particles, 183
neutralizing antibody, response in
cattle and pigs, 183
OVA and SWMII T cell sites, 184
peptide presentation, 179–182
protective immune response
requirements, 182–185
serotypes, 174
trypsin experiment, 178
VP1, 176
Fowlpox virus, 12
vaccines, 199
Foxes, rabies vaccine, 218, 222
Freund's adjuvant, *see also* Complete
Freund's adjuvant; Incomplete
Freund's adjuvant
killed BCG, 295
Fungi, recombinant DNA technologies,
118–119

G

gag gene, 148–149
protease, 157
Gastroenteritis
Salmonella, 274
transmissible gastroenteritis virus, 35–36
gB2 gene, 142–143
gD1 gene, 142–143
Gene cloning technologies, 111
Gene transfer, by marker rescue,
poxvirus, 214–218
Germinal center, cellular interactions,
97–99
gII gene, 144
gIII gene, 144
gIV gene, 144
Glucan, immunostimulators, 333
Glycoprotein
herpesvirus, 141–143
influenza virus, 66
RS virus, 255
Goatpox, 11, 199
Goats
anthrax, 37–38
brucellosis, 49, 291
caprine arthritis-encephalitis virus,
415–416
Corynebacterium pseudotuberculosis, 37